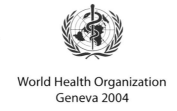

World Health Organization
Geneva 2004

ANTI-TUBERCULOSIS DRUG RESISTANCE IN THE WORLD

Third Global Report

The WHO/IUATLD Global Project on Anti-tuberculosis
Drug Resistance Surveillance
1999-2002

WHO Library Cataloguing-in-Publication Data

WHO/IUATLD Global Project on Anti-Tuberculosis Drug Resistance Surveillance.
Anti-tuberculosis drug resistance in the world: third global report/
the WHO/IUATLD Global Project on Anti-Tuberculosis Drug Resistance
Surveillance, 1999-2002.

1.Tuberculosis, Multidrug-resistant - epidemiology 2.Drug resistance, Bacterial - statistics
3.Bacteriological techniques 4.Data collection - methods
5.Cross-sectional studies I.Title.

ISBN 92 4 156285 4   (NLM classification: WF 360)   WHO/HTM/TB/2004.343

Designed and typeset in Italy
Printed in Singapore

WRITING COMMITTEE

Written by:
- Mohamed Abdel Aziz, M.D., M.P.H., M.B.T.Sc.,World Health Organization, Geneva, Switzerland
- Abigail Wright, M.P.H., World Health Organization, Geneva, Switzerland
- Aimé De Muynck, Ph.D., M.D., M.P.H., M.Sc., Consultant, World Health Organization, Geneva, Switzerland
- Adalbert Laszlo, Ph.D., World Health Organization, Geneva, Switzerland

With the contribution of:
- Françoise Portaels, Ph.D., Prince Léopold Tropical Institute Antwerp, Belgium
- Hans L. Rieder, M.D., M.P.H., International Union Against Tuberculosis and Lung Disease (The UNION), Kirchlindach, Switzerland
- Andrea Infuso, M.D., EuroTB, Institut de Veille Sanitaire, Saint-Maurice, France
- Armand Van Deun, M.D., Prince Léopold Tropical Institute, Antwerp, Belgium
- Andrea Luna, M.D., M.P.H., Instituto de Salud Pública de Chile, Santiago, Chile
- Sabine Rüesch-Gerdes, Ph.D., National Reference Centre for Mycobacteria, Borstel, Germany
- Karin Weyer, DSc., Medical Research Council, Pretoria, South Africa
- Francis Drobniewski, Ph.D. Health Protection Agency, Mycobacterium Reference Unit, London, UK
- Rose Liefooghe, M.Sc. Consultant, World Health Organization, Geneva, Switzerland
- Charles Wells, M.D., Division of TB Elimination, Centers for Disease Control and Prevention (CDC), Atlanta, GA, USA
- Brian Williams, Ph.D., World Health Organization, Geneva, Switzerland
- Kitty Lambregts, M.D., Ph.D., World Health Organization, Geneva, Switzerland
- Malgorzata Grzemska, M.D., Ph.D., World Health Organization, Geneva, Switzerland
- Paul Nunn, M.D., World Health Organization, Geneva, Switzerland
- Marcos Espinal, M.D., Dr.P.H., M.P.H., World Health Organization, Geneva, Switzerland
- Leopold Blanc, M.D., M.P.H., World Health Organization, Geneva, Switzerland
- Christopher Dye, DPhil, World Health Organization, Geneva, Switzerland
- Mario Raviglione, M.D., World Health Organization, Geneva, Switzerland

GLOBAL NETWORK OF SUPRANATIONAL REFERENCE LABORATORIES

- Département de Microbiologie, Unité de Mycobactériologie, Institut de Médicine Tropicale Prince Léopold, *Antwerp, Belgium* (Professor Françoise Portaels) *(Coordinating Centre, 1999-2004)*
- Laboratoire de la Tuberculose, Institut Pasteur d'Algérie-Alger, *Algiers, Algeria* (Dr Fadila Boulahbal)
- Queensland Mycobacterium Reference Laboratory, *Chermside, Australia* (Dr Chris Gilpin)
- National Institute of Public Health, *Prague, Czech Republic* (Dr Marta Havelkova)
- Instituto de Salud Pública de Chile, *Santiago, Chile* (Dr Andrea Luna)
- Centre national de Référence des Mycobacteries, Institut Pasteur, *Paris, France* (Dr Véronique Vincent)
- National Reference Centre for Mycobacteria, Forschungszentrum, *Borstel, Germany,* (Dr Sabine Rüesch-Gerdes)
- Kuratorium Tuberkulose in der Welt e.V., *Gauting, Germany* (Professor Knut Feldmann)
- Tuberculosis Research Centre (TRC), Indian Council of Medical Research, *Chennai, India* (Dr Chinnambedu N. Paramasivan)
- Laboratory of Bacteriology, Istituto Superiore de Sanità, *Rome, Italy* (Dr Graziella Orefici)
- Japan Anti-Tuberculosis Association, *Tokyo, Japan* (Dr Satoshi Mitarai)
- Instituto Nacional de Saúde, *Porto Codex, Portugal* (Dr Maria Filomena Rodrigues)
- Korean Institute of Tuberculosis, *Seoul, Republic of Korea* (Dr Gill-han Bai/ Dr Sang Jae Kim)
- Unit for Tuberculosis Operational and Policy Research, Medical Research Council, *Pretoria, South Africa* (Dr Karin Weyer)
- Servicio de Microbiologia, Hospital Universitari Vall d'Hebron, Autonomous University, *Barcelona, Spain* (Dr Nuria Martin-Casabona)
- Swedish Institute for Infectious Disease Control, *Solna, Sweden* (Dr Sven Hoffner)
- National Institute of Public Health and the Environment (RIVM), *Bilthoven, The Netherlands* (Dr Dick van Soolingen)
- Health Protection Agency, Mycobacterium Reference Laboratory Unit, King's College Hospital (Dulwich), *London,United Kingdom* (Dr Francis Drobniewski)
- Mycobacteriology / Tuberculosis Laboratory, Centers for Disease Control and Prevention (CDC) *Atlanta, GA, United States of America* (Dr Beverly Metchock)
- Department of Public Health, Massachusetts State Laboratory Institute, *Boston, MA, United States of America* (Dr Alexander Sloutsky)

CONTRIBUTING MEMBERS OF THE WORKING GROUP

•**Algeria:** Professor Fadila Boulahbal •**Andorra:** Dr Margarida Coll Armangue •**Argentina:** Dr Lucia Barrera, Omar Latini •**Australia:** Dr Richard Lumb •**Austria:** Dr John-Paul Klein •**Belgium:** Dr Maryse Wanlin, Dr An Aerts •**Bosnia and Herzegonia:** Dr Biljana Stefanovic, Professor Zehra Dizdarevic •**Botswana:** Dr Lisa J Nelson, Mr Gasekgale Moalosi, Mr Michael Mwasekaga •**Cambodia:** Dr Onazaki, Dr Kouske Okada •**Canada:** Melissa Phypers, Dr Edward Ellis •**Chile:** Dr Andrea Luna Heine, Dr Rosario Lepe •**China:** Dr Wu Xongrong, Dr Kai Man Kam, Dr Su Ya, Dr Du Changmei, Dr Daniel Chin •**Colombia:** Dr Clara Inés Léon Franco, Dr Martha Inírida Guerrero, Dr Claudia Sierra, Dr Nancy Naranjo, Dr Maria Consuelo Garzón •**Croatia:** Dr Ira Gjenero Margan •**Cuba:** Dr Ernesto Montoro, Dr Mária J. Llanes, Lic. Dihadenys Lemus •**Czech Republic:** Dr Vlasta Mazánková, Mr Jiri Holub •**Democratic Republic of Congo:** Professor Francoise Portaels, Dr Henrietta Wembanyama •**Ecuador:** Dr Judith Vaca, Dr Dolores Kuffo •**Egypt:** Dr Essam Elmoghazy •**El Savador:** Dr Julio Garay Ramos •**Estonia:** Dr Vahur Hollo •**Finland:** Dr Petri Ruutu •**France:** Dr Bénédicte Decludt, Jerome Robert •**Georgia:** Professor George Khechinashvili •**Germany:** Dr Walter Haas, Dr Michael Forßbohm •**Honduras:** Dr Noemi Paz de Zavala, Dr Hilda Membreño •**Iceland:** Dr Blöndal Thorsteinn •**India:** Dr Chinnambedu Paramasivan, Dr Lakhbir Singh Chauhan, Dr Reuben Granich •**Ireland:** Dr Joan O'Donnell •**Israel:** Dr Daniel Chemtob, Dr Zohar Mor •**Italy:** Dr Dina Caraffa de Stefano, Dr GB Migliori •**Japan:** Dr Chyoji Abe •**Kazakhstan:** Dr Rimma Agzamova, Dr Galemzhan Borankulovich Rakishev •**Latvia:** Dr Janis Leimans •**Lithuania:** Dr Edith Davidaciené, Dr Anaida Sosnovskaja, Dr Puneet Dewan •**Luxembourg:** Dr Pierrette Huberty-Krau, Dr Nobert Charlé •**Malta:** Dr Malcolm P Micallef •**Mongolia:** Dr Gombagaram Tsogt, Dr Naranbat Nymadawa •**Nepal:** Dr Dirgh Singh Bam, Dr Christian Gunnenburg •**Netherlands:** Dr Paul van Gerven, Dr Nico Kalisvaart •**New Zealand:** Dr Helen Heffernan •**Norway:** Dr Einar Heldal, Dr Brita Winje Askeland •**Oman:** Dr Suleiman Al-Busaidy •**Poland:** Dr Maria Korzeniewska-Kosela •**Puerto Rico:** Dr Ada Martinez •**Qatar:** Dr Zubaida Daham F. Al-Suwaidi •**Russian Federation (Orel):** Dr Paul Arguin, Dr Evgenia Nemtsova, Dr Boris Kazzeony, Helen Kiryanova •**Russian Federation (Tomsk):** Dr Irena Gelmananova, Dr Donna Barry, Professor Mikhail I. Perelman, Olga Sirotkina, Vera Pavlova •**San Marino:** Dr Antonella Sorcinelli •**Serbia and Montenegro:** Professor Dusan Popovac, Dr Radmila Curcic •**Singapore:** Dr Cynthia Chee •**Slovakia:** Dr Eva Rajecova, Dr Ivan Solovic •**Slovenia:** Professor Jurij Sorli •**South Africa:** Dr Karin Weyer •**Spain (Barcelona):** Dr Nuria Martin-Casabona •**Spain (Galicia):** Dr Elena Cruz Ferro, Dr Emma Fernández Nogueira, Dr María Luisa Pérez del Molino Bernal •**Sweden:** Dr Victoria Romanus •**Switzerland:** Dr Peter Helbling, Dr Ekkehardt Altpeter •**Thailand:** Dr Dhanida Rienthong •**The Gambia:** Dr Richard Adegbola, Dr Francis Drobniewski •**Turkmenistan:** Dr Babakuli Jumaev MSF, Dr Ashir Ovezov •**United Kingdom (England, Wales and Northern Ireland):** Dr John Watson, Dr Alistair Story, Dr Delphine Antoine •**Scotland:** Dr Jim McMenamin, Dr Fiona Johnston •**United States of America:** Dr Marisa Moore •**Uruguay:** Dr Valentin Cuesta, Dr Jorge Rodriguez •**Uzbekistan:** Dr Helen Cox, Dr Gulnoz Tulkunovna Uzakova, Dr Roy Male •**Venezuela:** Dr Raimond Armengol, Dr Albina Vasquez •**Zambia:** Dr Vincent Tihon •**WHO Regional Offices: •Africa:** Dr Daniel Kibuga, Dr Eugene Nyarko •**The Americas:** Dr Rodolfo Rodriguez Cruz, Dr Pilar Ramon-Pardo •**Eastern Mediterranean:** Dr Akihiro Seita, Dr Samiha Baghdadi •**Europe:** Dr Richard Zaleskis, Mr Jerod Scholten •**South-East Asia:** Dr Jai P. Narain, Dr Nani Nair •**Western Pacific:** Dr Dongil Ahn, Dr Marcus Hodge

ACKNOWLEDGEMENTS

This project was in part financially supported by the United States Agency for International Development. The Tuberculosis Coalition for Technical Assistance (TBCTA) funded laboratory training activities associated with this project. We are grateful to EuroTB for their participation and contribution of European drug resistance surveillance data. This project could not have succeeded without the support of national authorities and the institutions hosting each of the national and international laboratories. A special acknowledgement is due to Dan Bleed and Mehran Hosseini for technical support of data management.

CONTENTS

CONTENTS

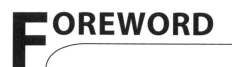OREWORD

The release of this third report of the WHO/IUATLD Global Project on Anti-tuberculosis Drug Resistance Surveillance marks the end of the first decade of activity. The three reports that have been produced are the result of unprecedented collaborative effort, and the Project itself serves as a model for surveillance, not only for tuberculosis (TB) but for many microbial diseases. Surveillance of resistance to anti-tuberculosis drugs is an essential component of a monitoring system. The benefits of surveillance are multiple: strengthening of laboratory networks, evaluation of programme performance, and the collection of data that inform appropriate therapeutic strategies. Most importantly, global surveillance identifies areas of high resistance and draws the attention of national health authorities to the need to reduce the individual or collective shortcomings that have created them.

This report makes two notable contributions to the discussion on surveillance: first, it addresses the importance of conducting surveillance on re-treatment cases, and second, it raises the issue of the role of the laboratory in TB control.

In the past, surveillance has focused on the prevalence of bacterial resistance among new patients – an extremely useful indicator for a TB programme. Prevalence of resistance among previously untreated patients reflects programme performance over a long period of time (the previous 10 years), and indicates the level of transmission within the community.

The prevalence of bacterial resistance among patients with a history of previous treatment has received less attention because surveillance of this population is a more complex process. Re-treatment patients are a heterogeneous group composed of chronic patients, those who have failed a course of treatment, those who have relapsed, and those who have returned after defaulting. In some settings, this population constitutes more than 40% of smear-positive cases. The association between drug resistance and re-treatment has been repeatedly demonstrated, both at the individual and the programme level; however, the prevalence of drug resistance varies greatly among subgroups of this population. Chronic cases and failures of a first treatment tend to be at greater risk of harbouring resistant and multidrug-resistant (MDR) bacilli. The other categories of patient (relapses and return after default) are more likely to have drug resistance than new cases, but are almost always at a lower risk for MDR than failures and chronic cases. This report therefore recommends that all subgroups of re-treatment cases be separately notified and their outcomes reported, and that surveillance of resistance be conducted on a representative sample of this population. This will make the comparison of resistance prevalence within and between countries more robust and will elucidate patterns of resistance among the subgroups, which will allow better definition of appropriate re-treatment strategies.

The second area I will touch on is that of the laboratory. It is clear that, while laboratory services are fundamental to TB control, they are often the weakest component of the system. High quality sputum smear microscopy, culture and drug susceptibility testing should be standard components of TB control everywhere, but unfortunately they are not. This lack of capacity in laboratories is already limiting the expansion of surveillance to settings that represent the most important gaps in our knowledge, and will undoubtedly adversely affect the ability of national TB programmes (NTPs) accurately to diagnose and treat MDR-TB.

It is now critical that we recognize the importance of the laboratory in the control of tuberculosis. National governments, health development agencies and partners must provide adequate financial and technical resources to radically improve diagnostic services in national TB laboratory networks.

We know from the experience of several countries, including my own, that the effective application of the internationally accepted DOTS strategy can prevent the emergence of drug resistance. Additionally, evidence is now emerging that the existing reservoir of resistant bacilli can be reduced through the supplementary application of DOTS-Plus, a strategy for the management of drug-resistant cases. Drug resistance surveillance, in conjunction with a functional laboratory network, must be expanded to help TB control programmes to identify problem areas for further support. After ten years, as this report points out, it is time to make surveillance a routine component of TB control. Only with improvement in laboratory capacity will this be possible.

Professor Pierre Chaulet
Algiers, Algeria

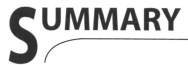
SUMMARY

1.   BACKGROUND AND METHODS

This is the third report of the WHO/IUATLD Global Project on Anti-Tuberculosis Drug Resistance Surveillance. The two previous reports were published in 1997 and 2001 and included data from 35 and 58 settings,[a] respectively. The main conclusions of the two previous reports were that drug-resistant tuberculosis (TB) was present in all settings surveyed, multidrug resistance (MDR) was identified in most settings, and that good TB control practices were associated with lower or decreasing levels of resistance. The goal of this third report is to expand knowledge of the prevalent patterns of resistance globally and explore trends in resistance over time.

This report includes new data from 77 settings or countries collected in the third phase of the project, between 1999 and 2002, representing 20% of the global total of new smear-positive TB cases. It includes 39 settings not previously included in the Global Project and reports trends for 46 settings.

Data were included if they adhered to the following principles: (1) the sample was representative of all TB cases in the setting under evaluation; (2) new patients were clearly distinguished from those with previous treatment;[b] and (3) optimal laboratory performance was assured and maintained through links with a supranational reference laboratory (SRL). Data were obtained through routine or continuous surveillance of all TB cases (38 settings) or from specific surveys of sampled patients, as outlined in approved protocols (39 settings). Data were reported on a standard reporting form, either annually or at the completion of the survey.

The Supranational Reference Laboratory Network (SRLN) was formed in 1994 to ensure optimal performance of the national reference laboratories participating in the Global Project. The network comprises 20 laboratories in five WHO regions and is coordinated by the Prince Léopold Institute of Tropical Medicine in Antwerp, Belgium. The coordinating centre ensures the quality of the SRLN by conducting annual proficiency testing, through the exchange of a panel of 30 pretested and coded isolates with resistance to any of the following four first-line drugs – isoniazid (INH), streptomycin (SM), rifampicin (RMP) and ethambutol (EMB).

2.   RESULTS

2.1   Magnitude and trends of anti-TB drug resistance
New cases

Data on new cases were available for 75 settings. In total, 55 779 patients were surveyed. The prevalence of resistance to at least one antituberculosis drug (any

---

[a] Setting is defined as a country or a subnational setting (i.e. province, district, or oblast).
[b] There are three exceptions; Australia, Democratic Republic of Congo, Kinshasa, and Scotland reported only combined cases.

resistance) ranged from 0% in some Western European countries to 57.1% in Kazakhstan (median = 10.2%). Median prevalences of resistance to specific drugs were as follows: SM, 6.3%; INH, 5.9%; RMP, 1.4%; and EMB, 0.8%. Prevalence of MDR ranged from 0% in eight countries to 14.2% in Kazakhstan (51/359) and Israel (36/253)[c] (median = 1.1%). The highest prevalences of MDR were observed in Tomsk Oblast (Russian Federation) (13.7%), Karakalpakstan (Uzbekistan) (13.2%), Estonia (12.2%), Liaoning Province (China) (10.4%), Lithuania (9.4%), Latvia (9.3%), Henan Province (China) (7.8%), and Ecuador (6.6%)[d].

Increases in prevalence of resistance can be caused by poor or worsening TB control, immigration of patients from areas of higher resistance, outbreaks of drug-resistant disease and variations in surveillance methodologies. Trends in drug resistance in *new cases* were determined in 46 settings (20 with two data points and 26 with at least three). Significant increases in prevalence of any resistance were found in Botswana, New Zealand, Poland, and Tomsk Oblast (Russian Federation). Cuba, Hong Kong SAR, and Thailand reported significant decreases over time. Tomsk Oblast (Russian Federation) and Poland reported significantly increased prevalences of MDR. Decreasing trends in MDR were observed in Hong Kong SAR, Thailand, and the USA.

Previously treated cases

Data on previously treated cases were available for 66 settings. In total, 8405 patients were surveyed. The median prevalence of resistance to at least one drug (any resistance) was 18.4%, with the highest prevalence, 82.1%, in Kazakhstan (262/319). Median prevalences of resistance to specific drugs were as follows: INH, 14.4%; SM, 11.4%; RMP, 8.7%; and EMB, 3.5%. The median prevalence of MDR was 7.0%. The highest prevalences of MDR were reported in Oman (58.3%; 7/12) and Kazakhstan (56.4%; 180/319). Among countries of the former Soviet Union the median prevalence of resistance to the four drugs was 30%, compared with a median of 1.3% in all other settings. Given the small number of subjects tested in some settings, prevalence of resistance among previously treated cases should be interpreted with caution.

Drug resistance trends in previously treated cases were determined in 43 settings (19 with two data points and 24 with at least three data points). A significant increase in the prevalence of *any resistance* was observed in Botswana. Cuba, Switzerland, and the USA showed significant decreases. The prevalence of MDR significantly increased in Estonia, Lithuania, and Tomsk Oblast (Russian Federation). Decreasing trends were significant in Slovakia and the USA.

Association of drug resistance with the quality of TB control

Multivariate analysis showed the proportion of cases being re-treated among the total number of cases was significantly associated with both MDR and any drug resistance. The percentage of re-treatment cases in a national TB programme is an indicator of programme performance.

2.2 MDR-TB

We estimated the annual incidence of MDR cases in 69 settings included in this report.[e] For most Western and Central European countries, the estimated incidence

---

[c] Data reported from Israel in subsequent years show a considerably lower prevalence of MDR.

[d] Data from Ecuador included in the analysis are preliminary.

[e] Estimates were generated by applying prevalences determined in surveys to reported notification figures for the corresponding population and thus are dependent upon case-finding in the country and quality of recording and reporting of the national programme.

was fewer than 10 cases each. Estonia, Latvia, Lithuania and two oblasts in the Russian Federation were estimated to have between 99 and 248 MDR cases. For Henan and Hubei Provinces of China, the figure was more than 1000 cases each, and for Kazakhstan and South Africa, more than 3000. In order to analyse the burden of MDR in a given setting, prevalence in new and re-treatment cases should be linked with relevant programme information, such as proportion and categories of re-treatment among all cases, as well as absolute case numbers.

Rifampicin resistance was evaluated as a predictor of MDR-TB, in order to explore the relevance of rapid rifampicin resistance testing to identify cases likely to have MDR-TB. This would allow the rapid initiation of infection control measures and effective treatment. The positive predictive value (PPV), a function of the sensitivity and specificity of RMP resistance testing and the prevalence of MDR and non-MDR rifampicin resistance, was highest among previously treated cases in settings with high MDR prevalence and low non-MDR rifampicin resistance.

2.3 Patterns and amplification 1994–2002

Analysis of almost 90 000 isolates representative of the most recent data from countries between 1994 and 2002 confirmed that, globally, more isolates were resistant to INH than to any other drug (range 0–42%). In general, INH and SM resistance were more prevalent than RMP or EMB resistance. HSRE[f] was the most prevalent pattern among previously treated cases and the proportions of isolates resistant to three or four drugs were significantly greater among this group than among new cases. This relationship holds globally as well as regionally and suggests amplification of resistance. It appears that monoresistance to either INH or SM is the main gateway to acquisition of additional resistance.

3. CONCLUSIONS

3.1 Scale of the epidemic of drug-resistant TB

1 Drug-resistant TB was found among TB patients surveyed in 74 of 77 settings between 1999 and 2002. As in the two previous surveys, drug-resistant TB, including multidrug-resistant TB, was found in all regions of the world. The prevalence of MDR-TB was exceptionally high in almost all former Soviet Union countries surveyed, including Estonia, Kazakhstan, Latvia, Lithuania, the Russian Federation, and Uzbekistan. Proportions of isolates resistant to three or four drugs were also significantly higher in this region. High prevalences of MDR-TB were also found among new cases in China (Henan and Liaoning provinces), Ecuador and Israel. Central Europe and Africa, in contrast, reported the lowest median levels of drug resistance.

2 The proportion of retreatment of all TB cases is an indicator of programme performance.[1,2] As in previous phases of the Global Project, a link was found between poor programme performance, or insufficient coverage of a good programme, and drug resistance. Previously treated cases, worldwide, are not only more likely to be drug-resistant, but also to have resistance to more drugs than untreated patients.

f HSRE = resistance to INH, SM, RMP, and EMB.

SUMMARY

SUMMARY

3　Significant increases in prevalence of any resistance and MDR were detected in a number of settings. Increases in MDR-TB are especially worrying, since such cases are significantly more difficult to treat, and mortality is higher than for drug-susceptible cases. Increases in prevalence of any resistance may reflect an environment that favours the acquisition of additional resistance and can lead to future increases in MDR.

4　Between 1994 and 2002, the Global Project surveyed areas representing over one-third of notified TB cases worldwide. However, enormous gaps still exist in many crucial areas, especially countries with a large TB burden or where available data strongly suggest that there may be a much larger problem, particularly China, India, and countries of the former Soviet Union.

5　The ability to conduct a drug resistance survey is indicative of a reasonable level of capacity of the TB control services, most importantly the laboratory service. Thus it is likely that TB control in some unsurveyed areas is worse than in those surveyed.

4.　RECOMMENDATIONS

4.1　Management of TB control

1　The findings of this phase of the Global Project emphasize the importance of strengthening TB control worldwide, by expanding DOTS[g] in order to prevent the emergence of further drug resistance. Existing cases need to be managed by national programmes, regardless of prevalence, through application of the DOTS-Plus strategy[h] and using the Green Light Committee[i] to ensure quality of second-line drugs and proper implementation and monitoring. Full adoption of DOTS is vital if the creation of MDR-TB cases is to be halted.

2　In light of the high frequency of resistance to three or four drugs in previously treated patients, the WHO Category II regimen for re-treatment should be re-evaluated in some settings and the re-treatment guidelines should be revised if necessary. A re-evaluation should also be conducted of the efficacy of both Category I and III regimens, in which INH is recommended in the continuation phase, in settings with a high prevalence of isoniazid resistance.

3　Standardized annual recording and reporting on all categories of re-treatment – relapse, failure and return after default – should be mandatory. Accurate reporting on this population will help in monitoring programme performance and developing re-treatment strategies, and provide the required information for survey sampling.

---

g Internationally adopted strategy to control tuberculosis.
h Strategy under development for the management of multi-drug resistant tuberculosis
i The Green Light Committee reviews project applications for DOTS Plus pilot projects. Projects accepted by the GLC are then granted access to preferentially priced second-line drugs.

4 Rapid testing for rifampicin resistance may provide a useful proxy for MDR, but only in situations of high MDR prevalence (with little or no non-MDR rifampicin resistance). Early identification of these patients would permit rapid isolation and initiation of appropriate treatment, thus avoiding acquisition of additional resistance, until results of further drug susceptibility testing (DST) are available.

4.2   Surveillance of drug resistance

1 Information on drug resistance is urgently needed from unsurveyed areas of China, India, and the former Soviet Union, in the light of the prevalence of resistance detected in those countries to date and given the high rate of DOTS expansion currently under way or planned. Information on anti-TB drug resistance is also needed from countries where no surveys have yet been conducted, particularly high-burden countries, such as Afghanistan, Bangladesh, Indonesia, United Republic of Tanzania, Pakistan and Nigeria. Drug resistance surveillance should be seen as an essential component of TB control programmes in these settings.

2 Continuous drug resistance surveillance, culture and drug susceptibility testing of every TB patient are desirable wherever resources permit. Where this is not feasible but there is survey capacity, periodic surveys with separate sampling of new and re-treatment cases should be undertaken. The different types of re-treatment cases should be identified, namely relapse, failure and return after default. This is essential for the planning of a treatment programme for those with known or suspected drug resistance (DOTS Plus).

3 In order to expand drug resistance surveillance, national governments and international partners need to invest, in a coordinated way, in the evaluation and strengthening of national laboratories. The Laboratory Strengthening Subgroup of the DOTS Expansion Working Group is well placed to assist in this task.

4 A comprehensive approach to drug resistance surveillance is necessary to accurately evaluate the course of drug resistance, particularly in settings with high MDR prevalence. Data collection from drug resistance surveillance and DOTS Plus projects, as well as routine collection of notifications and outcomes, should be linked in order to allow interventions to be evaluated.

5 The high proportions of resistance to three and four drugs among cases that have been previously treated emphasize the importance of developing new anti-TB drugs.

6 This report has raised some key questions regarding drug resistance that cannot be answered through routine surveillance. Operational research should be carried out to determine, among other things, the impact of HIV on the transmission of MDR-TB in certain settings, the impact of amplification

SUMMARY

of resistance at both the individual and population level, and the impact of private sector treatment policies on drug resistance. Financial support from the international community will be essential for such research.

▌NTRODUCTION

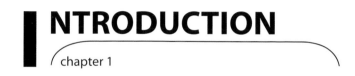

chapter 1

Since its inception in 1994, the scope and objectives of the WHO/IUATLD Global Project on Anti-Tuberculosis Drug Resistance Surveillance have expanded, on the basis of the many lessons learned over nine years of surveillance and the amount of epidemiological, laboratory and resistance data now available. These data have helped identify areas of high prevalence of drug resistance, as well as provided valuable information for policy development; but most importantly, they have served to raise key questions about the behaviour, emergence, and control of drug resistance. These questions can only be addressed through continued expansion of routine surveillance and well organized operational research.

Surveys of resistance to anti-tuberculosis (TB) drugs can be conducted at relatively low cost to a TB programme, and have the potential to yield many direct and indirect benefits to countries. The direct benefits come from measurements of the level of resistance in the population and thus quantification of the problem in terms of lives and cost, which allows appropriate interventions to be planned. Surveillance also provides a mechanism through which the effectiveness of the national TB programme can be monitored.[3] This information is instrumental in informing important policy decisions. The indirect benefits of surveillance may be even more substantial. The capacity of the national reference laboratory (NRL) is strengthened through surveillance activities, as are relationships within and outside the national TB control programme (NTP). Notably, surveillance activities have stimulated collaboration among peripheral laboratories, leading to the formation of functioning networks within countries, and have promoted synergism between the networks and care providers in the NTP.

The Global Project has actively catalysed changes in policies and programmes for TB control. DOTS-Plus, a strategy for the management of drug-resistant TB, was a result of Global Project findings, recognizing the need to mitigate the spread of drug resistance through the development of a strategy to treat resistant cases, supplementing DOTS expansion efforts. The results of the pilot phase of DOTS-Plus are now being evaluated and incorporated into the larger DOTS expansion strategy. The Global Project has also led to improvements in the capacity of many national reference laboratories and several peripheral networks through long-term relationships with supranational reference laboratories (SRLs) and participation in the proficiency testing and other external quality assurance (EQA) programmes. It has highlighted the importance of a strong laboratory network and contributed to the newly formed Laboratory Strengthening Subgroup under the WHO DOTS Expansion Working Group. The Laboratory Strengthening Subgroup draws upon the SRL network as its primary resource as it seeks to improve the overall functional capacity of each country's laboratory network, with an emphasis on smear microscopy.

Looking to the future, the Global Project is expanding the coverage of drug resistance surveillance, prioritizing high burden countries and those with suspected high levels of multidrug resistance (MDR). New surveys will study a sample of previously treated cases representative of the population in the area, and incorporate surveillance of HIV in TB patients wherever feasible. A greater emphasis will be placed on operational research using the SRL network and country capacity. On the laboratory side, the SRL network will be strengthened through recently developed performance criteria, and subnetworks will benefit from standardization of routine quality assurance (QA) as well as analysis of national reference laboratory proficiency results over time.

This report is based on the analysis of a quarter of a million isolates collected since 1994, in 109 geographical settings or 90 countries, representing over one-third of all notified TB cases. The report addresses the following areas:

- the most recent profile of antituberculosis drug resistance, looking at the latest data available for the period 1999–2002;
- the dynamics of antituberculosis drug resistance over time, or trends;
- the major determinants of drug resistance;
- evaluation of "hot spots" and how to define the burden of MDR-TB;
- the use of rifampicin resistance as a surrogate marker for MDR;
- the global profile of antituberculosis drug resistance, looking at the most recent data for each country or geographical setting surveyed since 1994, identifying prominent resistance patterns in regions and subregions, in regards to the evolution and amplification of resistance;
- results of proficiency testing of laboratories over time.

INTRODUCTION

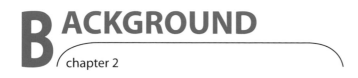

BACKGROUND
chapter 2

2.1 ANTIMICROBIAL RESISTANCE AND PUBLIC HEALTH

The emergence of resistance to antimicrobials is a natural biological occurrence. The introduction of every antimicrobial agent into clinical practice for the treatment of infectious disease in humans and animals has been followed by the detection in the laboratory of isolates of resistant microorganisms, i.e. microorganisms able to multiply in the presence of drug concentrations found in hosts receiving therapeutic doses. Such resistance may be either a characteristic associated with an entire species or acquired through mutation or gene transfer. Resistance genes encode information on a variety of mechanisms that microorganisms use to withstand the inhibitory effects of specific antimicrobials. These mechanisms can confer resistance to other antimicrobials of the same class and sometimes to several different antimicrobial classes.[4] With increasing antimicrobial use and misuse over the years, resistance to antimicrobial agents has emerged in viruses, bacteria, fungi and protozoa, posing new challenges for both clinical management and control programmes.[5,6,7,8,9,10,11]

2.2 MECHANISMS OF ANTI-TB DRUG RESISTANCE AND FACTORS ASSOCIATED WITH ITS EMERGENCE

Resistance of *Mycobacterium tuberculosis* to anti-TB drugs is man-made. Wild isolates of *M. tuberculosis* that have never been exposed to anti-TB drugs are virtually never clinically resistant.[12] There are a few exceptions, but these exceptions are not thought to contribute greatly to the overall burden of resistance. For instance, isolates of *M. tuberculosis* from Madras (Chennai), India, have been found to have a higher average level of resistance to para-aminosalicylic acid (PAS) than isolates from patients in the United Kingdom. Madras isolates of tubercle bacilli also have higher minimum inhibitory concentrations (MIC) of thioacetazone than British isolates and isolates from other parts of India.[13] This resistance is called natural resistance. Most bovine isolates are naturally resistant to PAS and pyrazinamide (PZA), and most mycobacteria other than tuberculosis (MOTT) are resistant to the standard antituberculosis drugs.[14]

Exposure to a single drug, whether as a result of poor adherence to treatment, inappropriate prescription, irregular drug supply, or poor drug quality, suppresses the growth of bacilli susceptible to that drug but permits the multiplication of pre-existing drug-resistant mutants.[15] The patient then develops ***acquired resistance***. Subsequent transmission of such bacilli to other persons may lead to disease that is drug-resistant from the outset, an occurrence known as ***primary resistance***. Because the terms are somewhat conceptual, the terms "resistance among new cases" and "resistance among previously treated cases" have been adopted as proxies.[16,17,18]

The emergence of drug-resistant *M. tuberculosis* has been associated with a variety of factors related to management, health providers and patients. In some countries, management factors may include the lack of a standardized therapeutic regimen, poor programme implementation, compounded by frequent or prolonged shortages of drugs, inadequate resources, political instability, or lack of political commitment. Use of anti-TB drugs of unproven quality[19] is an additional concern, as is the sale of these medications over the counter and on the black market. Moreover, incorrect management of individual cases, difficulties in selecting the appropriate chemotherapeutic regimen with the right dosage, and patient non-adherence to prescribed treatment also contribute to the development of drug resistance.[20,21,22,23,24,25,26,27,28]

2.3   THE THREAT OF DRUG RESISTANCE FOR TB CONTROL

Although tremendous efforts to control TB have been undertaken at the global and national levels over the past decade, almost 2 million patients still die every year. The forty-fourth World Health Assembly (WHA) in 1991 recognized the growing importance of TB and declared TB a public health emergency. In 1993, WHO formulated the DOTS strategy, which comprises five elements considered essential for global TB control:
- political commitment;
- case detection using sputum smear microscopy among persons seeking care for prolonged cough;
- standardized short-course chemotherapy under proper case-management conditions, including directly observed treatment;
- regular, uninterrupted drug supply;
- standardized recording and reporting system that allows assessment of individual patients as well as overall programme performance.

The DOTS strategy, if implemented correctly, is one of the most cost-effective public health interventions available.[32]

Data from the two previous global reports on resistance to anti-TB drugs have shown that drug resistance is present worldwide.[16,17,33,34] Studies have also indicated that drug-resistant TB is more difficult to cure. The cure rates among patients harbouring multidrug-resistant isolates range from 6% to 59%.[35] Owing to the complex nature of second-line drug treatment in terms of cost, toxicity, and delivery of appropriate regimens,[36] drug-resistant forms of tuberculosis present a real threat to TB control in some settings.

The management and control of drug resistance require a step-by-step approach. Countries can determine the magnitude of the problem through continuous surveillance or periodic surveys, and develop interventions accordingly. Surveys need a minimum set of conditions and criteria.[37] Among those criteria is the presence of an accurate recording and reporting system, a laboratory network capable of performing good quality sputum smear microscopy, a national reference laboratory performing high quality culture and drug susceptibility testing (DST), and the will to conduct a survey. Many countries that might be expected to have resistance problems do not yet have the infrastructure or political will to monitor the situation. The data obtained through the Global Project therefore reflect only the situation in countries with the capacity to carry out a survey.

2.3.1 Increased access to drugs

Recently, international efforts have resulted in the creation of a number of mechanisms that provide support to national TB programmes in their efforts to control TB. For instance, the Global TB Drug Facility (GDF) is a mechanism that aims to expand access to, and availability of, high-quality TB drugs to facilitate global DOTS expansion.[38,39] The

Green Light Committee (GLC) provides access to preferentially priced second-line drugs for the treatment of multidrug-resistant tuberculosis.[40,41] Access is granted to applicants who demonstrate compliance with DOTS-Plus project guidelines, validated by the GLC. The Global Fund to Fight AIDS, Tuberculosis and Malaria (GFATM) provides unprecedented financial resources to countries to combat these three major diseases. The long-term success of these initiatives will be enhanced by assurance that the increased distribution of antimicrobial drugs does not unduly accelerate the emergence of resistance. Thus, programmes to ensure the appropriate use of drugs and to monitor drug resistance should be put into place.

2.3.2 HIV

Data presented in the first and second global reports suggested that HIV infection is not an independent risk factor for the development of drug resistance. While some of the data available are contradictory,[42] evidence from many settings suggests that HIV-infected TB patients are not more likely to develop drug resistance than HIV-negative TB patients.[16,33,43,44] Outbreaks of MDR-TB among HIV-infected patients were observed in the USA,[45,46,47,48] Argentina,[49] and some European cities.[50,51] These outbreaks, occurring mainly in hospital settings[52], were associated with delays in diagnosis and high case-fatality rates. In areas of high HIV prevalence, the number of TB cases is increasing drastically and may indirectly lead to an increase in transmission of resistant as well as susceptible isolates. Thus, drug resistance in the context of HIV should be carefully monitored.

2.3.3 Private sector

Very little precise information is available on the number of TB patients managed in the private sector. Even with a good NTP information system, notification of TB cases from the private sector is rare especially among low- and middle-income countries. India, for instance, has the highest burden of TB and the largest private sector, which manages as many as half of all TB cases without notifying them to the NTP. TB cases managed by the private sector may account for almost a sixth of the global burden of TB.

The few available studies suggest that in many low-income TB-endemic countries with large private health sectors, a significant number of individuals with TB symptoms turn first to private physicians, traditional healers or private pharmacists.[53] This often results in a delayed diagnosis of TB and an increased likelihood of disease transmission. These studies also indicate that private practitioners commonly deviate from standard nationally and internationally recommended TB management practices. Although the settings of those studies varied greatly, the findings did not. Private practitioners in those countries placed an undue emphasis on chest radiography for diagnosis. They rarely used the initial and follow-up sputum examinations, and tended to prescribe inappropriate drug regimens, often with incorrect combinations, and inaccurate dosages for the wrong duration[54,55,56,57] In addition, there was little attention to maintaining records, notifying cases and evaluating treatment outcomes. The effect of TB case management in the private sector on drug resistance levels and patterns has not been clearly evaluated. However, in view of the large TB caseload in the private sector and evidence suggesting substandard case management, it can be expected that the private sector, in general, plays an important role in the evolution of anti-TB drug resistance.[20]

BACKGROUND

MATERIALS AND METHODS
chapter 3

3.1 METHODOLOGICAL FRAMEWORK

Methods used in the Global Project have been extensively described in the two previous reports. For this reason, methods common to the three reports are summarized here, while changes or novel methods are described in detail.[16,33]

The Global Project methodology for surveillance of drug resistance was developed by WHO/IUATLD and a working group in 1994, and laid out in *Guidelines for surveillance of resistance in tuberculosis*, published in 1994, revised in 1997 and updated in 2003.[18] The methodology operates on three main principles: (1) surveillance must be based on a sample of TB patients representative of all cases in the geographical setting under evaluation; (2) drug resistance must be clearly distinguished according to the treatment history of the patient (i.e. never treated or previously treated) in order to allow correct interpretation of the data; and (3) optimal laboratory performance must be attained through participation in a quality assurance programme, including the international exchange of isolates of *M. tuberculosis*.

3.2 DEFINITIONS OF DRUG RESISTANCE

3.2.1 Drug resistance among new cases (proxy for primary resistance)

Resistance among new cases is defined as the presence of resistant isolates of *M. tuberculosis* in patients who, in response to direct questioning, deny having had any prior anti-TB treatment (for as much as 1 month) and, in countries where adequate documentation is available, for whom there is no evidence of such a history.

3.2.2 Drug resistance among previously treated cases (proxy for acquired resistance)

Resistance among previously treated cases is defined as the presence of resistant isolates of *M. tuberculosis* in patients who, in response to direct questioning, admit having been treated for tuberculosis for 1 month or more or, in countries where adequate documentation is available, in a patient for whom there is evidence of such a history.

3.2.3 Combined prevalence of drug resistance

Combined prevalence of drug resistance is the prevalence of resistance in the population surveyed regardless of prior treatment. Despite the importance of the distinction between drug resistance among new and previously treated cases, the study of combined prevalence is relevant for the following reasons:
- In some countries and settings, such as Australia (2000), Belgium (1997), Democratic Republic of Congo (Kinshasa, 1998), Israel (1998 and 1999), the Netherlands (1995), and Scotland (2000), the history of prior treatment was not ascertained.

- In some countries and settings, patients were stratified in three groups: new, previously treated and unknown; the last group was numerically important in approximately 20% of the settings. Exclusion of this group would provide a partial (and probably biased) view of the overall occurrence of resistance.
- Given the risk of misclassification due to reporting bias by patients or health staff, the combined prevalence of anti-TB drug resistance represents a better approximation to the level of drug resistance in the community than the separate data for new and previously treated patients. In some countries, policy-makers are primarily interested in knowing the overall burden of resistance, regardless of treatment history.

The following approaches were used to obtain combined estimates of drug resistance:
- For settings reporting only combined cases, we took the data as reported by the national authorities.
- For countries conducting drug resistance *surveillance* of all their TB patients, we followed the strategy used in the two previous reports, i.e. we combined the individual data for patients with and without previous anti-TB treatment. We also added the data of the "unknown" group, where available. This is noted in individual country profiles.
- For countries that conducted *surveys*, we used an approach similar to that used in the previous reports, in which the prevalence found in the sampled new and previously treated cases was applied to the reference population data (national notifications of new and previously treated cases for the year of survey) to obtain a standardized estimate.

3.3 SURVEY AREAS AND SAMPLING STRATEGIES

New surveillance or survey projects presented in this report were carried out between 1999 and 2002, with the exception of the 1998–1999 survey in Venezuela, a 1998 survey in Kinshasa, Democratic Republic of Congo, and 1997 data for Japan. Final data from surveys in Colombia (1999) and Venezuela (1998–1999) are included, whereas only preliminary data on partial samples were included in the previous report. In previous reports, England and Wales, Northern Ireland, and Scotland submitted data separately. Since 1999, the United Kingdom submits data to EuroTB in two ways – for England, Wales and Ulster (Northern Ireland) together, either with or without Scotland. We have remained as consistent as possible with regard to area divisions in order to allow interpretation of trends, thus England, Wales and Ulster are combined for trend analysis, and Scotland remains separate. Cuba, France, Italy, and Japan operate sentinel networks for surveillance. All, with the exception of Italy, can be considered nationally representative. Italy's network covers nearly half the country and is expanding. The last two surveys in Italy are considered comparable; however, the survey appearing in the first report, which sampled only HIV-positive patients, has not been included in the trend analysis. Additionally, the two data points for Argentina are not comparable because two different sampling schemes were applied. Final data from Ecuador and Honduras were not available at the time of analysis for this report, and results should be considered preliminary. Final data from Ecuador are included in the country profile annex. Data from Chile and Mpumalanga Province, South Africa, were included after analysis was completed; therefore, these data have been included in the country profile and the estimate of MDR burden, but not in other analyses.

3.3.1 Surveillance terminology and target survey areas

For the purposes of this report it is important to distinguish between *surveys* and *surveillance*. The two can loosely be differentiated by the proportion and type of the population surveyed, the length of the intake period, and the frequency with which the process is repeated.

Surveillance, in this report, refers to either continuous or sentinel surveillance. Continuous surveillance requires DST to be routinely performed on all bacteriologically confirmed cases in the coverage area, and thus reflects the entire TB population – smear-positive, smear-negative, extrapulmonary – regardless of treatment status. Sentinel surveillance of drug resistance, in the context of this report, comprises reporting of DST results from all TB cases from a (random or non-random) sample of sites. Sentinel surveillance reports annual data from the same sites.

Surveys are periodic, and reflect the population of registered pulmonary smear-positive cases. Depending on the area surveyed, a cluster sampling technique may be adopted, or all diagnostic units included. While some countries, such as Botswana, repeat surveys every 3–5 years, for the purposes of this report they are considered as repeated surveys and not surveillance.

In both survey and surveillance settings, the coverage area is usually the entire country, but in some cases subnational units are surveyed. Large countries, such as China, India, the Russian Federation and South Africa, tend to survey large administrative units (e.g. province, state, district, oblast). Some countries have opted to limit surveys or surveillance to metropolitan areas, as in the case of Democratic Republic of Congo, Serbia and Montenegro, and Spain. Several countries (e.g. Cuba, France, Italy, and Japan) conduct sentinel surveillance. And some countries have restricted surveys to subnational areas because of the remoteness of certain provinces or to avoid conflict areas. Data for Denmark do not include Greenland and the Faroe Islands. This report includes survey data from 39 countries or geographical settings and surveillance data from 38 countries or geographical settings.

3.3.2 Sample size and sampling strategies

Calculation of sample size for surveys follows the principles outlined in the WHO/IUATLD *Guidelines for the surveillance of resistance in tuberculosis*.[18] Briefly, sample sizes are calculated on the basis of the number of new sputum smear-positive cases registered in the previous year and the expected prevalence of rifampicin (RMP) resistance in new TB cases based on previous studies or data available from the NTP. Some countries, particularly those conducting an HIV prevalence survey among TB patients at the same time as the drug resistance survey, cultured all specimens from suspects, as was the case in South Africa, where the sample size was based on the number of culture-positive TB cases. Ideally, separate sample sizes should be calculated for new cases and previously treated cases. However, the number of sputum-positive previously treated cases reported per year is usually small and, the intake period needed to achieve a statistically adequate sample size would generally be too long. Therefore, most countries have obtained an estimate of the drug resistance level among previously treated cases by including all previously treated cases who present at centres during the intake period. While this may not provide a statistically adequate sample size, it can nevertheless give a reasonable estimate of drug resistance among previously treated cases. In the future, it may be possible to conduct surveys with sufficiently large samples of previously treated cases, especially in areas where such cases comprise a large percentage of NTP case-holding. An alternative approach is to conduct surveillance of all re-treatment cases while performing surveys of new cases less frequently, e.g. every three years, as in the case of Chile.

Sampling strategies for monitoring of drug resistance include:
- countrywide, continuous surveillance of the population;
- surveys with sampling of all diagnostic centres during a specified period;
- surveys with randomly selected clusters of patients;
- surveys with cluster sampling proportional to the number of cases notified by the diagnostic centre.

3.4   BACTERIOLOGICAL METHODS

In survey settings, sputum smear microscopy using the Ziehl-Neelsen technique was used for diagnosis of TB and subsequent enrolment in the survey. In surveillance settings, a combination of smear and culture was used for initial diagnosis. The majority of laboratories used Löwenstein-Jensen (L-J) culture medium, and some used Ogawa medium. Identification of isolates was based on the niacin production test, the nitrate reduction test the para-nitrobenzoic (PNB) acid (500 mg/l) test,[58] and the thiophene-2-carboxylic acid hydrazide (TCH) (2mg/l) resistance test.[59] Some countries also used hybridization probes. Species other than the pathogenic species of *M. tuberculosis* complex were excluded from the analysis.

Drug resistance tests were performed using the simplified variant of the proportion method on L-J medium, the absolute concentration method, the resistance ratio method,[60,61] or the radiometric Bactec 460 method.[62] The proportion method was most frequently used (55% of participating settings) in this phase of the Global Project. Resistance was expressed as the percentage of colonies that grew on critical concentrations of the drugs tested (i.e. 0.2 mg/l for isoniazid (INH), 2 mg/l for ethambutol (EMB), 4 mg/l for dihydrostreptomycin sulfate and 40 mg/l for rifampicin (RMP) when L-J medium is used). The criterion used for drug resistance was growth of 1% or more of the bacterial population on media containing the critical concentration of each drug. The results of the tests were recorded on standardized forms.

Proficiency testing and quality control of survey results are two components of external[a] quality assurance. Briefly, proficiency testing requires the exchange of a panel of 20 (or more) pretested isolates between the SRL and the NRL. Results of this round determine, in part, whether the NRL is able to conduct DST for the survey or whether additional training is necessary. For QA of survey results, the NRL sends a percentage of both resistant and susceptible isolates to the SRL for checking. The percentage of isolates sent for checking is determined before the beginning of the survey. Performance criteria are currently being developed for NRL proficiency testing. Additionally, there are now efforts to standardize the panels circulated to countries for easier interpretation of results between countries and over time. To date, the results of national reference laboratory proficiency testing have been evaluated by the corresponding SRL and interventions have been based on the judgement of the SRL. In several instances testing has been repeated to ensure acceptable quality and, in a very few instances, surveys have been interrupted because of discordance between the NRL and the SRL.

MATERIALS AND METHODS

---

[a] In most cases, external quality control is international, as often the SRL is located outside of the country.

3.5 COLLECTION OF DATA

3.5.1 Patient eligibility and registration

For surveys, all newly registered patients with smear-positive TB were eligible for inclusion, including children, foreign-born persons, hospitalized patients, and those with known HIV coinfection. In surveillance settings, all TB patients were included. It was recommended that special groups likely to have higher levels of resistance, e.g. prisoners, were sampled separately in order not to artificially elevate overall rates of resistance. As in previous phases of the Global Project, HIV testing was not a mandatory component of these surveys; however, it has increasingly been incorporated in survey settings. Geographical settings that performed HIV testing as part of the survey were advised to follow international guidelines on counselling and confidentiality. In almost all settings, with the exception of Australia, Kinshasa, Democratic Republic of Congo, and Scotland, data were divided by treatment status. In some European countries, "unknown" was a category of treatment status; though this category is not displayed individually the cases are captured in the combined column. In a few countries, testing of streptomycin (SM) resistance is not systematically performed; where this is the case a footnote appears in the country profile.

3.5.2 Accuracy of information on prior TB treatment

It was recommended that reinterview and double-checking of patient histories be undertaken in survey settings to reduce the possibility of misclassification of previously treated cases. In geographical areas where people may be reluctant to reveal treatment status, verification of treatment status plays a particularly important role. In two Chinese provinces – Henan in 1996 and Liaoning in 1999 – rechecking took place after the completion of the survey because MDR among new cases appeared to be considerably higher than expected and misclassification was suspected.

3.5.3 Data management in individual countries

Since 1998, EuroTB, a project funded by the European Commission and based in Paris, France, has undertaken continuous collection and verification of drug resistance surveillance data in Western Europe and much of Central Europe. Since 2001, WHO and EuroTB have used a common collection form. All the data for Western Europe and much of that for Central Europe included in the present report were provided by EuroTB and conform to WHO/IUATLD Global Project standards. Other countries conducting surveillance have provided data either directly to WHO Headquarters or via WHO regional offices. All data files and epidemiological profiles have been returned to countries for verification before publication. In this phase of the Global Project, version 3 of the WHO software, *Surveillance of drug resistance in tuberculosis* (SDRTB 3.0), was used by many countries conducting surveys for data entry, management, and analysis at the local level.[63] However, most countries conducting continuous surveillance of drug resistance in all TB cases use their own software. The Global Project requests that survey protocols include a description of methods used for the quality assurance of data collection, entry, and analysis. However, to date there has been no systematic procedure to ensure that the methods described are actually employed at the country level.

3.6   STATISTICAL PROCEDURES – DATA ENTRY, CHECKING AND CLEANING

Recent data provided by national authorities or EuroTB for the Western and Central European regions were entered in a database to which all data from the first and second report were added, thus covering the whole study period 1994–2002.

The consistency and plausibility of the data have been checked through programmes written in Epi-Info 6 and SPSS/Windows 9.0. The data checking was not restricted to the third report, but included also the first and second reports. Inconsistencies and errors have been corrected if the available evidence allowed it. Where the analysis of the trends showed irregularities, verification was requested from the reporting parties. The final data sheets were submitted to the reporting bodies for their approval.

3.7   STATISTICAL ANALYSIS

3.7.1 Phase 3 of the Global Project (most recent data)

Analysis was conducted on drug resistance data for new cases, previously treated cases, and combined prevalence. The following patterns of drug resistance were highlighted: resistance to any TB drug, single-drug resistance, resistance to three or four drugs, MDR-TB, and resistance to any of the four first-line drugs (isoniazid, rifampicin, ethambutol, streptomycin). Descriptive statistics were calculated in Epi Info (version 6.04d) and SPSS/Windows 9.0. Arithmetic means, medians and ranges were determined as summary statistics for new, previously treated, and combined cases, for individual drugs and pertinent combinations. For geographical settings reporting more than a single data point since the second report, only the latest data point was used for the estimation of point prevalence. Chi-squared and Fisher exact tests were used to test the null hypothesis of equality of prevalences. All tests of significance were two-tailed and the alpha-error was kept at the 0.05 level in all inference procedures. Ninety-five percent confidence intervals were calculated around the prevalences and the medians.

The coverage of the Global Project was estimated using notified TB cases, notified new smear-positive cases, and population figures for the year 2001 reported to WHO.[64] For geographical settings reporting more than one data point, only the latest data point was used for these calculations. Reported notifications were used for each country that conducted a representative nationwide survey. For surveys carried out on a subnational level (states, provinces, oblasts), information representing only the population surveyed is included where appropriate.

3.7.2 Dynamics of resistance over time

Analysis was conducted on prevalence of drug resistance among new cases, among previously treated cases, and combined prevalence. In order to be comprehensive, all countries and settings with more than one data point were included in this exercise; thus some information from the second phase of the global project is repeated. The following patterns of drug resistance were highlighted: any drug resistance, MDR, any INH resistance, and any RMP resistance.

In geographical settings where only two data points were available since the start of monitoring, the prevalences were compared through the prevalence ratio (the first data point being used as the base for comparison), and through error bar charts, representing the 95% confidence interval around the prevalence ratio. The chi-squared test and Fisher exact two-tailed test were used to test the equality of prevalences, and 95% confidence intervals were set around the prevalence ratios.

For settings that reported at least three data points, the trend was determined visually as ascending, descending, flat or "saw pattern". The relative increase or decrease was expressed as a ratio, e.g. for MDR among new cases in Botswana: the MDR prevalence for 2002 was 1.3% and for 1995 0.2%; the ratio = 1.3/0.2, a 6.5-fold increase. Where the trend was linear, the slope was tested using a chi-squared test of trend. Where no linear trend was present, a chi-squared or Fisher exact test was used. The chi-squared test was applied to absolute numbers, not proportions.

3.7.3 Determinants of drug resistance (ecological analysis)

In order to study the factors associated with drug resistance, an ecological analysis was performed. The variables included were selected in function of their presumed impact on resistance and their potential for retrieval. A conceptual framework was developed that structured the retained variables along three axes: patient-related, health-system-related, and contextual factors. Prevalence of any resistance and MDR were retained as outcome variables.

3.7.3.1 Sources of information

All countries participating in Global Project surveys received a standardized form to collect relevant data. Several countries did not report on specific ecological variables, thus reducing the impact of the analysis. Ecological analysis was performed at the country level, thus the indicators reflect national information. Data on the incidence of TB and the TB programme information were taken from the WHO report, *Global tuberculosis control: surveillance, planning, financing.*[64] The information on the contextual and health-system-related factors was obtained from various sources: UNDP's *Human Development Report* for 2002,[67] *The World Health Report 2000*,[72] and *The World Health Report 2002*.[71] Efforts were made to fill in gaps in information, but for some settings not all relevant data were available. To avoid the elimination of those settings from the multivariate analysis, the "hot-deck" technique[65] was applied, substituting the missing values with the mean value for the particular WHO region or subregion.

3.7.3.2 Statistical analysis of the aggregate data

A bivariate analysis was carried out by means of the Spearman rank correlation. Multiple linear regression analysis was carried out with SPSS/Windows 9.0, and mainly backwards approaches were used. The significant variables were retained for the multivariate analysis and a multiple regression technique was used.

The arcsin transformation of the square root of the outcome variables was carried out as a normalization procedure to safeguard the requirements of the multiple linear regression modelling. This procedure stabilizes the variances when the outcome variable is a rate, and is especially useful when the value is smaller than 30% or higher than 70%, which is the case for both outcome variables. The impact of weighting on the regression results was explored, taking sample sizes at country level as weights. However, the differences between the weighted and unweighted regressions were trivial and the results given are those of the unweighted multiple linear regression. In the model, only factors with a P value <0.10 were retained. All tests of significance were two-tailed. The most parsimonious models were retained as final models, for which the normal plot for standardized residuals complied best with the linearity requirements.

MATERIALS AND METHODS

3.7.4 **MDR projections**

The validity of a statistical cut-off point for an MDR "hot spot" was examined in relation to the distribution of the most recent data points from settings included in the Global Project since 1994. The criterion of "outlier" in the ranked MDR prevalences was used as the basis for the proposition of this point.

The burden of MDR at the country/geographical setting level was estimated epidemiologically, by determining the expected total number of combined MDR cases. For countries implementing surveys, the figure was estimated by applying the prevalence of MDR among new cases to the reported number of notified new sputum smear-positive cases and the prevalence of MDR among previously treated cases to the number of notified re-treatment cases. Notifications included in the WHO TB report[64] were used, or from national TB programmes for subnational settings. This approach is highly dependent on case-finding in the country and the quality of recording and reporting of the national programme. For countries conducting surveillance, new and previously treated MDR cases were added to generate a total population. Ninety-five percent confidence limits around proportions were determined using the Fleiss quadratic method in Epi Info (version 6.04d).

3.7.5 **Patterns of resistance**

Patterns of resistance were studied at the level of isolates. Almost 90 000 isolates, representative of the most recent data point for every country surveyed between 1994 and 2002, were included in the analysis. Patterns were determined for prevalence (in relation to total number of isolates tested) and for proportion (in relation to the total number of isolates showing any resistance).

3.7.6 **Resistance to RMP: a good surrogate marker for MDR?**

In determining whether rifampicin resistance is a good surrogate marker for MDR, the pertinent question is as follows: "What is the probability that an isolate testing resistant to RMP is, also resistant to INH?" The question is best addressed using the positive predictive value (PPV). The calculation of PPV is usually based on a 2 x 2 table. However, the use of RMP resistance as a surrogate for MDR should be addressed using a 2 x 3 table, to account for the sensitivity and specificity of the test and the range of non-MDR rifampicin resistance, such as resistance only to RMP (monoR), to RMP and EMB (RE), to RMP and SM (RS), and to RMP, EMB and SM (RES).

	Any R +		Any R-	Total
	MDR+	MDR-		
R+	R+/MDR+	R+/MDR-	R+/AnyR-	∑ R+
R-	R-/MDR+	R-/MDR-	R-/AnyR-	∑ R-

Where:
MDR + = reported HR, HRS, HRE, HRSE resistant cases;
MDR - = reported monoR, RE, RS, RES resistant cases;
AnyR - = all reported non-rifampicin-resistant isolates in the sample (i.e. all susceptible isolates).
The total of MDR+, MDR- and AnyR- cases = total sample population.

The values inside the boxes are calculated as follows :
R+/MDR+ = the number of MDR+ cases multiplied by the sensitivity;
R+/MDR- = the number of MDR- cases multiplied by the sensitivity;
R+/AnyR- = the number of AnyR- cases multiplied by [1- specificity].

Sensitivity and specificity values were calculated from the cumulative results of 5 rounds of SRLN proficiency testing[66] PPV was then calculated as (R+/MDR+) / ∑R+. The PPV was graphically represented as a scatter plot against the MDR prevalence.

3.8 VALIDITY OF THE FINDINGS

Surveillance and survey data are prone to errors that may to some extent invalidate the findings. Those errors, or biases, may be related to the selection of subjects, the data-gathering or the data analysis.

3.8.1 Selection bias

Where cases are sampled only for a short period or in a restricted geographical area, the sample may not be fully representative of the total eligible population. This was the case in Italy in 1994, when only HIV-infected patients were studied. As a result, in the first report, these data were excluded from the analysis; we have also excluded the Italian data from the trend analysis. Selection bias may also occur when only a particular subgroup of TB patients is included in the sample, as was the case in a number of settings that included only MDR cases in the previously treated cases. For these settings, the analysis was restricted to new cases only.

3.8.2 Observation and information bias

Distinguishing accurately between new and previously treated cases is not always possible, as this depends on the patients' willingness to disclose a history of prior anti-TB treatment and on the training and motivation of the staff. For various reasons, patients may be unaware of their treatment antecedents, or prefer to conceal this information. Consequently, in some survey settings, a certain number of previously treated cases were probably misclassified as new cases. (Misclassification in the opposite direction is considered unlikely.) The impact of this misclassification may result in an overestimation of the resistance rates among new cases; it is difficult, however, to estimate the magnitude of this bias. It is important to mention that the prevalence of resistance rates will be biased only if the correctly classified and misclassified TB patients have different risks for drug resistance.

Test bias

Another bias, which is often not addressed in field studies, is the difference between the true prevalence and the observed or "test" prevalence. That difference depends on the magnitude of the true prevalence in the population, and the performance of the test under study conditions (i.e. its sensitivity and specificity). In practice, no test is completely accurate. Therefore reported prevalence will either over- or underestimate the true prevalence in the population. In the context of anti-TB drug resistance surveillance, where prevalence of MDR is relatively low, an overestimation of prevalence rates is more likely even with relatively high sensitivity and specificity of the DST.[66] Theoretically, underestimation of the prevalence rates could also occur, when tests of low sensitivity are used in situations of high endemicity.

Representativeness of rates

Some settings reported a small number of resistant cases, and a few settings reported a small number of total cases examined. There were a number of possible reasons for these small denominators in various participating geographical settings, ranging from small absolute populations in some surveillance settings to feasibility problems in survey settings. This was particularly true for previously treated cases. The resulting reported prevalences thus lack stability and important variations are seen over time, though most of the variations are not statistically significant. Where there were

MATERIALS AND METHODS

serious doubts concerning the representativeness of the sample of previously treated cases, the data were not included in the final database.

Analysis of trends

Although serious efforts have been made to obtain data that are as reliable as possible, some residual irregularities were detected in a number of settings. Such irregularities may be caused by diagnostic misclassification, changes in coverage, or reporting errors. They may also be a result of selective migration. However, most are minor and do not invalidate the observations.

Ecological fallacy

Whenever data to be analysed consist of summaries at group level, as is the case here, there is risk of ecological fallacy,[a] where observed relationships at one level do not hold true at another level. As an example, TB programme indicators (coverage, functionality, effectiveness) were not found to be related to the resistance rates at the aggregate level. There is, however, substantial evidence that a good DOTS programme prevents the emergence of drug resistance among new cases, at the individual patient level.

The estimation of the MDR burden

In settings where exhaustive surveillance was carried out, the population data produced a straightforward estimate of the MDR burden in all pulmonary and extrapulmonary TB cases in the area. With survey data, the estimation was based on the sample rates and new and re-treatment notifications. Upper and lower estimates were based on the assumption of reasonable representativeness of the sample and parent populations.

Patterns

The analysis included only the isolates examined at the most recent data point. The advantage of this approach is the avoidance of excessive weighting of crude results by those settings with several data points and a large sample size.

MATERIALS AND METHODS

---

[a] Ecological fallacy: an error in inference due to failure to distinguish between different levels of the factors involved. A correlation between variables based on group (ecological) characteristics is not necessarily reproduced between variables based on individual characteristics. An association at one level may disappear or even be reversed by grouping the data.

TABLE 1. WHO/IUATLD network of supranational laboratories and associated national reference laboratories (1994-2003)

SRL	Country	Setting	Year	Status
Tuberculosis Research Centre, Chennai, India				
	India	North Arcot District, Tamil Nadu State	1999	Completed
	India	Raichur District, Karnataka State	1999	Completed
	India	Wardha District, Maharashtra State	2001	Completed
	Myanmar		2002	Completed
	Indonesia		*	*Planned*
	India	*State (to be determinated)*	*	*Planned*
	India	*State (to be determinated)*	*	*Planned*
Swedish Institute for Infectious Disease Control (SIIDC), Stockholm, Sweden				
	Sweden		*	Surveillance
	Latvia		*	Surveillance
	Estonia		*	Surveillance
	Finland		*	Surveillance
	Norway		*	Surveillance
	Lithuania		*	Surveillance
	Romania		*	*Ongoing*
	Islamic Republic of Iran		*	*Planned*
	Russian Federation	*Additional Oblasts*	*	*Planned*
Reference Laboratory Mycobacteriology, Statens Serum Institut (SSI), Denmark under SIIDC, Sweden				
	Denmark		*	Surveillance
	Iceland		*	Surveillance
	Lithuania		*	Surveillance
NIPH, Norway under SIIDC, Sweden				
	Mozambique		1999	Completed
Servicio de Microbiologia, Hospital Universitaris Vall d'Hebron, Barcelona, Spain				
	Spain	Barcelona	*	Surveillance
	Spain	Galicia	2002	Completed
Research Institute of Tuberculosis (RIT), Tokyo, Japan				
	Cambodia		2001	Completed
	Islamic Republic of Iran		1998	Completed
	Singapore		*	Surveillance
	Mongolia		1999	Completed
	Japan		1997	Completed
	Malaysia	Peninsular Malaysia	1997	Completed
Queensland Mycobacterium Reference Laboratory, Australia				
	Australia		*	Surveillance
	New Zealand		*	Surveillance
	India	Tamil Nadu State	1997	Completed
	India	Delhi State	1995	Completed
Health Protection Agency, Mycobacterium Reference Unit, London, UK (formerly PHLS)				
	Belgium		*	Surveillance
	Northern Ireland		*	Surveillance
	Ireland		*	Surveillance
	France	Sentinel sites	*	Surveillance
	Switzerland		*	Surveillance
	Malta		*	Surveillance
	Switzerland		*	Surveillance
	The Gambia		2000	Completed
	Kenya	Nearly countrywide	1995	Completed
	Israel		*	Surveillance
	United Kingdom	Scotland	*	Surveillance

MATERIALS AND METHODS

SRL	Country	Setting	Year	Status
	United Kingdom		*	Surveillance
	Kenya		*	*Ongoing*
	Russian Federation	*Additional Oblasts*	*	*Planned*
Prince Leopold Institute of Tropical Medicine, Antwerp, Belgium				
	Belgium		*	Surveillance
	D.R. Congo	Kinshasa	1999	Completed
	Romania		1995	Completed
	Georgia		*	*Planned*
	Brazil	*Nationwide, by state*	*	*Planned*
	BAS Congo		*	*Planned*
	Rwanda		*	*Planned*
	Peru		*	*Planned*
National Reference Center for Mycobacteria, Borstel, Germany				
	Germany		*	Surveillance
	Bosnia and Herzegovina		*	Surveillance
	Slovenia		*	Surveillance
	Turkmenistan	Aral Sea	2002	Completed
	Uzbekistan	Aral Sea	2002	Completed
	Serbia and Montenegro		*	Surveillance
	Kazakhstan		2001	Completed
	Zimbabwe		1995	Completed
	Croatia		*	Surveillance
	Slovakia		*	Surveillance
	Kyrgyzstan		*	*Planned*
	Armenia		*	*Planned*
	Azerbaijan		*	*Planned*
	Russian Federation	*Additional oblasts*	*	*Planned*
National Institute of Public Health, Prague, Czech Republic				
	Slovakia		*	Surveillance
	Czech Republic		*	Surveillance
National Institute of Public Health and the Environment (RIVM), Bilthoven, The Netherlands				
	Poland		1997, 2001	Completed
	Netherlands		*	Surveillance
	Ethiopia		*2004*	*Ongoing*
Medical Research Council (MRC) National TB Research Programme, South Africa				
	South Africa	Eastern Cape Province	2002	Completed
	South Africa	Gauteng Province	2002	Completed
	South Africa	Kwazulu-Natal Province	2002	Completed
	South Africa	Limpopo Province	2002	Completed
	South Africa	North West Province	2002	Completed
	South Africa	Western Cape Province	2002	Completed
	South Africa	Free State Province	2002	Completed
	South Africa	Mpumalanga	1997, 2002	Completed
	Swaziland		1995	Completed
	Lesotho		1995	Completed
	Zambia		2000	Completed
	United Republic of Tanzania		*	*Planned*
	Malawi		*	*Ongoing*
	Nigeria	*3 states*	*	*Planned*
Massachusetts State Laboratory, Boston, United States of America				
	Russian Federation	Tomsk Oblast	*	Surveillance
*Laboratory Centre for Disease Control, Ottawa, Canada, (Since 1999, National Reference Centre for Mycobacteriology, Winnipeg, Canada)				
	Dominican Republic		1995	Completed
	Canada		*	Surveillance

MATERIALS AND METHODS

SRL	Country	Setting	Year	Status
Laboratoire de la Tuberculose, Institut Pasteur d'Algérie-Alger, Algiers, Algeria				
	Benin		1997	Completed
	Egypt		2002	Completed
	Algeria		2001	Completed
	Syria		*2004*	*Ongoing*
	Jordan		*2004*	*Ongoing*
Kuratorium Tuberkulose in der Welt E.V., Gauting, Germany				
	Nepal		1996, 99, 01	Completed
	Ukraine	*Donetsk Oblast*	*	*Planned*
Korean Institute of Tuberculosis (KIT), Seoul, Republic of Korea				
	China	Hong Kong SAR	*	Surveillance
	China	Shandong Province	1997	Completed
	China	Henan	1996, 2001	Completed
	China	Guandong	1999	Completed
	China	Hubei	1999	Completed
	China	Zhejiang	1999	Completed
	China	Liaoning	1999	Completed
	Republic of Korea		1994, 1999	Completed
	Thailand		1997, 2001	Completed
	Viet Nam		1997	Completed
	China	*Xinjiang*		*Planned*
	China	*Hunan*	*	*Ongoing*
	China	*Beijing City*	*	*Planned*
	China	*Shanghai City*	*	*Planned*
	China	*Chongqing*	*	*Planned*
	China	*Heilongjiang*	*	*Planned*
	China	*Inner Mongolia*	*	*Ongoing*
* indicates Hong KongTuberculosis Laboratory, Hong Kong Special Administrative unit acts is acting SRL				
Istituto Superiore di Sanità, Rome, Italy				
	Italy		*	Surveillance
	Qatar		*	Surveillance
	Oman		*	Surveillance
	Mozambique		*	*Planned*
	Turkey		*	*Planned*
	Kosovo		*	*Planned*
*Instituto Panamericano de Proteccion de Alimentos y Zoonosis (INPPAZ) Buenos Aires, Argentina				
	Chile		1997	Completed
	Uruguay		1997	Completed
	Brazil		1996	Completed
	Cuba		*	Surveillance
	Argentina		1994, 1999	Completed
	Peru		1996	Completed
	Nicaragua		1998	Completed
	Bolivia		1996	Completed
Instituto Nacional de Saúde,Porto, Portugal				
	Portugal		1995	Completed
Instituto de Salud Pública de Chile, Santiago, Chile				
	Chile		2001	Completed
	Colombia		2000	Completed
	El Salvador		2001	Completed
	Venezuela		1999	Completed
	Ecuador		2002	Ongoing

MATERIALS AND METHODS

MATERIALS AND METHODS

SRL	Country	Setting	Year	Status
	Uruguay		1999	Completed
	Cuba		*	Surveillance
	Honduras		2002	Ongoing
	Paraguay		*2003*	*Ongoing*
	Guatemala		*2003*	*Ongoing*
	Bolivia		*2003*	*Ongoing*
	Panama		*	*Planned*
Institut Pasteur, Centre National de Référence des Mycobactéries, Paris, France				
	Guinea	Sentinel sites	1998	Completed
	Russian Federation	Ivanovo Oblast	1998	Completed
	Côte d'Ivoire		1996	Completed
	Central African Republic	Bangui	1998	Completed
	France	Sentinel sites	*	Surveillance
	New Caledonia		1996	Completed
	Oman		*	Surveillance
	Algeria		2001	Completed
	Senegal		*	*Planned*
	Lebanon		*	*Planned*
Centers for Disease Control and Prevention (CDC), Atlanta, United States of America				
	Botswana		1996, 1999, 2002	Completed
	United States		*	Surveillance
	Puerto Rico		*	Surveillance
	Russian Federation	Orel Oblast	2002	Completed
	Mexico	Baja California, Sinaloa, Oaxaca	1997	Completed
*Armauer Hansen Institut, Würtzburg, Germany				
	Sierra Leone	Nearly countrywide	1996	Completed
	Uganda	3 GLRA Zones *	1997	Completed
*indicates the laboratory has either closed or is no longer part of the network				

Figure 1. Estimated coverage of the Global Project, 1994-2002*

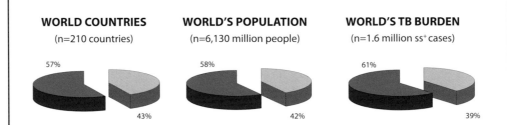

WORLD COUNTRIES
(n=210 countries)

57%
43%

WORLD'S POPULATION
(n=6,130 million people)

58%
42%

WORLD'S TB BURDEN
(n=1.6 million ss+ cases)

61%
39%

* Coverage, depicted in grey, was estimated using population figures and notified TB incidence in 2001. For subnational administrative units (state, province, oblast) denominators include population and TB incidence from those units only.

Table 2. Coverage of the Global Project by WHO region, 1994–2002

WHO region	Parameter	Total in region (2001)	Project total	(%)
AFR	Total settings	-	24	-
	Total countries	46	17	37
	Population	655,515,000	217,418,000	33
	TB cases (ALL)	811,172	394,785	49
	TB cases (new ss+)	375,997	186,139	50
AMR	Total settings	-	18	-
	Total countries	44	18	41
	Population	842,442,000	802,922,000	95
	TB cases (ALL)	229,873	218,603	95
	TB cases (new ss+)	129,536	119,926	93
EMR	Total settings	-	5	-
	Total countries	23	5	22
	Population	496,422,000	174,076,000	35
	TB cases (ALL)	165,060	11,480	7
	TB cases (new ss+)	68,924	8,022	12
EUR	Total settings	-	39	-
	Total countries	51	39	71
	Population	874,221,000	476,395,000	54
	TB cases (ALL)	368,136	121,552	33
	TB cases (new ss+)	86,012	41,107	48
SEAR	Total settings	-	6	-
	Total countries	10	3	30
	Population	1,559,819,000	166,100,000	11
	TB cases (ALL)	1,414,845	156,999	11
	TB cases (new ss+)	561,901	79,363	14
WPR	Total settings	-	17	-
	Total countries	36	11	31
	Population	1,702,487,000	730,926,000	43
	TB cases (ALL)	824,023	400,105	49
	TB cases (new ss+)	379,783	193,017	51
WORLD	Total settings	-	109	-
	Total countries	210	90	43
	Population	6,130,906,000	2,567,837,000	42
	TB cases (ALL)	3,813,109	1,303,524	34
	TB cases (new ss+)	1,602,153	627,574	39

* Denominators include notified TB cases and specific population of the setting surveyed

MATERIALS AND METHODS

MATERIALS AND METHODS

WHO / IUATLD Global Project Coverage, 1994-2002

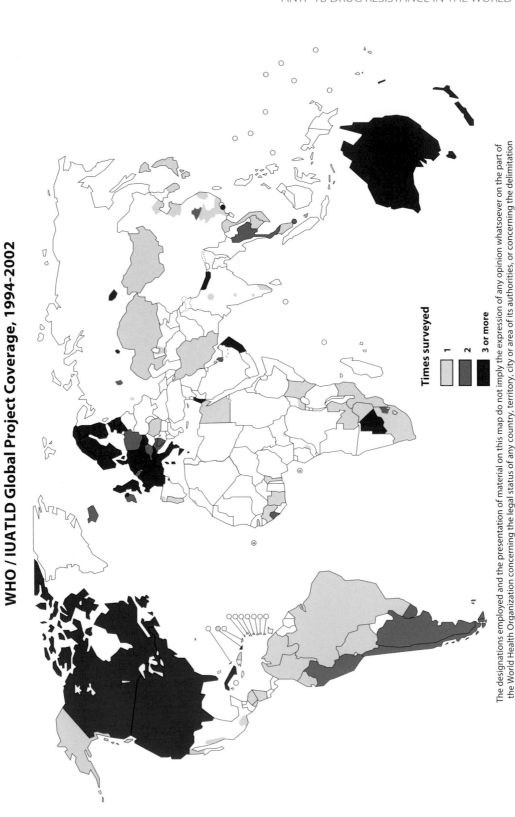

Times surveyed

1

2

3 or more

The designations employed and the presentation of material on this map do not imply the expression of any opinion whatsoever on the part of the World Health Organization concerning the legal status of any country, territory, city or area of its authorities, or concerning the delimitation of its frontiers or boundaries. Dashed lines represent approximate border lines for which there may not be full agreement

RESULTS
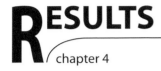

chapter 4

Phase 3 of the Global Project provides the most recent data on antituberculosis drug resistance, from 77[a] geographical settings in 62 countries. Of these, 39 settings have never previously provided data. Two settings have not been included in the analysis: Mpumalanga Province, South Africa, and Chile.

Subnational surveys, i.e. at the provincial, district, or city level, account for the discrepancy between the number of geographical settings and the number of countries. Six countries had results for 21 projects: eight in South Africa covering the entire country (the provinces of Eastern Cape, Free State, Gauteng, Kwazulu-Natal, Limpopo, North West, Mpumalanga, and Western Cape), four in China (the provinces of Henan, Hubei, and Liaoning, and Hong Kong Special Administrative Region), three in India (North Arcot District, Tamil Nadu State; Raichur District, Karnataka State; and Wardha District, Maharashtra State), two in the Russian Federation (Orel and Tomsk Oblasts), two in Spain (Barcelona and Galicia Provinces), and two in the United Kingdom (England, Wales, and Northern Ireland; and Scotland).

Types of data

The most recent anti-TB drug resistance profile contains data from 77 settings:[b]
- 65 settings provided information on drug resistance among *new, previously treated* and *combined* cases;
- 9 settings reported drug resistance information on *new cases* only;
- 3 settings (Australia, Kinshasa (Democratic Republic of Congo) and Scotland) reported drug resistance information on *combined* cases only.

Thus analyses were possible for: new cases (74 settings); previously treated cases (65 settings); and combined cases (69 settings).[c]

4.1 PREVALENCE OF DRUG RESISTANCE

4.1.1 Drug resistance among new cases of tuberculosis

Full details of the prevalence of drug resistance among new cases for the period 1999–2002 are given in Annex 1. Countries and geographical settings are stratified by WHO Region. The median number of cases tested per setting was 459. The number of cases tested ranged from 3 (Andorra) to 9751 (USA).

---

[a] Data from 77 settings are included in the analysis; 79 settings have been included in the country profile annex, representing 63 countries.
[b] Data from the following settings are still preliminary: Ecuador, Honduras.
[c] This is the sum of the 65 settings reporting new, previously treated and combined cases, plus the three settings that reported only combined data, plus the combined data for Puerto Rico. Puerto Rico reported only new cases in 2001, but new, previously treated and combined cases from 1997 until 2000. We therefore included the combined data of Puerto Rico for 2000.

Any resistance among new cases

Seventy-four countries/geographical settings provided data on the prevalence of drug resistance among new cases of TB. The overall drug resistance ranged from 0% (Andorra, Iceland, Malta) to 57.1% (Kazakhstan), with a median of 10.2% (95% CI: 8.8–11.6%). Thirteen settings reported a prevalence of any resistance higher than 25%. Of these, nine reported prevalences near 30%, and four reported substantially higher levels: Kazakhstan (57.1%), Karakalpakstan, Uzbekistan (48.1%), Liaoning Province, China (42.1%) and Tomsk Oblast, Russian Federation (37.3%) (Figure 2).

Figure 2: Countries/settings with prevalence of any resistance higher than 25% among new cases, 1999–2002

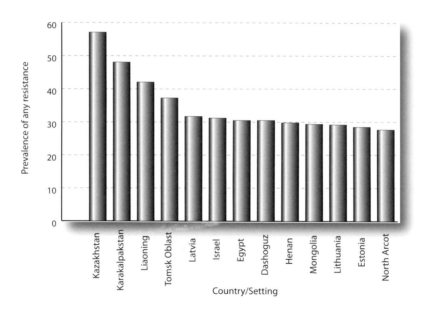

Prevalence of any drug resistance among new TB cases, 1994-2002

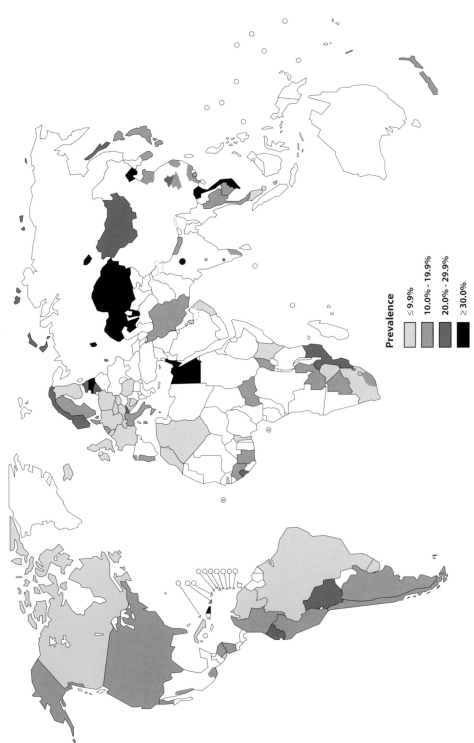

Prevalence

≤ 9.9%

10.0% - 19.9%

20.0% - 29.9%

≥ 30.0%

The designations employed and the presentation of material on this map do not imply the expression of any opinion whatsoever on the part of the World Health Organization concerning the legal status of any country, territory, city or area of its authorities, or concerning the delimitation of its frontiers or boundaries. Dashed lines represent approximate border lines for which there may not be full agreement

RESULTS

MDR among new cases

Prevalence of MDR ranged from 0% (Andorra, Cambodia, Iceland, Luxembourg, Malta, New Zealand, Oman, Scotland, Slovenia, and Switzerland) to 14.2% (Kazakhstan and Israel[a]). The median was 1.1%. Ten settings had an MDR prevalence higher than 6.5% (Figure 3).

Figure 3: Countries/settings with MDR prevalence higher than 6.5% among new cases 1999-2002

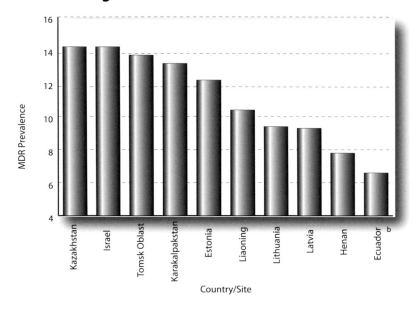

Resistance among new cases according to number of drugs

Prevalence of monoresistance (resistance to a single drug) ranged from 0% to 21.7% (Egypt) with a median of 7.0% (Annex 1Annex 1). Nine settings reported rates higher than 15%: Egypt (21.7%); Liaoning, China (21.6%); Dashoguz, Turkmenistan (21%); Mongolia (18.3%); North Arcot District, India (16.7%); Henan Province, China (15.6%); Raichur District, India (15.5%); Wardha District, India (15.2%); and Norway (15.0%). Resistance to two drugs ranged from 0% to 17.8% (Kazakhstan), with a median of 2.2%. Resistance to three or four drugs was less than 2% in 80% of the settings. Six settings had rates over 10%: Kazakhstan (25.3%); Karakalpakstan, Uzbekistan (19.8%); Israel (14.6%); Estonia (13.4%); Tomsk Oblast, Russian Federation (13.1%); and Latvia (10.3%).

[a] Data reported from Israel in subsequent years (2001 and 2002) show a considerably lower prevalence of MDR.
[b] Data reported from Ecuador are preliminary.

Prevalence of MDR-TB among new TB cases, 1994-2002

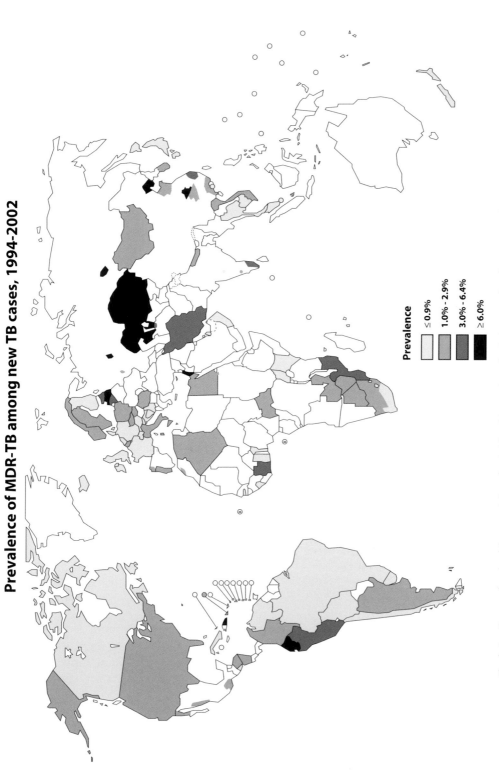

Prevalence

≤ 0.9%

1.0% - 2.9%

3.0% - 6.4%

≥ 6.0%

The designations employed and the presentation of material on this map do not imply the expression of any opinion whatsoever on the part of the World Health Organization concerning the legal status of any country, territory, city or area of its authorities, or concerning the delimitation of its frontiers or boundaries. Dashed lines represent approximate border lines for which there may not be full agreement

RESULTS

Any resistance among new cases by individual drug

Annex 2 shows the prevalence of any resistance to each of the four drugs among new cases. The highest prevalence of any resistance to each drug was observed in Kazakhstan (INH, 42.6%; RMP, 15.6%; EMB, 24.8%; SM, 51.5%). The distributions of resistance are illustrated as boxplots in Figure 4.

Figure 4: Prevalence of any resistance to INH, RMP, EMB and SM among new cases, 1999–2002

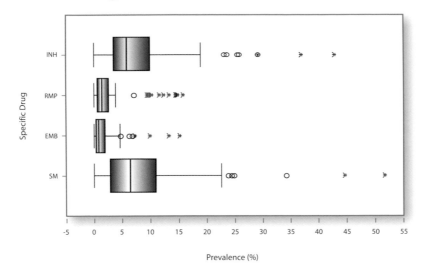

A boxplot is a summary graphical display, showing the median, quartiles, outliers and extreme values. The box represents the interquartile range, which contains 50% of the observations, and shows the median value and adjusted 25th and 75th percentiles. The whiskers are lines extending from the box to the highest and lowest values that are not outliers. A line across the box indicates the median. Circles represent outliers and stars extreme values. Outliers and extreme values are so low or so high that they stand apart from the data batch. They merit attention as they present valuable information about epidemiological clues or data validity.

Outliers are values between 1.5 and 3 box lengths from the upper or lower edge of the box. Extreme values are more than 3 box lengths from the upper or lower edge of the box.

Any INH resistance. The median prevalence of resistance to INH was 5.6%. Several outliers were observed: Tomsk Oblast, Russian Federation (29.1%); Latvia (29.0%); Israel (25.7%); Lithuania (25.4%); Liaoning Province, China (25.3%); North Arcot, India (23.4%) and Estonia (22.9%). Extreme high values were found in Karakalpakstan, Uzbekistan (37.0%), and in Kazakhstan (42.6%).

Any RMP resistance. The median prevalence of resistance to RMP was 1.4%. One outlier was observed (Egypt, 7.0%) and ten settings reported extreme values: Latvia (9.3%); Lithuania (9.8%); Henan, China (9.7%); Ecuador (10.2%); Liaoning Province, China (11.4%); Estonia (12.2%); Karakalpakstan, Uzbekistan (13.2%); Tomsk Oblast, Russian Federation (14.3%); Israel (14.6%); and Kazakhstan (15.6%).

Any EMB resistance. The median prevalence of resistance to EMB was 0.8%. Outliers were observed in Orel Oblast, Russian Federation (4.7%); Latvia (6.2%); Norway (6.9%); and Lithuania (7.3%). Extreme values were observed in Kazakhstan (24.8%); Karakalpakstan, Uzbekistan (15.1%); Estonia (13.2%); and Israel (9.9%).

Any SM resistance. The median prevalence of resistance to SM was 6.3%. Outliers were observed in Egypt (23.6%), Mongolia (24.2%), Latvia (24.4%), Dashoguz, Turkmenistan (24.8%), Tomsk Oblast, Russian Federation (34.1%) and Liaoning Province, China (34.1%). Extreme high values were reported in Karakalpakstan, Uzbekistan (44.3%), and Kazakhstan (51.5%).

New cases resistant to INH but susceptible to RMP

In fifteen settings, more than 10% of cases were resistant to INH but susceptible to RMP (Figure 5). The highest values were observed in Kazakhstan (28.4%) and Karakalpakstan (23.6%).

Figure 5: Settings with more than 10% of new cases showing resistance to INH but sensitivity to RMP, 1999–2002

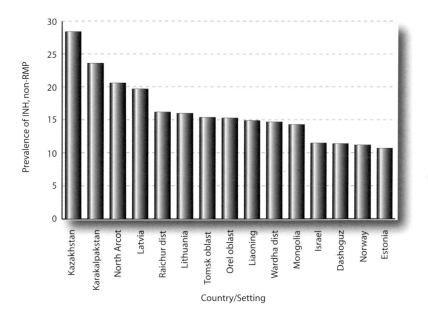

4.1.2 Drug resistance among previously treated cases

Data on the prevalence of drug resistance among previously treated cases were available for 66 countries/geographical settings (Annex 3 and 4). The number of cases tested ranged from 1 (Malta and Iceland) to 668 (Poland) with a median of 100 cases per setting. Several settings reported a small number of cases tested (1–19 cases in 6 settings; 20–49 cases in 14 settings; 50–99 cases in 11 settings).[a]

---

[a] In view of the smallness of the denominator in these settings, their observed rates can be labelled as "unstable"; not too much importance should be attached to their level and variations.

Any resistance among previously treated cases

The median prevalence of any resistance among previously treated cases was 18.4%. There was no resistance reported in the Gambia, Iceland, Malta and Luxembourg, where the number of previously treated cases was very small. In contrast, Kazakhstan and Karakalpakstan, Uzbekistan, showed tremendously high prevalences of any resistance – 82.1% and 79.4%, respectively. In 11 settings, prevalence of any resistance was higher than 50% (Figure 6).

Figure 6: Countries/settings with a prevalence of any resistance higher than 50% among previously treated cases, 1999–2002

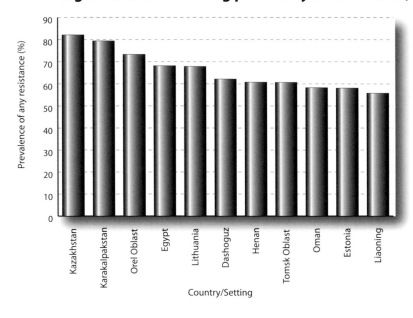

RESULTS

Prevalence of any drug resistance among previously treated TB cases, 1994-2002

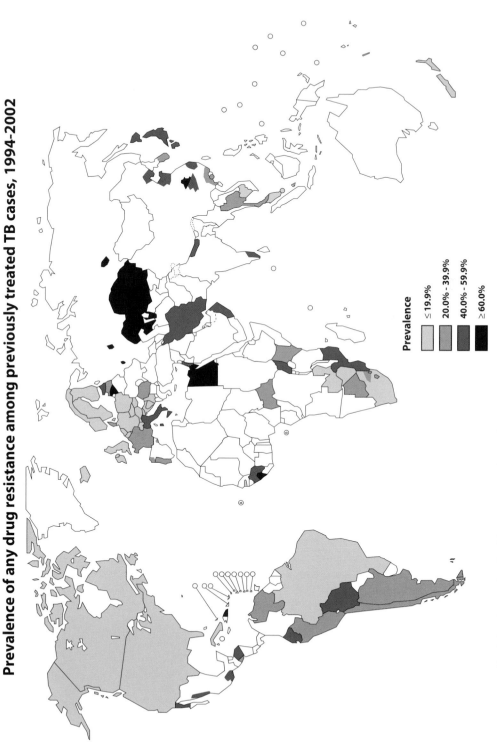

Prevalence

≤ 19.9%

20.0% - 39.9%

40.0% - 59.9%

≥ 60.0%

The designations employed and the presentation of material on this map do not imply the expression of any opinion whatsoever on the part of the World Health Organization concerning the legal status of any country, territory, city or area of its authorities, or concerning the delimitation of its frontiers or boundaries. Dashed lines represent approximate border lines for which there may not be full agreement

RESULTS

MDR among previously treated cases

The median prevalence of MDR was 7.0%. No MDR was reported in the Gambia, Iceland, Luxembourg, Malta, New Zealand, Norway, Belgrade (Serbia and Montenegro), and Slovenia. Kazakhstan (56.4%) and Oman (58.3%) reported the highest prevalences of MDR.

Figure 7: Countries/settings with prevalence of MDR higher than 30% among previously treated cases, 1999–2002

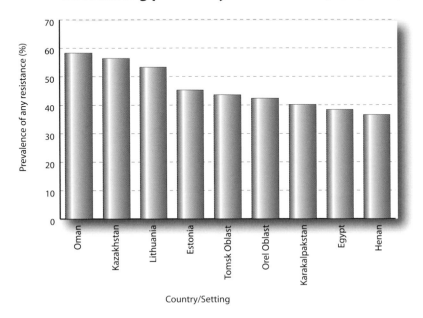

Resistance among previously treated cases according to number of drugs

Resistance to a single drug ranged from 0% in the Gambia, Iceland, Luxembourg, Malta and Oman, to 27.6% in Honduras and 23.5% in Dashoguz, Turkmenistan. The median prevalence of monoresistance was 8.7%. The median prevalence of resistance to two drugs was 4.5%, with the highest prevalences reported by Denmark (21.2%) and Liaoning Province, China (20.9%). The median prevalence of resistance to three or four drugs was 4.5%. Twelve settings reported no resistance to three or four drugs (Belgrade, Finland, the Gambia, Iceland, Ireland, Luxembourg, Malta, New Zealand, Norway, Sweden, Switzerland, and Zambia). The highest prevalences of resistance to three or four drugs were reported in Orel Oblast, Russian Federation (52.9%), Oman (58.3%) and Kazakhstan (62.3%).

Prevalence of MDR-TB among previously treated TB cases, 1994-2002

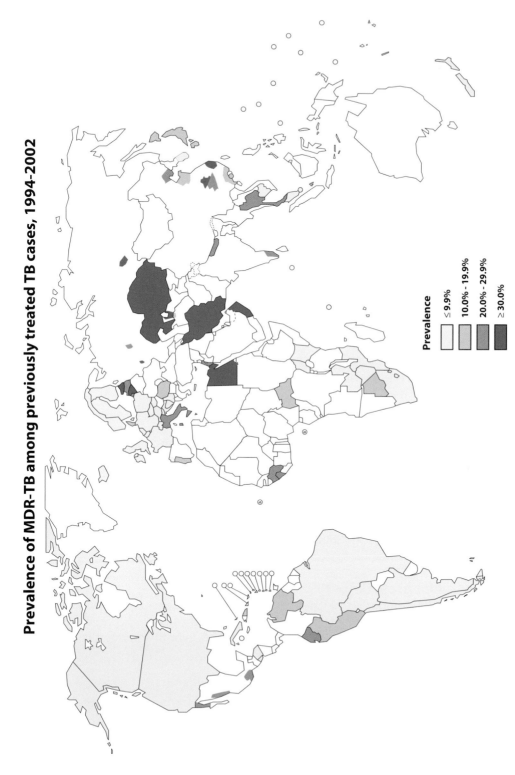

Prevalence

≤ 9.9%
10.0% - 19.9%
20.0% - 29.9%
≥ 30.0%

The designations employed and the presentation of material on this map do not imply the expression of any opinion whatsoever on the part of the World Health Organization concerning the legal status of any country, territory, city or area of its authorities, or concerning the delimitation of its frontiers or boundaries. Dashed lines represent approximate border lines for which there may not be full agreement

RESULTS

Resistance among previously treated cases by individual drug

Annex 4 shows the prevalence of any resistance to each of the four drugs among previously treated cases. The distribution of the prevalence rates is shown in Figure 8.

Figure 8: Prevalence of any resistance to INH, RMP, EMB and SM among previously treated cases, 1999–2002

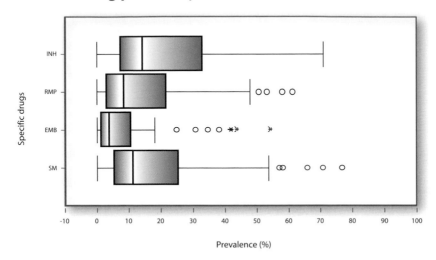

Any INH resistance. The median prevalence of resistance to INH was 14.4%. The range was wide: from 0% to 71.0% (Orel Oblast). No outliers were observed.

Any RMP resistance. The median prevalence of resistance to RMP was 8.7%. Four outliers were observed: Egypt (50.7%); Lithuania (53.3%); Oman (58.3%); and Kazakhstan (61.4%).

Any EMB resistance. The median prevalence of resistance to EMB was 3.5%. Outliers were observed in Oman and Puerto Rico (25%), Egypt (30.9%), Karakalpakstan, Uzbekistan (34.6%), and Lithuania (38.0%). Extreme high values were identified in Estonia (41.9%), Orel Oblast, Russian Federation (43.8%), and Kazakhstan (54.2%).

Any SM resistance. The median prevalence of resistance to SM was 11.4%. Outliers were observed in Tomsk Oblast, Russian Federation (57.3%), Oman (58.3%), Lithuania (58.6%), Orel Oblast, Russian Federation (66.2%), Karakalpakstan, Uzbekistan (71.0%), and Kazakhstan (77.1%).

4.1.3 Combined prevalence of drug resistance

Data on the combined prevalence of drug resistance were available for 69 geographical settings. Full details of drug resistance prevalence among combined cases for the period 1999–2002 are given in Annex 5 and Annex 6. In both annexes, the settings are stratified by WHO region.

Any resistance among combined cases

The overall prevalence of drug resistance ranged from 0% (Andorra, Iceland and Malta) to 63.9% (Karakalpakstan, Uzebekistan). The median was 10.4% (95% CI: 8.2–13.0%). Figure 9 shows the ten countries/settings with combined prevalence of any resistance higher than 30%. The absence of any setting in the Region of the Americas is worthy of note.

Figure 9: Countries/settings with combined prevalence of any resistance higher than 30%, 1999–2002

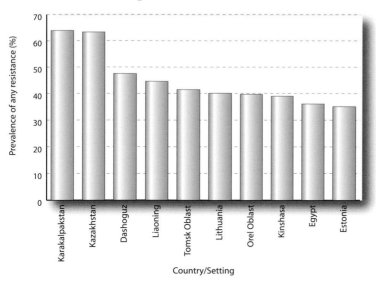

MDR among combined cases

Combined prevalence of MDR ranged from 0% (Andorra, Luxembourg, Iceland, Malta, New Zealand, Scotland and Slovenia) to 26.8% in Karakalpakstan, Uzbekistan. The median prevalence of MDR among combined cases was 1.7%. Figure 10 illustrates the eleven countries/settings with MDR prevalence higher than 10%.

Figure 10: Countries/settings with combined MDR prevalence higher than 10%, 1999–2002

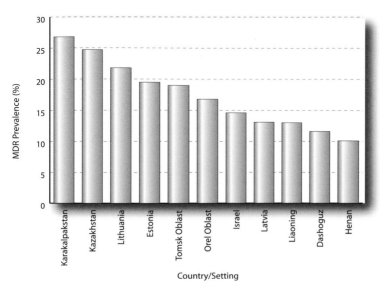

RESULTS

Resistance among combined cases according to number of drugs

Prevalence of monoresistance ranged from 0% to 22.3% (Dashoguz, Turkmenistan) with a median of 6.9% (Annex 5). Prevalences ≥ 15% were observed in six settings: Dashoguz, Turkmenistan (22.4%); Liaoning Province, China (21.4%); Egypt (21.2%); Kinshasa, Democratic Republic of Congo (18.5%); Karakalpakstan, Uzbekistan (16.4%); and Henan Province, China (15.4%). Resistance to two drugs ranged from 0% to 15.5% (Karakalpakstan, Uzbekistan) with a median of 2.3%. Resistance to three or four drugs was less than 2% in almost two-thirds of the settings, with a median of 1.3%. Seven settings reported prevalences higher than 15%: Kazakhstan (34.5%); Karakalpakstan, Uzbekistan (31.9%); Lithuania (27.6%); Orel Oblast, Russian Federation (22.8%); Estonia (20.1%); Tomsk Oblast, Russian Federation (18.6%); and Dashoguz, Turkmenistan (15.3%).

Any resistance among combined cases by individual drug

Annex 6 shows the prevalence of any resistance to each of the four drugs among combined cases. The highest prevalence of resistance to all four drugs was observed in Kazakhstan. The distribution of the prevalence of resistance to each individual drug is illustrated in figure 11.

Exceptionally high prevalences and outliers were found in many countries/ settings.

Figure 11: Prevalence of resistance to specific TB drugs among combined cases, 1999–2002

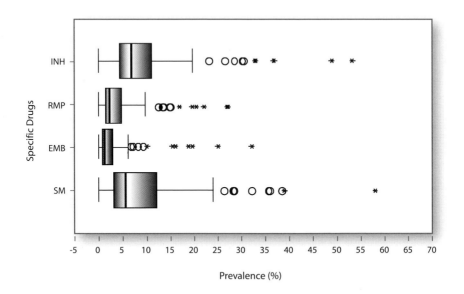

Any INH resistance. The median prevalence of resistance to INH was 6.6%. While Andorra, Iceland and Malta showed no resistance to INH, high levels of resistance were observed in Estonia (30%), Latvia (30.3%), Dashoguz, Turkmenistan (32.8%), Tomsk Oblast, Russian Federation (33.1%), Lithuania (36.7%), Orel Oblast, Russian Federation (36.8%), Karakalpakstan, Uzbekistan (53.1%), and Kazakhstan (58.8%).

Any RMP resistance. The median prevalence of resistance to RMP among combined cases was 2.2%. Andorra, Iceland, Luxembourg, Malta, Scotland and Slovenia showed no resistance to RMP, while high values were observed in Dashoguz, Turkmenistan (12.2%), Henan Province, China (12.3%), Latvia (13.1%), Ecuador (13.1%), Egypt (13.4%), Liaoning Province, China (14.6%), Israel (14.9%), Orel Oblast, Russian Federation (16.8%), Estonia (19.5%), Tomsk Oblast, Russian Federation (20.3%), Lithuania (22%), Karakalpakstan, Uzbekistan (26.8%), and Kazakhstan (27%).

Any EMB resistance. The median prevalence of resistance to EMB was 1.3%. High EMB resistance among combined cases was observed in Lithuania (16%), Orel Oblast, Russian Federation (18.7%), Estonia (19.5%), Karakalpakstan, Uzebekistan (24.9%), and Kazakhstan (32.1%).

Any SM resistance. The median prevalence of resistance to SM was 6.1%. High values were observed in Lithuania (32.1%), Liaoning Province, China (35.5%), Orel Oblast, Russian Federation (35.8%), Tomsk Oblast, Russian Federation (38.3%), Dashoguz, Turkmenistan (38.9%), Karakalpakstan, Uzebekistan (57.8%), and Kazakhstan (57.9%).

4.2 PREVALENCE OF DRUG RESISTANCE BY REGION

4.2.1 Drug resistance among new cases

The medians of the main parameters (any resistance, MDR, resistance according to the number of drugs, and resistance to individual drugs) for the various WHO regions were generally close, with only a few exceptions. However the range of resistance prevalence varied considerably within regions (Figure 12).

The medians of any drug resistance were between 7.1% and 11.4% for all regions except South-East Asia, where the median was much higher (19.8%). The ranges in the Western Pacific Region and especially in the European region were much wider than for the other regions. The European Region has one outlier: Kazakhstan (57.1%).

The medians of MDR were similar in all regions (0.9 to 2.2%), but there were ten outliers and extreme values: Ecuador (6.6%) in the Americas; Henan (7.8%) and Liaoning (10.4%) Provinces, China in the Western Pacific; Latvia (9.3%), Lithuania (9.4%), Estonia (12.2%), Karakalpakstan, Uzbekistan (13.2%), Tomsk Oblast, Russian Federation (13.7%), Israel (14.2%), and Kazakhstan (14.2%) in the European Region.

The medians of any resistance to individual drugs were to a large extent similar in all WHO regions, with the exception of South-East Asia, which had a much higher median of any resistance to INH. The range of any resistance to each of the four drugs was by far the widest in the European region. The medians of monoresistance to RMP, EMB and SM were similar for all regions. The medians for INH monoresistance ranged from 1.8% to 3.7%, except in South-East Asia, which had a median 3–5 times higher (10.7%).

RESULTS

Figure 12: Prevalence of any resistance among new cases, by WHO region, 1999–2002

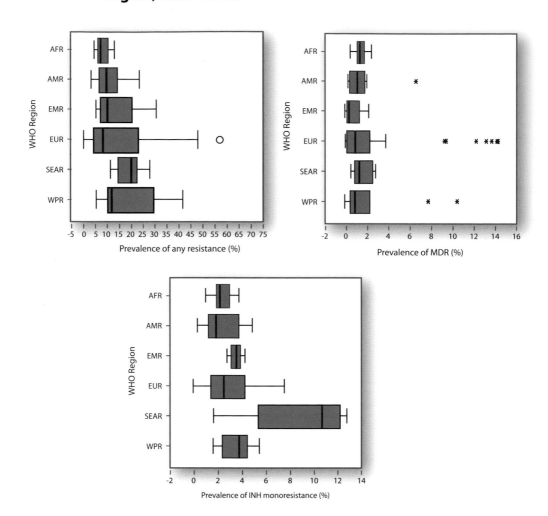

4.2.2 Drug resistance among previously treated cases

Because of the small number of countries reporting results for previously treated cases in the Eastern Mediterranean and South-East Asia, both regions have been left out of the analysis. Figure 13 summarizes the most salient features of resistance among previously treated cases in the WHO regions. The medians of most parameters for the African and European Regions were around the same level, while the median values for the Americas were somewhat higher, and those in the Western Pacific Region substantially higher, with the exception of RMP monoresistance. The ranges of values for the African Region and the Americas were quite narrow, those of the Western Pacific Region wider, while the widest are observed in the European Region, reflecting the diversity of the resistance prevalence. The median prevalences of any resistance in the Regions of Africa, the Americas and Europe were around 20%, while the median prevalence in the Western Pacific Region reached 32.6%. MDR medians fluctuated around 5%, except in the Western

Pacific Region (15.5%); the European Region had a very wide range, with two important outliers: Lithuania (53.3%) and Kazakhstan (56.4%). This was also true for the prevalence of resistance to 3 or 4 drugs, where Kazakhstan was an outlier (62.4%). The Puerto Rico outlier (25%) is an artefact caused by the small sample size (n = 4).

Figure 13: Prevalence of resistance among previously treated cases, stratified by WHO region, 1999–2002

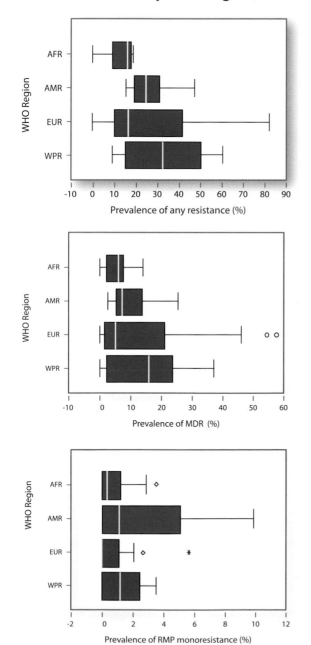

RESULTS

RMP monoresistance showed a different pattern: the European Region had the lowest median, followed by the African Region; the Western Pacific Region and the Americas had similar medians, but the latter had the widest range. Two outliers were present: Limpopo Province, South Africa (3.4%), in the African Region and the Czech Republic (2.6%) in the European Region. Italy (5.6%) in the European Region had an extreme high value. For most of the parameters the African Region had the lowest medians as well as the smallest ranges.

4.2.3 A closer look at the European Region
In the European Region, the very wide ranges observed for all parameters suggest an important heterogeneity. We therefore explored stratification in three geographical subregions – Western, Central and Eastern Europe (Table 3).

Table 3: European subregions

WESTERN EUROPE	CENTRAL EUROPE	EASTERN EUROPE
Andorra	Bosnia and Herzegovina	Estonia
Austria	Croatia	Kazakhstan
Belgium	Czech Republic	Lithuania
Denmark	Poland	Latvia
Finland	Slovakia	Russian Fed. (Orel Oblast)
France	Slovenia	Russian Fed. (Tomsk Oblast)
Germany	Serbia and Montenegro	Turkmenistan (Dashoguz)
Iceland		Uzbekistan (Karakalpakstan)
Ireland		
Israel		
Italy		
Luxembourg		
Malta		
Netherlands		
Norway		
Spain (Barcelona)		
Spain (Galicia)		
Sweden		
Switzerland		
United Kingdom		

As a general observation for both new and previously treated cases, most median values were lowest in the Central Europe subregion, somewhat higher in Western Europe, and highest in Eastern Europe. This was also true for the ranges of the parameters – narrow for Central Europe, somewhat wider for Western Europe, and widest for the Eastern European subregion.

Figure 14: MDR prevalence among new and previously treated cases by European Subregion, 1999–2002

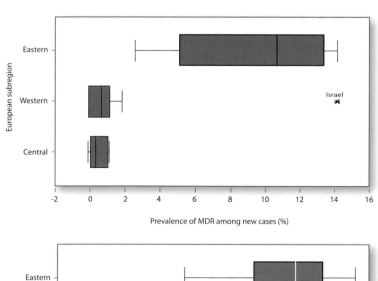

Prevalence of MDR among new cases (%)

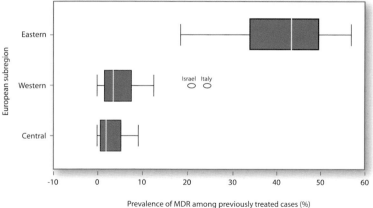

Prevalence of MDR among previously treated cases (%)

In the Western European subregion, Israel is an outlier for prevalence of any resistance and MDR among new, as well as previously treated, cases (Figure 14). A high rate of immigration from areas with a higher prevalence of resistance, such as countries of the former Soviet Union, is one possible reason. Italy is an outlier for MDR among previously treated cases.

4.3 DYNAMICS OF DRUG RESISTANCE PREVALENCE OVER TIME (1994-2002)

The Global Project has collected data from 109 countries/geographical settings, representing 90 WHO Member States and territories. The following analysis includes data from the three global reports, as well as data provided between the publication of reports. It thus reflects both published and previously unpublished data.

RESULTS

4.3.1 Dynamics of drug resistance among new cases

The second Global Report[16] presented information on 24 settings with more than one data point.[a] For most settings, only two data points were available. The present report examines time trends for resistance in new cases in 46 settings: 20 settings provided two data points and 26 three or more data points (Table 4).

Table 4: Number of data points per setting for new cases, by WHO region, 1994–2002

WHO Region	No. of data points							Total
	1	2	3	4	5	6	7	
Africa	21	1	1					23
Americas	11	3	1	1		2		18
Eastern Mediterranean	3	1	1					5
Europe	10	11	11	5	1			38
South-East Asia	4	1	1					6
Western Pacific	11	3				1	1	16
TOTAL	60	20	15	6	1	3	1	106

Dynamics in settings reporting two data points

Of the 20 settings that reported two data points, three (Andorra, Iceland and Malta) had no resistant cases. Twelve showed only slight variations in prevalence, while significant changes were observed in five settings: Poland, Peru, Argentina,[b] Henan Province (China),[c] and Thailand. An increase was observed in all resistance parameters (any resistance, monoresistance, any INH and any RMP resistance) in Poland.

Changes in prevalence over time have been summarized through the prevalence ratio (PR), i.e. the ratio of the prevalence at the second data point to that at the initial data point. For example, for Ivanovo Oblast: MDR prevalence in 1998 was 9.0%; MDR prevalence in 1995 was 4%; thus PR = 9.0/4.0 = 2.25. This shows a potentially important increase. The 95% confidence interval (1.07–4.67) confirms that the increase is at least 1.07 times, and at most 4.67 times, the baseline prevalence. When the 95% CI includes 1 (marked by the horizontal line), the null hypothesis of no significant change cannot be rejected (Figure 15).

[a] Each reporting period is defined as a "data point". Most data points cover a year, although some cover longer or shorter periods.

[b] It is important to note that differences in prevalence of drug resistance in Argentina are almost certainly due to a change in sampling methodology.

[c] It is important to note that, because of misclassification and other problems in the first survey, the observed decrease in most resistance parameters in Henan may not be very meaningful.

Figure 15: Prevalence ratios of any resistance among new cases, 1994–2002

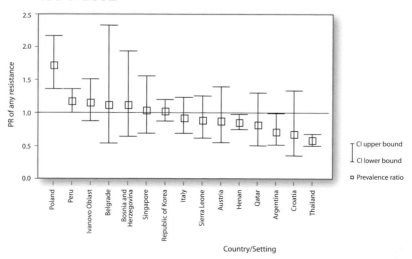

Eight settings showed a decrease in prevalence of any resistance. In three of these settings (Argentina, Henan (China), and Thailand) the decrease was significant. Some settings had a wide CI around the prevalence ratio, e.g. Belgrade, Serbia and Montenegro. Two settings, Ireland (PR=1.4) and Uruguay (PR=1.92), with extremely broad confidence intervals (0.28–7.95 and 0.77–4.81, respectively) are not included in the figure. A wide CI is generally due to the smallness of the sample.

Figure 16 presents the prevalence ratios for MDR and their confidence intervals for 16 countries/geographical settings. The CI in most settings was very wide. Only five settings showed a significant change. Two showed a significant decrease: Argentina and Thailand. The decrease in Henan, China, was of only borderline significance. Seven settings showed an increase over time, of which only Poland and Ivanovo Oblast were significant.

Figure 16: Prevalence ratios of MDR among new cases, 1994–2002

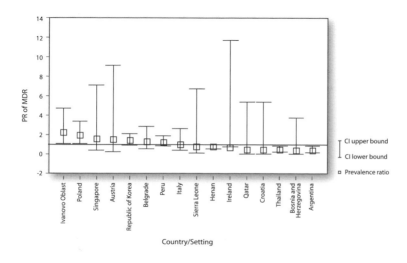

Trends in settings reporting three or more data points

For the 26 settings that reported at least three data points, time trends could be determined. The details are given in Annex 7, Annex 8, Annex 9 and Annex 10. Regarding any resistance (Annex 7), seven settings reported significant changes. New Zealand and Norway reported a doubling and Botswana a tripling of the prevalence. Tomsk Oblast, (Russian Federation) also showed significant increases. Cuba, Germany, and Hong Kong SAR showed significantly decreasing trends. Figure 17 depicts the trend of prevalence of any resistance among new cases in Botswana.

Figure 17: Confidence-bounded trend in any resistance among new cases in Botswana

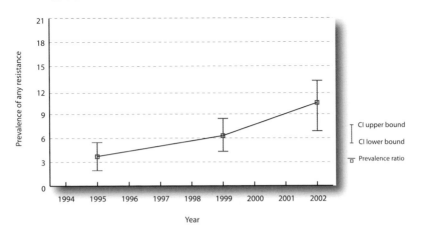

Regarding MDR (Annex 8), a significant increasing trend was found in Tomsk Oblast, Russian Federation. Lithuania presented a non-significant increase (Figure 18). MDR in Estonia (Figure 19) increased until 1999, but decreased in 2000.[a] Latvia, USA, and Hong Kong SAR reported significantly decreasing trends.

Figure 18: Confidence-bounded trend in MDR among new patients in Lithuania

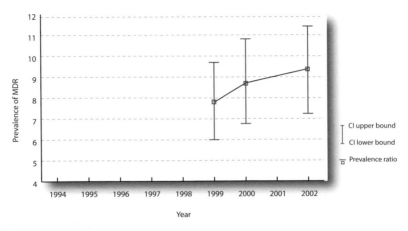

[a] Preliminary data for 2001 and 2002 indicate an increase in MDR to levels similar to those observed in 1999.

Figure 19: Confidence-bounded trend in MDR among new patients in Estonia

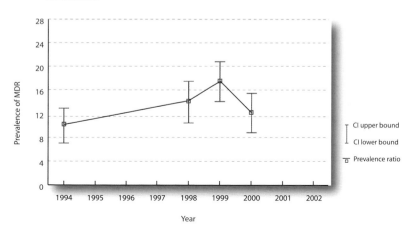

With regard to prevalence of any INH resistance (Annex 9), a decrease was significant in Finland and Germany.[a] Prevalence of any INH resistance more than tripled in Botswana since the first survey in 1995. Tomsk Oblast (Russian Federation) showed a steady and significant increase, reaching a level of resistance 1.5 times higher in 2002 than in 1998. Sweden presented a significant increase.

Regarding trends in prevalence of any RMP resistance (Annex 10), significant decreases were observed in Hong Kong SAR, Latvia and the USA. Tomsk Oblast, Russian Federation, and Slovakia both reported significant increases.

4.3.2 Dynamics of drug resistance among previously treated cases

More than half of the settings provided only one data point, 19 provided at least two, and 23 provided three or more data points (Table 5).

Table 5: Number of data points per setting for previously treated cases, by WHO region, 1994–2002

WHO Region	No. of data points							Total
	1	2	3	4	5	6	7	
Africa	18	1	1					20
Americas	10	2	1	1	1	1		16
Eastern Mediterranean	2	1						3
Europe	11	11	10	5	1			38
South-East Asia	2	1						3
Western Pacific	9	3				1	1	14
TOTAL	**52**	**19**	**12**	**6**	**2**	**2**	**1**	**94**

[a] Data from 2001 and 2002 report higher prevalences of INH resistance among new cases; however this may be linked to changes in surveillance methodology.

RESULTS

Dynamics in settings reporting two data points

Of the 19 settings reporting two data points, four had no resistant cases; consequently, only 15 settings were retained for analysis. Regarding any resistance among previously treated cases (Figure 20), a significant decrease was observed in Argentina, Ivanovo Oblast, Russian Federation, Peru and the Republic of Korea. The decrease was borderline in Henan Province (China) and Italy. Only Nepal showed a significant increase. For all other settings, the changes were not significant.

Figure 20: Prevalence ratios of any resistance among previously treated cases, 1994–2002

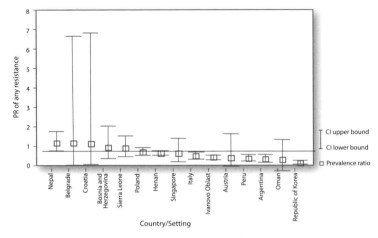

With regard to changes in prevalence of MDR (Figure 21), in most settings the confidence intervals for the PR were very wide, as a result of the small number of MDR cases. There are only two significant decreases (Argentina and the Republic of Korea) and one significant increase (Nepal). All other settings showed no statistically significant change.

Figure 21: Prevalence ratios of MDR among previously treated cases, 1994–2002

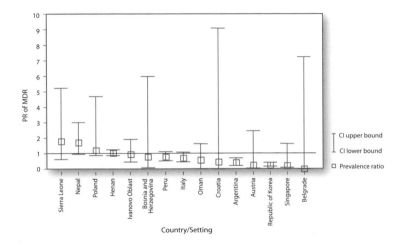

Regarding any INH resistance (Figure 22), five settings showed a significant decrease: Argentina, Italy, Peru, the Republic of Korea and Ivanovo Oblast, Russian Federation, the last being borderline. Nepal and Sierra Leone showed a borderline increase. All other settings showed variations with large confidence intervals; the upper limit for Belgrade, Serbia and Montenegro, reached 27.3 and for Croatia 8.9.

Figure 22: Prevalence ratios of any INH resistance among previously treated cases, 1994–2002

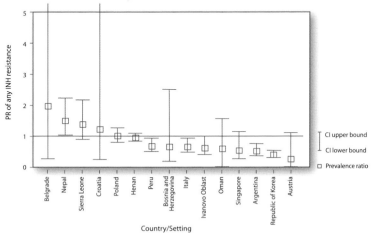

Trends in settings reporting three or more data points

Four settings – Cuba, Switzerland, Latvia and USA – showed a significant decrease in prevalence of any resistance (Annex 11). All other settings showed only slight variations that were not significant.

F   MDR (Annex 12), three settings showed a significant decrease (Latvia, Slovakia, and USA). Three settings showed a significant increase; Estonia, Lithuania, and Tomsk Oblast (Russian Federation). The variations in all 17 other settings were not significant. Annex 13 presents trends in prevalence of any RMP resistance.

4.3.3 Dynamics of drug resistance among combined cases

More than half of the settings provided only one data point, 20 provided two, and 26 settings provided three or more data points (Table 6).

Table 6: Number of data points per setting for combined cases by WHO region, 1994–2002

WHO Region	No. of data points							Total
	1	2	3	4	5	6	7	
Africa	19	1	1					21
Americas	10	1	1	1	1	1		15
Eastern Mediterranean	2	1						3
Europe	8	12	11	6	1			38
South-East Asia	2	1						3
Western Pacific	9	3				1	2	15
TOTAL	**50**	**20**	**13**	**7**	**3**	**2**	**1**	**96**

Of the 20 settings reporting two data points for prevalence of any resistance, three had no resistant cases (Andorra, Iceland, Malta); the remaining 17 were included in the analysis. Surveillance data from nine settings are displayed in Figure 23 and Figure 24, which show the prevalence ratios and 95% confidence intervals. Data from the remaining eight settings originated from surveys. As these data had to be adjusted, no confidence intervals could be calculated and, consequently, the level of significance of any increase or decrease could not be determined.

Dynamics in settings reporting two data points

Figure 23: Prevalence ratios of any resistance among combined cases, 1994–2002

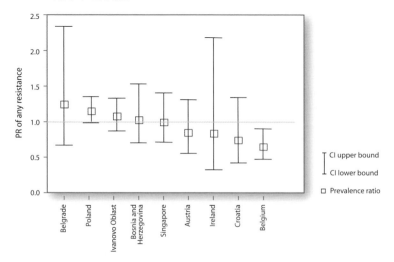

With regard to prevalence of any resistance (Figure 23) only one setting, Belgium, showed a significant decrease over time. Poland showed a borderline increase. No other survey settings reported statistically significant changes over two data points.

Figure 24: Prevalence ratios of MDR among combined cases, 1994–2002

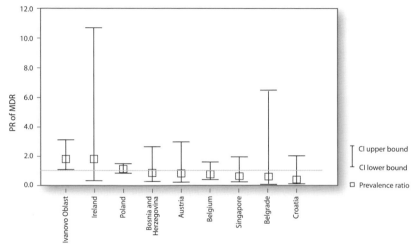

Figure 24 shows the prevalence ratios of MDR in surveillance settings. The confidence intervals in some settings were very wide. A borderline significant increase was observed in Ivanovo Oblast (Russian Federation). Six settings showed minor decreases.

Annex 14 shows trends in combined prevalence of any resistance. Significant increases were observed in Israel, Lithuania, New Zealand and Norway. Significant decreases were observed in the Netherlands and Hong Kong SAR (China), the latter illustrated in Figure 25.

Figure 25: Confidence-bounded trend in any resistance among combined patients in Hong Kong SAR, China

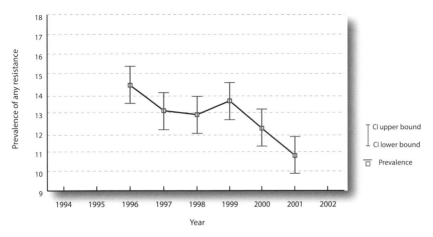

Figure 25 shows trends in combined prevalence of MDR. A significant increase in MDR prevalence was observed in Israel, Lithuania and Tomsk Oblast (Russian Federation), the latter depicted in Figure 27. An initial decrease followed by a stabilization of prevalence was seen in Latvia (Figure 26). Decreasing trends were observed in Hong Kong SAR and USA.

Figure 26: Confidence-bounded trend in MDR among combined patients in Latvia

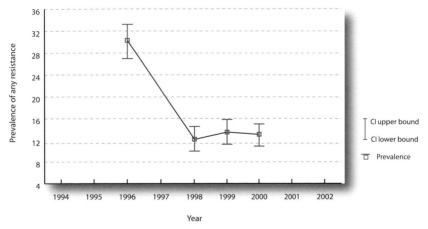

RESULTS

Figure 27: Confidence-bounded trend in MDR among combined patients in Tomsk Oblast

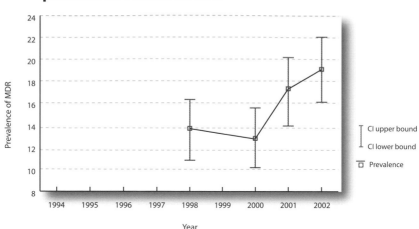

With regard to prevalence of any INH resistance (Annex 16), significant increases were observed in Israel, Lithuania, Tomsk Oblast (Russian Federation), and Sweden. Decreasing trends were significant in Canada and the Netherlands.

Prevalence of any RMP resistance (Annex 17) significantly increased in Israel, Tomsk Oblast (Russian Federation), and Lithuania. Significant decreases were observed in Hong Kong SAR and the USA.

4.4   POTENTIAL DETERMINANTS OF DRUG RESISTANCE

In order to assess the impact of potential risk factors for drug resistance on resistance rates, an ecological analysis was performed.

4.4.1 Variables included in the ecological analysis

A conceptual framework (Figure 28) was developed, which structures the retained variables along three axes: patient-related, health-system-related and contextual factors.

The following patient-related factors were retained: level of education[67] and purchasing power. Preferences for the private sector could not be included as a factor, as no aggregate data were available. The human poverty index[67] and the out-of-pocket expenditure,[68] as a percentage of total health expenditure, measure the purchasing power.

The following contextual factors were retained: notified TB incidence rate,[68] HIV rate[69] and percentage of TB cases with HIV, gross domestic product (GDP),[70] health expenditure (expressed as percentage of GDP),[68] the human development index,[67] and the GINI equity index.[67]

Health system factors relate to the functioning of the health system and the NTP. The latter was explored in terms of the percentage of re-treatment cases, the year of introduction of RMP, and through different aspects of the DOTS programme: percentage coverage of DOTS, the proportion of sputum positive cases treated under DOTS, the detection rate under DOTS, and the success rate among patients treated under DOTS.[64] The functionality of the health system[71] was evaluated by the DALE (disability adjusted life expectancy). Although the model included the fairness index[a,72] (the responsiveness of the health system relative to people's expectations[b]) as a measurement of functionality, it could not be included in the final analysis.

Figure 28: Conceptual model of ecological factors affecting TB drug resistance

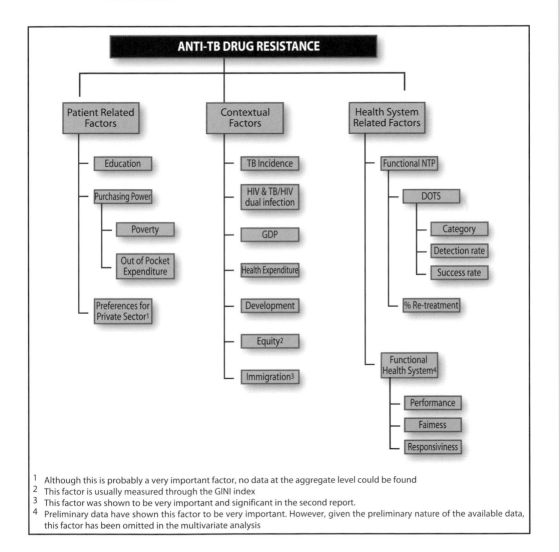

1 Although this is probably a very important factor, no data at the aggregate level could be found
2 This factor is usually measured through the GINI index
3 This factor was shown to be very important and significant in the second report.
4 Preliminary data have shown this factor to be very important. However, given the preliminary nature of the available data, this factor has been omitted in the multivariate analysis

a The fairness concept implies that the health system responds equally well to everyone, without discrimination. This means that the cost of episode of illness is distributed according to the patient's ability to pay rather that the illness itself.
b Two aspects were distinguished: the level and distribution of the health system.

RESULTS

4.4.2 Bivariate analysis

The details of the Spearman correlation coefficients are given in Annex 18, Annex 19, Annex 20, and Annex 21. Two outcome variables were selected, i.e. any resistance and MDR prevalence. The correlation analysis was stratified for new and combined cases, and in each stratum, the analysis was carried out for all countries and for the subgroup of the low- and middle-income countries (GDP < US$18 000).

For the new cases, the three major arms of the conceptual model (Figure 28) – patient-related, contextual and health-system-related factors – were significantly correlated with the outcome variables. This correlation also holds for the low- and middle-income countries. Similar results were obtained for the combined cases.

Among all new cases, the notified TB incidence rate was positively correlated with both any resistance and MDR. Percentage of re-treatment cases and the human poverty index were correlated with MDR only. Among new cases in the stratum of low- and middle-income countries, the notified TB incidence rate was correlated with any resistance and the percentage of re-treatment cases was correlated with MDR.

Among all combined cases, the notified TB incidence and the human poverty index were correlated with both any resistance and MDR. The human development index (HDI) and health expenditure were negatively correlated with MDR only. Among combined cases in the stratum of low- and middle-income countries, the percentage of re-treatment cases was positively correlated, and health expenditure negatively correlated, with both outcome variables.

4.4.3 Multivariate analysis[a]

The results of the multilinear regression modelling were stratified by new and combined cases. In each stratum, a subanalysis was carried out for the low- and middle-income countries. The multivariate analysis showed that the most significantly correlated factor with both overall resistance and MDR was the percentage of re-treatment cases. Economic factors (GDP, poverty index, and human development index) were also correlated. Direct programme indicators (DOTS coverage, TB incidence rates, and percentage of TB cases with HIV infection) were not significantly correlated with prevalence of resistance, at the aggregate level.[b]

For the countries that were eligible for the regression analysis, only one factor contributed significantly to the regression of both outcome variables in both new and combined cases – percentage of re-treatment cases. GDP was negatively correlated with MDR among new and combined cases and with any resistance among combined cases. Among the countries belonging to the subgroup of low- to middle-income countries, percentage of re-treatment cases was also the most significant factor, though GDP was also negatively correlated with any resistance in new and combined cases and with MDR among new cases.

---

[a] Given recent uncertainty about the reliability of the responsiveness and the fairness indices, they have not been included in the model.
[b] The results of ecological analyses have to be interpreted with caution, as the findings at aggregate level are not necessarily valid at the level of each individual country, province, district or oblast. Another possible reason for the lack of significant contribution of programme indicators could be the lack of reliability or robustness of the programme data.

4.5   MAGNITUDE OF THE MDR-TB PROBLEM

4.5.1 MDR-TB "hot spots"
In the first Global Report, the term "hot spot" was used to refer to areas with a high prevalence of MDR-TB among new cases. The second Global Report introduced a reference point of 3% prevalence of MDR-TB among new cases, as an indication of high MDR prevalence. Over time, a 3% prevalence of MDR among new cases became the customary threshold to define a "hot spot". Because many factors determine the extent to which MDR is a problem in a given country or geographical setting, we examined several aspects of MDR burden. The first was the statistical validity of a cut-off point or threshold.

A stem-and-leaf plot analysis shows the distribution of MDR prevalence for recent data points from 74 settings with data on new cases (Figure 29) This distribution shows that 6.6% is the natural departure point for "extreme values", a much higher value than would be expected from the normal distribution of data. In looking at the distribution of MDR prevalences from earlier data points (1994–1998) (Figure 30), an almost identical distribution can be observed, with outliers situated above 6.5%.

Table 7 shows the settings from the third phase of the Global Project with MDR prevalence among new cases higher than 6%. There was only one setting that fell between 3% and 6% – Dashoguz Velayat, Turkmenistan.

Figure 29: Stem-and-Leaf plot of MDR prevalences in new cases, 1999–2002

Frequency	Stem & Leaf	
24.00	0	000000000011222333344444
13.00	0	5577778889999
13.00	1	0111111223334
6.00	1	677788
5.00	2	00234
3.00	2	568
0.00	3	3
1.00	3	8
10.00	**Extremes**	**(≥6.6)**
Stem width:	1.0	
Each Leaf:	1 case(s)	

Figure 30: Stem-and-Leaf plot of MDR prevalences in new cases,1994–1998

Frequency	Stem & Leaf	
31.00	0	00000000003333344555566778888899
10.00	1	0012224579
10.00	2	1111335788
4.00	3	0357
3.00	4	469
1.00	5	3
6.0	**Extremes**	**(≥6.5)**
Stem width:	1.0	
Each Leaf:	1 case(s)	

Table 7: Countries/settings with MDR-TB prevalence higher than 6.5%, 1999–2002

Setting	Survey Year	MDR Prevalence %	No. of MDR-TB cases in sample
Ecuador	2002	6.6	26
Henan	2001	7.8	95
Latvia	2000	9.3	83
Lithuania	2001	9.4	77
Lianoning	2002	10.4	85
Estonia	2000	12.2	50
Uzbekistan	2000	13.2	14
Tomsk Oblast	2002	13.7	73
Israel	2001	14.2	36
Kazakhstan	2000	14.2	51

Dynamics of the hot spots (1994–2002)

Table 8 shows the 22 settings that at some point had a prevalence of MDR higher than 3% among new cases. There were two settings in the African Region; four in the Americas; two in the Eastern Mediterranean; nine in the European Region; two in South-East Asia; and three in the Western Pacific. Twelve of the 22 settings had MDR prevalence above 6.5% (shown in bold in Table 8). According to the stem-and-leaf analysis, these are outliers and can be considered as extreme values.

Figure 31 shows settings with an MDR prevalence among new cases ≥3%, and that have reported at least two data points. Of the ten settings, two showed an important increase (Ivanovo and Tomsk Oblasts); Estonia showed an increase, followed by a decrease; and Latvia showed a decrease, followed by stabilization of prevalence. Henan province, China, showed a decrease. It is of note that, of the six survey settings with at least two data points and reporting prevalences of MDR ≥ 6.5%, none has yet decreased below 6.5%.

Figure 31: Evolution of MDR Hot Spots, 1994–2002

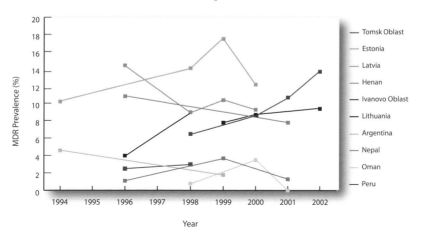

Table 8: Settings/countries presenting an MDR prevalence ≥ 3.0% at least once between 1994 and 2002

Country	Year of observation								
	1994	1995	1996	1997	1998	1999	2000	2001	2002
Africa									
Côte d'Ivoire		5.3							
Mozambique					3.5				
Americas									
Argentina	4.6					1.8			
Dominican Republic	6.6								
Ecuador									6.6
Peru		2.5				3.0			
Eastern Mediterranean									
Islamic Republic of Iran				5.0					
Oman					0.8		3.5	0.0	
Europe									
Estonia	10.2				14.1	17.5	12.2		
Israel							14.2		
Kazakhstan							14.2		
Latvia			14.4		9.0	10.4	9.3		
Lithuania						7.8	8.7		9.4
Russian Fed. (Ivanovo Oblast)	4.0				9.0				
Russian Fed. (Tomsk Oblast)					6.5		8.6	10.7	13.7
Turkmenistan - Dashoguz							3.8		
Uzbekistan - Karakalpakstan							13.2		
South-East Asia									
India (Tamil-Nadu)				3.4					
Nepal			1.1						
Western Pacific									
China (Henan)			10.8					7.8	
China (Liaoning)						10.4			
China (Zhejiang)					4.5				

RESULTS

4.5.2 Burden of MDR-TB

The burden of MDR-TB can be described in terms of prevalence, but also in terms of the absolute number of cases and, most importantly, the capacity of the country to address the problem. In many countries where the population of TB cases is low, a high MDR prevalence does not necessarily reflect high absolute numbers of cases. Conversely, a low prevalence of MDR in high-burden countries, such as China or India, could reflect a considerable number of MDR cases that the national TB programme must treat and cure. To take the absolute number correctly into consideration, the sample findings need to be extrapolated. Annex 24 contains estimates of the numbers of new MDR cases per year for the countries included in the most recent phase of the Global Project. The 95% confidence limits show the lower and upper boundaries of the estimation.

South Africa and Kazakhstan were estimated to have the highest MDR burden in terms of absolute numbers, with around 3000 MDR cases each, followed by three provinces in China (Hubei, Henan and Liaoning). Luxembourg, Andorra, Malta, Iceland, Slovenia, New Zealand and Scotland had the fewest MDR cases. The status of applications to the Green Light Committee is detailed in Annex 25.

4.5.3 Resistance to RMP: a good surrogate marker for MDR?

It has been widely observed that rifampicin resistance is very frequently accompanied by isoniazid resistance, and it has therefore been suggested that rifampicin resistance may be a good surrogate marker for MDR.[73,74] If so, a future rapid test for rifampicin resistance may be useful for early identification of MDR cases, allowing rapid implementation of infection control measures, further DST and, where feasible, adjustment of treatment regimens. Whether resistance to RMP is a good surrogate marker for MDR is largely dependent on two factors: the internal validity, or the ability to detect true rifampicin resistance in the population; and the external validity, i.e. the likelihood that isolates with rifampicin resistance will also be resistant to isoniazid in a given setting. The conventional test for rifampicin resistance will yield reliable results if performed correctly, and therefore the ability of RMP resistance to act as a surrogate marker for MDR is related predominantly to the likelihood ratio or positive predictive value.

Figure 32: Scatterplot of positive predictive value of RMP resistance test by MDR prevalence in new cases, for latest data point, 1994–2002

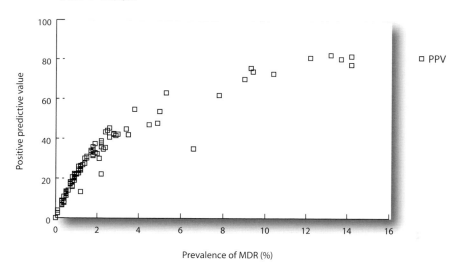

Figure 32 shows that the positive predictive value for the RMP resistance test among new cases was no greater than 90% at the highest measured MDR prevalence (14.2%). Positive predictive values around the 6.5% MDR outlier value fluctuated between 50% and 70%.

Figure 33: Scatterplot of positive predictive value of RMP resistance test by MDR prevalence in previously treated cases, for latest data point, 1994–2002

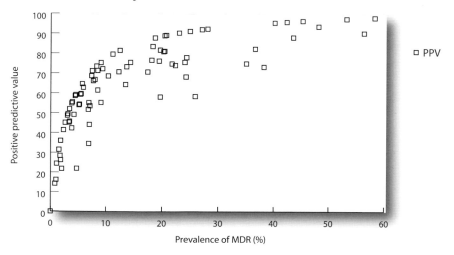

Figure 33 shows that the positive predictive value of the RMP resistance test among previously treated cases reached the 90% level at an MDR prevalence of around 20% and reached values close to 100% in settings with an MDR prevalence between 40% and 60%.

RESULTS

Traore and colleagues[75] have shown that the reliability of rapid RMP resistance detection methods as a surrogate marker of MDR-TB depends on the sensitivity and specificity of the test and the prevalence of RMP monoresistance. The above analysis is in agreement with their finding, although our analysis included all non-MDR rifampicin resistance – monoresistance, resistance to RMP and EMB (RE), to RMP and SM (RS), and to RMP, EMB, and SM (RES). The analysis of these results allows us to conclude that rifampicin resistance is not a good surrogate marker for MDR-TB in new cases of tuberculosis, where such a marker would be most useful. However, the use of rifampicin resistance as a surrogate marker of MDR-TB may be appropriate in certain settings,[76] for example, among previously treated cases where the prevalence of MDR-TB is 40% or above, and non-MDR rifampicin resistance is low. Although detection of MDR-TB is of the utmost importance, rifampicin mono-resistance has also been linked with treatment failure and is thus of clinical and public health relevance[35].

4.6 DRUG RESISTANCE PATTERNS
(relationships between new and previously treated cases, amplification, and major pathways of drug resistance creation)

Resistance to anti-TB drugs has so many dimensions and measurements, that distinguishing its main patterns is a challenging task. In this section, we attempt to discern patterns at the isolate level and track how they might have evolved by comparing new and previously treated cases, globally as well as by WHO region. Based on the relative prevalence of the 15 combinations of drug resistance possible with four drugs and the four resistance modes, i.e. mono, double, triple and quadruple resistance, we draw inferences as to how the most frequent types might have interacted and how the four resistance modes might have progressed under the selective pressure of drug treatment. We also try to cast light on the most probable pathways for the creation of drug resistance.

Drug susceptibility test results to the four main antituberculosis drugs were obtained for 90 080 cases (77 175 new cases and 12 905 previously treated cases). The mean proportion of previously treated cases in the sample was 14.3%, with regional subsamples ranging from 10.3% in South-East Asia to 19.2% in the European Region. Table 9 depicts the global and WHO regional distribution of the 15 different drug-resistant types and the 4 resistance modes found among new and previously treated cases.

Drug resistance data were first analysed by taking as denominator the total number of cases examined in order to determine rates, expressed as percentages to allow a better understanding of the overall picture of TB drug resistance. In order to learn more about drug resistance patterns within the drug-resistant subset of isolates and to be able to compare differences between new and previously treated case groups, due to possible amplification, we also analysed the data taking as denominator the total number of drug-resistant cases in order to determine proportions, which are also expressed as percentages.

From analysis of the data using *the total number of cases examined* as denominator, we can make the following general statements:
- Among new cases, the most frequent drug-resistant types globally are H (3.4%), S (3.8%), SH (2.4%), HRS (0.7%) and HSRE (0.7%).
- A similar frequency of drug-resistant types H, S, and HS was found in the African, European, and South-East Asian Regions. Streptomycin monoresistance was the most

prevalent type of resistance in the Americas, the Eastern Mediterranean, and the Western Pacific Region.

- Among previously treated cases, the most frequent type of drug resistance was quadruple resistance, globally and in all WHO regions except Africa and the Americas, where the most frequent type was isoniazid monoresistance.
- Globally, any resistance was 12.9% among new cases, compared with 32.7% among previously treated cases, a 2.5-fold difference.
- The corresponding differences in the WHO regions ranged from 1.9 in Africa and the Americas, to 2.6 in South-East Asia and the Western Pacific, 3.1 in the Eastern Mediterranean, and 3.9 in the European Region.

From the analysis of the data using *the total number of drug-resistant cases* as denominator, we can make the following general statements:

- Among new cases globally, monoresistance represented the majority of the drug resistance problem (60.9%), followed by double resistance (24.9%), triple resistance (8.8%) and quadruple resistance (5.3%).
- Among previously treated cases globally, monoresistance was only 35%, double resistance 25%, triple resistance 20.4%, and quadruple resistance 19.6%.
- Lower proportions of isolates monoresistant to isoniazid or streptomycin account for most of the difference in the monoresistant proportion in previously treated cases.
- Among new cases, the three most frequent drug-resistant types globally as well as regionally were H, S and SH. These types, together with SHR and SHRE, accounted globally for 84.9% of all resistant cases. These proportions were essentially similar in all WHO regions (range 83.3% to 86.8%) except the Eastern Mediterranean where the proportion was 78.3%.
- Among previously treated cases the most frequent drug resistance type was HRSE, both globally and in all WHO regions except Africa and the Americas.

RESULTS

Table 9: Global patterns of resistance: isolates from latest data point in countries surveyed between 1994 and 2002

Patterns of resistance	PREVALENCE OF DRUG RESISTANCE					
	New Cases			Previously treated cases		
	N	%	%	N	%	%
Strains resistant to 1 drug	6071	7.9	60.9	1476	11.4	35.0
Strains resistant to 2 drugs	2486	3.2	24.9	1052	8.2	25.0
Strains resistant to 3 drugs	877	1.1	8.8	860	6.7	20.4
Strains resistant to 4 drugs	530	0.7	5.3	828	6.4	19.6
TOTAL RESISTANCE	**9964**	**12.9**	**100.0**	**4216**	**32.7**	**100.0**
Strains susceptible to 4 drugs	67211	87.1		8689	67.3	
TOTAL STRAINS TESTED	**77175**	**100.0**		**12905**	**100.0**	
MONORESISTANCE	**6071**	**7.9**	**60.9**	**1476**	**11.4**	**35.0**
- Isoniazid (INH)	2591	3.4	26.0	754	5.8	17.9
- Rifampicin (RMP)	323	0.4	3.2	193	1.5	4.6
- Ethambutol (EMB)	226	0.3	2.3	84	0.7	2.0
- Streptomycin (SM)	2931	3.8	29.4	445	3.4	10.6
DOUBLE RESISTANCE	**2486**	**3.2**	**24.9**	**1052**	**8.2**	**25.0**
- INH + RMP	382	0.5	3.8	423	3.3	10.0
- INH + EMB	109	0.1	1.1	34	0.3	0.8
- INH + SM	1833	2.4	18.4	492	3.8	11.7
- RMP + EMB	27	0.0	0.3	18	0.1	0.4
- RMP + SM	72	0.1	0.7	70	0.5	1.7
- EMB + SM	63	0.1	0.6	15	0.1	0.4
TRIPLE RESISTANCE	**877**	**1.1**	**8.8**	**860**	**6.7**	**20.4**
- INH + RMP + EMB	95	0.1	1.0	101	0.8	2.4
- INH + RMP + SM	574	0.7	5.8	647	5.0	15.3
- INH + EMB + SM	196	0.3	2.0	93	0.7	2.2
- RMP + EMB + SM	12	0.0	0.1	19	0.1	0.5
QUADRUPLE RESISTANCE	**530**	**0.7**	**5.3**	**828**	**6.4**	**19.6**
ANY RESISTANCE						
- Isoniazid (INH)	6310	8.2	63.3	3372	26.1	80.0
- Rifampicin (RMP)	2015	2.6	20.2	2299	17.8	54.5
- Ethambutol (EMB)	1258	1.6	12.6	1192	9.2	28.3
- Streptomycin (SM)	6211	8.0	62.3	2609	20.2	61.9

RESULTS

Figure 34 illustrates the above data for each WHO region. The proportions of triple and quadruple resistance have been combined to facilitate interpretation. The following general statements can be made about the regional picture:

- The comparison of drug resistance proportions between new and previously treated cases shows that, in all six WHO regions, there was a consistently lower level of monoresistance in previously treated cases, with a concomitantly higher combined triple and quadruple resistance. Double resistance proportions fluctuate without significant differences.

- In accordance with the nature of this analysis, the lower proportion of monoresistance and double resistance is equivalent to the higher proportion of the combined triple and quadruple resistance.

- The amplification shift towards triple/quadruple proportions is more accentuated in the Eastern Mediterranean, European, South-East Asian and Western Pacific Regions than in Africa and the Americas.

Figure 34: Proportion of resistance in new and previously treated cases by WHO region

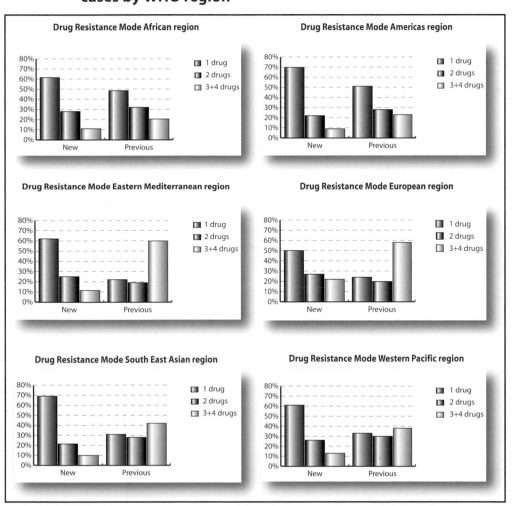

RESULTS

81

4.7 PROFICIENCY TESTING IN THE SUPRANATIONAL LABORATORY NETWORK, 1994-2002

Nine rounds of proficiency testing were carried out between 1994 and 2002. The first five rounds were undertaken under the coordination of the National Reference Centre for Tuberculosis of Health-Canada, Ottawa, a WHO Collaborating Centre for Tuberculosis Bacteriology. The last four were under the coordination of the Mycobacteriology Unit of the Prince Léopold Institute of Tropical Medicine, Antwerp, Belgium. Susceptibility testing was done for INH, RMP, SM, and EMB. The following results reflect the overall performance of all laboratories that took part in this proficiency testing exercise from 1994 to 2002.

Table 10 shows the accuracy and reproducibility of DST for all four antituberculosis drugs obtained by all laboratories that participated in the SRL network activities throughout the nine rounds of testing. The cumulative sensitivity was 99% for isoniazid, 98% for rifampicin, and 91% for both streptomycin and ethambutol. The cumulative specificity was 98% for both rifampicin and isoniazid, 93% for ethambutol, and 91% for streptomycin. Efficiencies of 100% were found for rifampicin and isoniazid, 97% for ethambutol, and 92% for streptomycin. Intralaboratory reproducibility of results in the two identical pairs of 10 isolates tested was 98% for isoniazid and rifampicin, 96% for ethambutol, and 91% for streptomycin. These results are almost identical to those reported in 2002 by Laszlo et al.[66] where only the fourteen laboratories that participated in the first five rounds of proficiency testing were evaluated.

Table 10: Average results (%) of nine rounds of proficiency testing in all participating SRL network laboratories 1994-2002

	INH	RMP	EMB	SM	HR	INH	RMP	EMB	SM	HR
	Sensitivity					Efficiency				
1994	98.7	93.5	65.1	88.7	92.3	99.4	96.2	91.4	92.1	91.7
1995	94.4	99.3	75.4	92.0	93.7	92.8	99.2	80.8	90.0	87.0
1996	96.9	98.0	89.8	96.2	95.0	97.5	99.0	94.2	93.2	92.6
1997	100.0	99.5	97.0	90.9	99.5	100.0	99.1	91.4	93.2	99.5
1998	100.0	99.5	95.4	97.1	99.5	99.8	99.5	96.5	92.4	99.3
1999	100.0	100.0	92.5	87.4	100.0	99.5	98.0	95.0	93.2	99.5
2000	100.0	87.5	89.5	85.1	87.5	100.0	94.7	91.1	81.5	87.5
2001	99.6	89.5	82.9	97.4	89.1	98.9	89.7	90.7	96.6	88.2
2002	99.3	100.0	95.5	87.1	99.3	99.5	100.0	96.5	88.7	98.8
Cumulative*	**98.7**	**97.2**	**89.3**	**90.8**	**95.9**	**98.6**	**97.0**	**92.1**	**92.3**	**94.6**

	INH	RMP	EMB	SM	HR	INH	RMP	EMB	SM	HR
	Specificity					Reproducibility				
1994	100.0	96.5	98.0	100.0	96.5	98.1	94.4	93.1	89.4	94.7
1995	86.1	98.6	83.8	81.9	84.9	97.8	98.3	90.6	96.7	83.0
1996	100.0	100.0	96.1	91.3	100.0	98.0	98.0	98.5	91.5	98.0
1997	100.0	98.6	89.0	95.5	98.6	100.0	99.1	96.4	95.5	98.6
1998	98.9	99.5	98.3	89.2	98.4	98.6	98.2	96.8	95.0	97.0
1999	98.8	92.5	96.0	99.0	91.4	99.0	98.0	97.0	96.5	90.5
2000	99.5	99.6	92.1	98.7	99.1	99.7	97.9	97.9	90.5	98.8
2001	98.0	89.7	98.4	96.0	87.9	97.4	96.8	97.4	97.4	85.6
2002	100.0	100.0	98.0	91.2	100.0	97.4	97.1	92.6	92.1	97.4
Cumulative*	**98.5**	**96.8**	**94.0**	**93.9**	**95.3**	**98.5**	**97.6**	**95.7**	**95.0**	**93.9**

D ISCUSSION

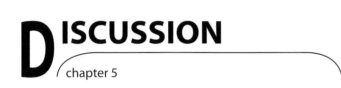

chapter 5

For over nine years, the Global Project has collected data from areas representing 39% of the world's sputum-positive TB cases. The number of countries participating in the project has increased nearly threefold since the first report. Performance criteria for the Supranational Laboratory Network have been developed, four new laboratories are candidates to join, and nine rounds of proficiency testing have been completed. Guidelines for the surveillance of drug resistance in tuberculosis have been revised, and a fourth version of software to analyse drug resistance has been developed. Most importantly, global results of the project are fuelling discussions about policy implications.

While coverage of the project is increasing on the whole, it varies widely. The areas represented in this project are those with at least the minimum requirements to conduct surveillance, and it is likely that the worst situations have not yet been uncovered. While the majority of countries surveyed report low to moderate levels of resistance, several countries have serious drug resistance problems that may jeopardize the control of TB. Paramount to the success of TB control is the expansion of good TB control policies worldwide, accompanied by expanded surveillance of drug resistance to identify areas that require directed initiatives to manage resistance.

The data reported in this third phase of the Project have reinforced many of the conclusions drawn in its first and second reports, and contribute to a more in-depth analysis of dynamics and trends. The median prevalences of any resistance and MDR among new cases of TB in this phase of the project were 10.2% and 1.1%, respectively. Despite the inclusion of different countries in each phase of the project, the medians for most resistance parameters were similar in all reports, but the outliers varied. MDR was again found to be highly prevalent in several areas of the Russian Federation and other countries of the former Soviet Union (Kazakhstan, Aral Sea regions of Uzbekistan and Turkmenistan, Estonia, Latvia, and Lithuania) as well as in some areas outside of this region, including Israel, Ecuador, and Liaoning and Henan Provinces of China. While it is important to follow trends in prevalence of MDR-TB, other resistance patterns must also be watched and closely monitored, as they are potential precursors of MDR. A prevalence of non-MDR INH resistance greater than 10% was found in fifteen countries. High prevalence of non-MDR RMP resistance were less frequent, but also of concern.

Though the Global Project has been operating since 1994 very few countries have reported data for all nine years. Thus, for many countries, it is too early to interpret trends. Data from repeated surveys employing comparable methodologies over several years are essential to determine with any certainty in which direction prevalence of drug resistance is moving.

It is also important to note that data reflect TB programmes at various stages of implementation; thus trends must be interpreted in the context of additional relevant programme indicators. Programme improvement can affect the prevalence of resistance in several ways. A better programme can result in the reduction of the overall number of re-treated cases; however, difficult (resistant) cases may persist. Thus, in some instances an increase in MDR prevalence in a population may reflect a stable number of MDR cases but a decrease in the overall re-treatment population. It is also possible that, as systems improve, coverage and reporting of culture and DST may be more regular resulting in increases in reported case numbers. Improvement in laboratory proficiency, particularly the sensitivity and specificity of drug susceptibility testing, may also affect the observed prevalence of resistance. The scenarios outlined above highlight the importance of evaluating trends in prevalence of drug resistance within the context of relevant programme developments.

5.1   MAGNITUDE OF RESISTANCE BY REGION

AFRICAN REGION

All WHO regions were represented in this phase of the Global Project. In the African region, areas representing 49.5% of new smear positive TB patients and 37% of countries have been surveyed since 1994. The African region has the fewest settings for which trends can be identified. Only Botswana, Sierra Leone, and Mpumalanga Province, South Africa, have carried out repeat surveys. In general, drug resistance in the region is low, but the trends in Botswana and Mpumalanga Province in South Africa indicate that it is increasing. Botswana in particular showed a significant increase in prevalence of any resistance. Though drug resistance was not significantly associated with HIV in the most recent survey, given the high prevalence of HIV in Botswana, even relatively small increases in resistance could have a significant impact on the population if patients with HIV infection become coinfected with drug-resistant *M. tuberculosis*.[77] In Botswana the number of TB cases notified almost doubled between 1995 and 2001; the case detection of smear-positive TB cases reached 75% in 2001 and the treatment success rate was 77%. According to these indicators, Botswana should be able to reach WHO targets for TB control; however increasing incidence, as well as drug resistance, may jeopardize efforts to control TB in the country. In this regard, it will be extremely important to monitor the prevalence of drug resistance in Botswana over time, as an indicator of resistance behaviour in sub-Saharan African countries with high HIV prevalence.

Sierra Leone, with two data points in the first and second reports, showed very little change in prevalence of resistance. However, in view of the social unrest in the country, it is possible that the NTP may have had difficulty implementing a high quality DOTS programme, and this may have affected the prevalence of resistance. Reported prevalence of resistance from recent surveys in Algeria and the Gambia was very low, and only slightly higher in Zambia, confirming the low levels of resistance in the region reported in previous phases in the project. A survey in the city of Kinshasa, Democratic Republic of Congo, reported results for combined cases only. However, the prevalence of MDR appeared to be relatively high for the region with 39% prevalence of any resistance and three-quarters of MDR cases resistant to all four drugs. It will be important to conduct a nationwide survey, as urban centres in general report higher prevalence of resistance than the national average. A survey is planned in Bas-Congo.

In 2001 and 2002, South Africa conducted a nationwide survey by province. Each province adopted a multistage cluster sampling strategy and samples were representative of the entire province. Results of this survey indicated moderate levels of MDR-TB, ranging from 0.9% to 2.6% among new cases, with an increase in Mpumalanga Province, the only province surveyed more than once in the Global Project. Prevalence of MDR-TB in new patients in Mpumalanga province increased from 1.5% in 1997 to 2.6% in 2001, while in re-treated patients prevalence increased from 8.1% in 1997 to 13.9% in 2001. During this same period, performance indicators for TB control have progressively declined and cure rates in Mpumalanga are currently among the lowest in South Africa. Regular reports of drug shortages and high default rates from treatment over this period have given further evidence of conditions for increasing drug resistance. In contrast, data from a previous province-wide survey in Western Cape, not included in the Global Project but following the accepted methodology, indicated relatively stable levels of drug resistance. Prevalence of resistance found in the 2001–2002 survey was nearly the same as those reported in the 1993 survey.[78] The TB programme in the Western Cape is currently among the best performing programmes in South Africa, which may partly explain the stable MDR-TB prevalence figures. In addition, the Western Cape was the first province in South Africa to systematically treat MDR-TB patients (since the mid-1980s). In the recent survey, it was the only province where there was not significant under detection of retreatment cases, i.e. the numbers estimated from the survey tallied with the numbers reported by the TB control programme. The above findings, when compared with those in Mpumalanga, illustrate two points: the potential impact of poor TB control, and the importance of regional surveys in large countries and countries with a high TB burden. The findings would have been obscured in a survey of South Africa as a whole. The nationwide survey in South Africa incorporated surveillance of HIV among TB patients. Prevalence of HIV among TB patients was 55.3 % nationwide, but ranged from 28.2% in the Western Cape Province to 71.9% in the Free State Province. Surveillance of HIV among TB patients in the context of a drug resistance survey is of particular importance, in order to study the relationship between the transmission of drug-resistant TB and HIV over time. Since 2001, drug susceptibility testing is conducted on all re-treatment, failure and non-converting cases and a standardized treatment regimen is provided to MDR-TB cases. Currently there are about 4000 MDR-TB patients receiving treatment. The standardized treatment regimen is priced at about US$ 3400 (non-GLC price) per patient for drugs alone.

Nationwide surveys are underway in Ethiopia and Kenya. Results should be available in 2004. Mozambique, which had one of highest prevalences of MDR (3.5%) in the region in its 1998-1999 survey, is preparing a repeat survey. Senegal and Rwanda will start surveys shortly. Nationwide data from the United Republic of Tanzania, Nigeria, and Democratic Republic of Congo should be prioritized on the agenda of TB control programmes in these high-burden countries in order to detect and address emerging MDR. Surveys in Côte d'Ivoire and Uganda should be repeated in the near future.

REGION OF THE AMERICAS

In the Americas, areas representing 92.6% of all smear positive cases and 41% of countries have been covered by the project. The high population coverage is largely a result of strong laboratory networks, good surveillance coverage of the countries with higher TB burden, and commitment to surveillance in the region. To a great extent, as found in previous reports, the prevalence of MDR is low in the region as a whole; however, there are important outliers.

In North America, Canada has shown a relatively steady prevalence of drug resistance among both new and previously treated cases. TB case notification has decreased since 1997 and prevalence of MDR has never risen above 1.0% among new cases, or 4% among previously treated cases. The USA has shown decreases in overall TB notifications as well as overall numbers of drug-resistant cases since 1995. Decreases in MDR and any rifampicin resistance were significant among new cases, and decreases in any resistance, MDR, any rifampicin and any isoniazid resistance were significant among previously treated cases. Cuba, a country with a history of good TB control, reported significant decreases in any resistance among both new and previously treated cases. Argentina showed a decrease in almost all resistance parameters between surveys. However, the first survey in 1994 sampled a cluster of HIV patients, among whom an outbreak of MDR had recently occurred, which probably biased the survey results. The 1999 survey reflected a change in sampling methodology adopted to minimize bias, and the lower prevalences reported in this survey are probably a more accurate representation of actual levels in the country. Uruguay showed a slight increase in all resistance parameters; however, the magnitude of overall resistance in the country is, to date, the lowest reported in the region. Preliminary results were available from Honduras and Ecuador. The sample from Honduras indicated that prevalence of drug resistance is similar to that in the majority of countries surveyed in the region. Ecuador was an extreme outlier for the region (MDR 4.92% among new cases). The high prevalence of MDR in Ecuador is most likely a result of late and partial implementation of DOTS. Interestingly, in Ecuador, MDR constitutes a higher proportion of any resistance in both new and previously treated cases than in any other country in the region. This is in contrast to Bolivia, which has a relatively high prevalence of any resistance, only a small proportion of which is MDR. Chile, which saw only slight and non-significant increases in resistance between 1997 and 2001, has employed one of the most innovative surveillance policies in the region, which may prove to be a useful model for other countries. Chile performs continuous surveillance of all previously treated patients, and conducts a survey on a representative sample of new cases every three years, thus obtaining accurate information on both populations, strengthening routine patient history interviews, and identifying resistance patterns of previously treated patients early in treatment. This model can perform well in countries with long-standing TB control; however, in new programmes where patient interviews have not been well established, the risk of misclassification may be a concern. A survey in Paraguay is almost completed. Brazil, Colombia, Costa Rica, Dominican Republic, Mexico, Panama, and Peru will commence surveys shortly. A repeat survey in the Dominican Republic will be particularly useful, since an MDR prevalence of 6.6% was reported in the first survey; however, the decade lapse between surveys presents an obstacle to useful comparison of results. A second survey in Mexico will be nationwide and not partial as in the 1997 survey. Brazil will shortly undertake a nationwide survey by state, sampling separately new and previously treated populations and incorporating surveillance of HIV in TB patients. A primary objective of this survey will be the strengthening of the TB laboratory network in the country.

EASTERN MEDITERRANEAN REGION
The Eastern Mediterranean Region has both the lowest coverage of new smear-positive cases (11.6%) and the lowest proportion of countries surveyed (21.7%). Trends are available only for the Gulf States of Oman and Qatar, both with small numbers of total cases and low to moderate levels of resistance, much of which is imported. Trends are

difficult to interpret because of the small numbers of cases, though drug resistance does not appear to be a problem in either of these countries. The survey recently conducted in Egypt showed moderate levels of MDR among new cases (2.2%) but unusually high prevalences of any and RMP monoresistance. Data on resistance to rifampicin must be interpreted with some caution as quality assurance procedures have not yet been finalized by the corresponding SRL. Surveys are under way in Jordan, Lebanon, and the Syrian Arab Republic, and the Islamic Republic of Iran and Morocco are preparing for repeat surveys, with nationwide coverage in Morocco. Other Gulf States, such as Bahrain, Kuwait, and United Arab Emirates, conduct routine drug resistance surveillance of all TB patients but this information has not been yet made available and annual proficiency testing with an SRL is not currently carried out.

EUROPEAN REGION

In the European Region, areas representing 47.8% of all smear-positive cases, and 70.6% of countries have been surveyed. The high coverage of countries in the region is primarily a result of continuous surveillance of bacteriologically confirmed TB cases in much of Western Europe and parts of Central Europe. The European region displays the greatest heterogeneity of resistance parameters in the world, including both the highest and the lowest prevalences.

Because of the varied history of TB control within the region, it is important to discuss the three subregions separately (Western, Central, and Eastern). In general, drug resistance is not a public health problem in Western Europe. Drug resistance prevalence is low, evidenced by an MDR median prevalence below 1%, much of which has been attributed to imported isolates and localized outbreaks. In Germany, higher proportions of any resistance and MDR were reported among new and previously treated cases in 2001 and 2002[a] following changes in the national surveillance system in 2001. Before 2001, drug resistance data in Germany were based on a nationally representative sample covering 55% of local health departments that had elected to report drug susceptibility test results, contributing 50.2% of all reported cases. Since 2001, results of drug susceptibility testing are notifiable by law and are analysed centrally; the higher proportions observed in 2001 and 2002, therefore, do not necessarily reflect an increase over time, but may be due to the methodological change. In France, most resistance parameters among new cases are stable, and resistance in the country is relatively low. Resistance to any drug is increasing significantly in Barcelona, but individual parameters are difficult to interpret. When data were stratified by origin of birth, resistance was higher in the foreign-born population. This, coupled with an increase in immigration in Barcelona since 2000, suggests that the rising prevalence of resistance may be linked to immigration. Israel is an outlier, presenting the highest levels of resistance for most parameters. The situation of this country is unique, because of the high levels of immigration from areas of the former Soviet Union.[79,80,81] Between 80% and 85% of TB patients in Israel are foreign-born, mainly from Ethiopia and countries of the former Soviet Union.[82] Data from 2001 and 2002 indicate that MDR among new cases dropped to 5.8% and 2.0% respectively. Total notifications of TB cases remain low ranging from 281 to 340 cases per year, while total number of MDR cases has fluctuated between 41 in 2000 and 17 in 2002.

Data from countries in Central Europe show relatively low prevalences of drug resistance, with indications of an increase in resistance in a few countries. Though based

a Based on unpublished data from Robert Koch Institute in Germany.

on only two data points, Poland showed a significant doubling in all resistance parameters among new cases; however, the prevalence of MDR-TB remains low at 1.2% among newly detected cases. Slovenia shows stable prevalence of any resistance with very few MDR cases detected. Slovakia has shown steady but non-significant increases in resistance parameters since reporting began in 1998. Both countries have long histories of good TB control. The Czech Republic reported a steady but non-significant increase in prevalence of any resistance and a recent, non-significant increase in MDR among new cases. In general, overall drug resistance does not appear to be a problem at this time; prevalence is low and total MDR cases are very few. It is likely that resistance will continue to be low in Central Europe.

Considerably higher prevalences of drug resistance, including MDR-TB, have been reported in Eastern Europe. The first phase of the Global Project identified drug resistance as a major public health problem in areas of the former Soviet Union. The second report reiterated these findings, and evidence from the third phase indicates that drug resistance is of serious magnitude and extremely widespread, and that there are high proportions of isolates resistant to three or four drugs.

The prevalence of MDR among new cases in Estonia increased between 1994 and 1999, as did case numbers, and significantly decreased in 2000; however, preliminary data from 2001 and 2002 indicate a slight increase in MDR among new cases. This increase, coupled with decreasing overall notifications of new cases, results in a prevalence similar to that observed in 1999, around 17%. MDR case numbers appear to be relatively steady, and translate to fewer than 70 new MDR cases per year. Recent data also indicate a further decrease in MDR among previously treated cases, both in prevalence and total case numbers, appearing to reflect a real sustained decrease over three years. This is encouraging and may be the result of well implemented DOTS in the recent past and national DOTS Plus coverage, though only a sustained decrease over the coming years will confirm this. With a high prevalence of MDR in the population, it is expected that interrupting the chain of transmission to produce a decrease in prevalence of resistance will take some time. Lithuania showed steady and important increases in most resistance parameters; however, only increases in MDR among previously treated cases and any resistance, any INH, and MDR among combined cases were significant. Additionally, overall re-treatment notifications have almost doubled since 1999. DOTS is implemented in 95% of the country, and Lithuania has plans to apply to the GLC once DOTS coverage is complete. In Latvia, new case notifications have increased steadily since 1996 as have total number of cases with any drug resistance; this is reflected in a slight but steady increase in prevalence of any resistance since 1998. Prevalence of MDR has fluctuated slightly since 1998 showing a small decrease in 2000; however, the total number of reported new cases with MDR was relatively steady from 1998 through 2000. Both the total number of re-treatment cases and the number of cases with drug resistance including MDR decreased in Latvia until 1999 and then increased in 2000. This may be a result of more complete reporting of DST results of all re-treatment cases; prior to 2000, only DST results for relapse cases were reported.

Surveys have been implemented in 3 oblasts of the Russian Federation. Tomsk Oblast presented a high prevalence of MDR among new cases with significant and increasing trends in most resistance parameters. Though prevalence of MDR appears to be increasing among previously treated cases, decreases in the total number of re-treatment cases since the first survey in 1998 were reported in 2002, while numbers of MDR cases fluctuated slightly over time. Trends must be interpreted with caution, as surveillance methodologies have changed over the years (methods of case detection and involvement of rural areas), and implementation of DOTS has increased. In order to determine drug resistance trends with any certainty, surveillance of drug resistance must continue. DOTS Plus was begun in Tomsk in late 2000. Data from the second Global Report indicated that prevalence of MDR was increasing in Ivanovo Oblast, and recent unpublished data from 2002 further support this trend.

Kazakhstan recently undertook a nationwide survey, which found a very high prevalence of MDR (14.2%) among new cases, with the majority of these cases resistant to four drugs. The sample size was based on new cases; however, during the survey intake period approximately equal numbers of new and previously treated cases presented at diagnostic units, and 47% of the total sample was composed of previously treated cases. This scenario suggests that there are at least 3000 MDR patients diagnosed in the country each year, 70% of whom are resistant to four first-line antituberculosis drugs. DOTS was implemented from 1998, and while notification rates continue to rise, TB mortality rates have steadily decreased. The use of second-line drugs appears to be extensive and a clear management strategy for MDR cases needs to be developed. A survey of the Aral Sea region in DOTS-covered areas of Uzbekistan and Turkmenistan indicate a very high prevalence of MDR in Karakalpakstan, Uzbekistan, and a moderately high prevalence of MDR in Dashoguz Velayat, Turkmenistan. Both areas reported high proportions of previously treated cases, with most MDR cases resistant to three or four drugs.

Very high prevalences of drug resistance have now been confirmed in Estonia, Latvia, Lithuania, Tomsk and Ivanovo Oblasts in the Russian Federation, Kazakhstan and the Aral Sea regions of Dahoguz Velayat, Turkmenistan, and Karakalpakstan, Uzbekistan. Preliminary evidence suggests even higher prevalences in other areas of the former Soviet Union. TB control following international guidelines must be given high priority, and immediate action must be taken to increase the coverage of drug resistance surveillance in the former Soviet Union. Currently, surveys are being planned in Kyrgyzstan, Moldova, Georgia, Donetsk (Ukraine), Armenia and Azerbaijan as well as a nationwide survey in Uzbekistan. The Russian Federation is developing a plan to systematically survey all oblasts. Currently protocols are being developed for 10 oblasts. In addition to routine national surveillance, it will be of the utmost importance to begin to gather data on the crossover of HIV and MDR, in order to implement proper infection control measures.[84] One of the identified obstacles to surveillance in the region is the lack of internationally quality controlled laboratories. In order to obtain reliable data from these areas, proficiency testing of national or regional reference laboratories must be carried out immediately. Of the highest priority is the proper implementation or expansion of DOTS and DOTS-Plus both to control MDR in areas of known high prevalence and to avoid an epidemic of potentially catastrophic proportions that could destabilize TB control in the region.

SOUTH-EAST ASIAN REGION

The South-East Asian Region also has a low survey coverage of new smear-positive cases (areas representing 14.1% of all smear-positive cases), largely as a result of low coverage of Bangladesh, India, and Indonesia. Sparse data make it difficult to assess the regional scenario with any accuracy. Resistance in the countries surveyed (Nepal, Thailand, and a few settings in India) is reportedly moderate, but with large numbers of total TB cases making the actual burden of resistant cases much higher. Additionally, a large and unregulated private sector and over-the-counter access to a wide range of TB drugs in many South-East Asian countries provides a conducive environment for the

DISCUSSION

development of drug resistance. Increasing surveillance coverage should be considered a regional priority. Recently, district surveys were carried out in India, in the states of Maharashtra, Tamil Nadu, and Karnataka. Data from two surveys in Tamil Nadu (one at the state and one at district level) indicate prevalences of MDR among new cases of around 3%, representing an enormous number of MDR-TB cases. Additionally, many states in the country report high proportions of re-treatment cases in the NTP, though very little is known about prevalence of drug resistance among this population. Only well designed state level surveys, sampling new and previously treated cases separately, will be able to assist in ascertaining a baseline prevalence in these populations at the state level. India is developing a plan to conduct nationwide surveillance of drug resistance by state, starting with two states this year and gradually adding and re-surveying states over time, as has been done in China and is planned in Brazil. Another objective of nationwide surveillance of drug resistance in India is the strengthening of laboratory networks, through the implementation of an external quality assurance system for smear microscopy and QA of culture and DST in state laboratories. The plan is ambitious and will require concerted political commitment to succeed. Nepal has conducted three surveys with mixed results. Prevalences of resistance among new cases from the first and third surveys were similar; however, the second survey found considerably higher prevalence of resistance among new cases. Resistance among previously treated cases (surveyed only in the last two surveys) decreased. The reasons for the fluctuations in resistance prevalence between surveys are unknown; further surveys will be helpful in confirming the prevalence of MDR-TB. Thailand showed significant decreases in prevalences of MDR and any resistance between 1997 and 2001, though notifications of all TB cases increased considerably during this time. It is possible that the decrease in drug resistance in Thailand is a result of good TB control and will be sustained in the future; however, at this time, there are not sufficient data to predict this with any certainty. It will be important to keep surveillance of drug resistance on the agenda in order to evaluate the progress of DOTS under recent health care reforms and to follow trends in high-risk populations identified in the course of the surveys.[85] Myanmar is finalizing a nationwide drug resistance survey and Indonesia has plans to conduct a partial survey in 2004. Bangladesh constitutes another important gap in drug resistance information in the region and nationwide surveillance there should be a priority. The human and financial capacity of the national reference laboratory needs to be enhanced before proficiency testing can take place and a nationwide survey implemented.

WESTERN PACIFIC REGION

The Western Pacific Region has very high surveillance coverage of new smear-positive cases (areas representing 50.8% of smear positive cases), in part because of the broad coverage of China and a strong commitment to surveillance in the region. China has a progressive surveillance policy and has surveyed six of 31 provinces in the country, with a repeat survey completed in Henan, and repeat surveys planned in Guangdong, Zhejiang, and Shandong provinces. New surveys are under way in Inner Mongolia and Hunan, surveys of Beijing and Shanghai cities are due to start shortly, and surveys are planned in Xinjiang, Heilongjiang, and Chongqing. Hong Kong SAR conducts continuous surveillance. Prevalence of drug resistance ranges from low in Hong Kong SAR to extremely high in Henan and Liaoning. The decrease in any resistance among new cases in Hong Kong SAR was significant and supports documented evidence of this trend.[86] Liaoning province reported an extremely high prevalence of MDR (10.8%) among new cases; however, patient reinterviews indicated an estimated 25–30% misclassification of previously treated cases as new cases, indicating that prevalence of MDR is more likely to be around 8%. Henan experienced a similar misclassification in 1996 (MDR adjusted from 16% to 10.8%). Though prevalence of MDR in the subsequent 1999 survey (7.8%) was lower than the adjusted figure reported in 1996, methodological problems preclude the acceptance that there was any real reduction in prevalence. In both settings, misclassification was difficult to avoid because of previous policies, and this underlines the importance of rechecking records and reinterviewing patients during the course of a survey. Of particular note in China is the well designed QA system that has evolved in conjunction with drug resistance surveillance. Proficiency testing of provincial laboratories that have conducted or are preparing to conduct surveys takes place annually, even after the survey has been completed. Annual PT of provincial laboratories should remain a priority; in this way China is taking steps to establish a long-term QA system for DST in the country.

Data from other countries surveyed indicate that anti-TB drug resistance elsewhere in the region is low in magnitude. Japan provided data from a 1997 nationwide sentinel survey and Mongolia from a 1999 nationwide survey, both showing relatively low prevalences of drug resistance. Singapore, which conducts surveillance of all culture-positive TB cases, also reported low prevalence of resistance. The 2001 survey in Cambodia indicated a very low prevalence of resistance in the population, which is important in view of the high number of TB cases and high HIV prevalence in the country, and may in part be a result of late introduction of rifampicin. Given the high prevalence of INH resistance, and somewhat moderate prevalence of MDR reported in the last survey, and results from recent municipal surveys in Viet Nam, it will be important to follow the prevalence of resistance in this country. Resistance in Australia, New Zealand, and the South Pacific islands appears to be largely of foreign origin and low in magnitude at this time.

5.2   ECOLOGICAL ANALYSIS

The ecological analysis reiterated findings of the first two phases of the project, namely that re-treatment is strongly associated with drug resistance. This finding highlights the importance of giving greater attention to this group of patients in terms of treatment, reporting, and representative drug resistance surveillance. In general, the ecological analysis was inconclusive with the exception of the above finding. Despite the inherent weakness in ecological analysis of aggregate data, the conceptual model can constitute a step forward for more reliable and individual data collection.

5.3   BURDEN OF MDR

In many countries with relatively few TB cases, a high prevalence of resistance does not reflect high absolute numbers of cases. Conversely, a low prevalence of MDR applied to high-burden settings, such as South Africa or some provinces in China, could reflect a considerable number of MDR cases. In South Africa, 2.9% of all TB sputum-positive cases are MDR, while in Kazakhstan one in every four smear-positive pulmonary TB case is MDR. Kazakhstan has a lower burden of disease and South Africa a lower prevalence of MDR, yet both countries have an enormous burden of 3000 or more MDR cases diagnosed each year. Nepal, Thailand and Estonia are other examples. Nepal and Thailand have 3.8% and 1.8% MDR prevalence among combined cases, respectively, but have about 5 times as many MDR cases as Estonia with 19.5% MDR. Ultimately the magnitude of the problem rests on the ability of a country to treat patients effectively.

The international community and partners must prioritize both technical and financial support to countries with an identified MDR-TB problem. Failure to do so will result in a situation where a substandard level of care and irrational use of second-line drugs will continue to perpetuate the transmission of, and potentially amplify further, highly drug-resistant isolates of tuberculosis. A critical mass of resistant cases has great potential not only to halt the progress of TB control but to reverse it. DOTS-Plus is a comprehensive management strategy for MDR-TB that includes the five tenets of the DOTS strategy. By definition, it is impossible to conduct DOTS-Plus in an area without having an effective DOTS-based TB control programme in place. Therefore the international community must also be willing to reject GLC applications from countries/ settings where basic TB programmes are suboptimal or not fully in place, in order to prevent further amplification of resistance. Fortunately, a number of funding mechanisms, such as the Global Fund to Fight AIDS, Tuberculosis and Malaria, now require all requests for the funding of second-line TB drugs to go through the GLC for approval.

5.4   SRLN

The network of supranational laboratories currently comprises 20 laboratories in five regions; three laboratories have closed since the beginning of the project and four are candidates to join. The network has completed nine rounds of proficiency testing since 1994; cumulative results over the nine rounds generally indicate overall high performance of the network. Results of proficiency testing at the NRL level are subject to scrutiny by the corresponding SRL and then shared with the Global Project. Following an evaluation by the supranational laboratory, a decision is made on whether to carry out the survey or repeat proficiency testing. The Global Project, partners and the SRLN itself have proposed performance criteria for the network at different stages of the project in order to address substandard performance and maintain a high level of quality to ensure reliable survey results. None of these proposals has ever been strictly adopted. Therefore, it was proposed that the SRLN develop criteria for network and NRL standards, with the following components: quantitative and qualitative indicators for admission into the network, assessment of performance, and contribution to the network of existing members, and type and timing of remedial action when substandard performance is detected. The network has recently agreed such criteria and details will be published in the coming year. In the future, performance criteria for NRLs will also be developed and agreed upon by the network.

Borderline isolates detected in two rounds of proficiency testing affected the overall performance of the network in those rounds and made reproduction of those isolates for PT of NRLs virtually impossible. The SRLN agreed that efforts should be made to exclude borderline isolates from quality assurance exercises, and borderline isolates that were included in previous panels should not be included in standard calculations of sensitivity and specificity for the purposes of evaluating individual laboratories. Preliminary research has shown that at least one of the apparently borderline isolates was in fact a mixed culture containing one drug-resistant and one susceptible isolate; however, further exploration is warranted.

The contribution of the Supranational Laboratory Network to the Global Project has been paramount in achieving the high quality and coverage of surveillance of drug resistance to date. While the WHO/IUATLD Global Project coordinates the SRLN and covers a small portion of operational costs, the supranational laboratories invest their own time and resources to assist in this global endeavour. There is a need for these costs to be met internationally to stabilize and enhance the network. Recently members of the SRLN have further contributed their time and experience to several regional DST training courses. Additionally, the majority of SRLN members along with partners have become involved in a Laboratory Strengthening Subgroup organized by the DOTS Expansion Working Group. The Laboratory Strengthening Subgroup seeks to assess and develop plans for improvement of entire national laboratory networks, with an emphasis on sputum smear microscopy. A recent meeting of the SRLN and the Subgroup agreed to develop a comprehensive workplan for the coming two years, and to engage the international community in putting laboratory network improvement firmly on the TB control agenda. Improved laboratory networks will translate into improved diagnostic and treatment capacity, and more accurate surveillance of drug resistance.

5.5 DRUG RESISTANCE PATTERNS

Among the advantages of being able to analyse DST results obtained from 1994 till 2002, from over 90 000 isolates and over 100 sites on all continents, is that even the most infrequent drug resistance types (combinations) can be detected with a high degree of sensitivity. This is not always true of the data from individual sites, where the number of cultures examined is less than 1000, given that some drug resistance types show prevalences of 0.1% or even lower. The total number of isolates examined is sufficiently high to guarantee statistical significance of both new cases and previously treated cases, even though all settings within some regions such as the Eastern Mediterranean and South-East Asia are not necessarily representative of the regions as a whole. The consistency of the findings argues for the robustness of the following conclusions.

Increase in drug resistance rates

Clinical TB drug resistance develops as a result of spontaneous genetic mutations in *M. tuberculosis*, which are selected if antituberculosis drugs are used inconsistently or inappropriately, e.g. if monotherapy is applied. In patients with drug-resistant tuberculosis, additional drug resistance may develop if a prescribed multidrug regimen includes the drugs these patients are already resistant to. In this situation, some of these patients may end up effectively receiving monotherapy. In this respect the findings of worldwide drug resistance surveys are revealing, in that the prevalence of drug resistance is significantly higher among previously treated patients than among new patients in all regions. The only logical inference is that present treatment practices create significant numbers of new resistant cases and amplify already present resistance.

This analysis shows a remarkable consistency, both globally and regionally, in the distribution of the major drug resistance types, as well as in the increase in drug resistance prevalence among previously treated cases relative to new cases. It should be noted that prevalence of drug resistance observed in previously treated cases is higher than in new cases in all regions. However, the size of the difference varies between regions. Since this difference is in great part directly related to the quality of drug treatment, this apparent characteristic could well lead to the development of an indicator that would measure the quality of treatment practices.

Amplification of drug resistance proportions

It is well understood that the creation of drug resistance follows a sequential process, i.e. monoresistance —> double resistance —> triple resistance —> quadruple drug resistance. The addition of a new drug to a failing drug regimen is an effective way of amplifying the drug resistance problem. Monoresistance can only be selected in the presence of a drug concentration leading to the selection of pre-existing mutant bacilli, whereas resistance to two drugs cannot be created simultaneously in the presence of effective concentrations of two drugs. This is because the number of bacilli present in the lesions (10^8) is usually much lower than the theoretically required bacillary load needed to produce double resistance, i.e. in the case of SM and INH, 2.29×10^{-8} and 2.56×10^{-8} respectively or 10^{-16}. Results obtained in this study show that the proportions of monoresistance are lower in patients having re-treatment, whereas double resistance remains essentially unchanged. Triple and quadruple resistance are higher by about the same proportion as monoresistance is lower. Amplification caused by re-treatment is the easiest way to interpret these changes, i.e. the selective pressures of treatment create double resistance from mainly monoresistant H/S cases. The absence of a significant change in double resistance proportions can be explained by selective pressure, leading to an increase in triple and quadruple drug resistance modes thus balancing the inflow from the monoresistance mode. Since resistance in re-treatment cases mostly reflects the quality of recent treatment, these results could lead to the development of an indicator, based on the extent of amplification. The difference between previously treated and new case triple and quadruple resistance proportions could constitute such an indicator. More analysis is needed to validate this proposed indicator.

Major drug resistance pathways

Lastly, we have seen that monoresistant H/S, double resistant HS, triple resistant HSR and quadruple resistant HSRE cases account for about 85% of all resistant cases. This suggests that, globally as well as in most regions, the main pathway of drug resistance amplification is H, S —> HS —> HSR —> HSRE. Other pathways can and do exist but their contribution to the drug resistance problem is relatively minor. We can therefore state that monoresistance to H or to S is the foundation for the acquisition of additional drug resistance.

Implications

The above analysis has shown that there is circumstantial but compelling evidence that either monotherapy or "effective" monotherapy, or both, are more widespread than commonly thought. These results corroborate recently emerging evidence that standard re-treatment regimens containing first-line drugs for failures of standard treatment should be abandoned in some settings. In a recent study, Quy et al[87] showed the limitations of the 2SRHZ/6HE regimen in preventing the amplification effect even in patients with primary resistance other than MDR-TB, including single drug resistance. From the analysis of the above data, there might also be wider implications for the standard 2SRHZ/6HE regimen at least in those countries with high rates of H/S monoresistance and HS double resistance. One possible way of breaking the amplification juggernaut would be to replace S in standard regimens and/or to add a third drug to the continuation phase.

ANNEXES

Annex 1: Prevalence (%) of drug resistance among new TB cases, by country/geographical setting and WHO region (1999-2002)

COUNTRY/SETTING	Year	No. of PATIENTS TESTED	OVERALL		RESISTANCE[a] TO:			Poly- resistance	MDR
			Susceptible	Resistant	1 Drug	2 Drugs	3+Drugs		
Africa									
Algeria	2001	518	93.8	6.2	4.1	1.0	1.2	1.0	1.2
Botswana	2002	469	86.4	13.6	9.0	3.4	1.3	3.4	1.3
The Gambia	1999	210	95.7	4.3	3.8	0.5	0.0	0.0	0.5
South Africa - Eastern Cape	2001	506	88.7	11.3	7.9	2.8	0.6	2.4	1.0
South Africa - Free State	2001	414	91.4	8.6	5.5	1.5	1.5	1.3	1.8
South Africa - Gauteng	2001	592	93.4	6.6	4.1	1.5	1.0	1.2	1.4
South Africa - Kwazulu-Natal	2001	595	93.4	6.6	3.7	1.0	1.8	1.2	1.7
South Africa - Limpopo	2001	451	92.9	7.1	2.9	2.4	1.8	1.8	2.4
South Africa - North West	2001	631	91.9	8.1	4.4	1.8	1.8	1.3	2.2
South Africa - Western Cape	2001	427	94.4	5.6	3.1	2.3	0.2	1.6	0.9
Zambia	2000	445	88.5	11.5	8.5	2.0	0.9	1.1	1.8
**South Africa - Mpumalanga	2001	702	90.6	9.4	5.6	2.1	1.1	1.3	2.6
Median		469	92.9	7.1	4.1	1.8	1.2	1.3	1.4
Americas									
Argentina	1999	679	89.8	9.7	7.5	1.2	1.5	0.9	1.8
Canada	2000	1244	91.5	8.5	5.8	1.8	0.7	1.9	0.7
Colombia	1999	1087	84.5	15.5	9.4	4.6	1.6	4.7	1.5
Cuba	2000	377	95.0	5.0	3.7	1.3	0.0	1.1	0.3
Ecuador	2002	394	76.6	23.4	12.9	8.4	2.0	3.8	6.6
El Salvador	2001	611	94.3	5.7	4.9	0.8	0.0	0.5	0.3
Honduras	2002	169	82.8	17.2	11.2	4.7	1.2	4.1	1.8
Puerto Rico	2001	100	88.0	12.0	6.0	5.0	1.0	4.0	2.0
Uruguay	1999	315	96.8	3.2	2.9	0.3	0.0	0.0	0.3
United States of America	2001	9751	87.3	12.7	8.8	2.8	1.1	2.7	1.1
Venezuela	1998	769	92.5	7.5	4.9	2.2	0.4	2.1	0.5
**Chile	2001	867	89.5	11.7	8.2	2.7	0.8	2.7	0.7
Median		554	90.3	9.7	6.0	2.2	1.0	2.1	1.1
Eastern Mediterranean									
Egypt	2002	632	69.5	30.5	21.7	6.5	2.4	6.6	2.2

COUNTRY/SETTING	Year	No. of PATIENTS TESTED	OVERALL		RESISTANCE[a] TO:			Poly-resistance	MDR
			Susceptible	Resistant	1 Drug	2 Drugs	3+Drugs		
Oman	2001	171	94.7	5.3	4.7	0.6	0.0	0.6	0.0
Qatar	2001	284	90.1	9.9	7.0	2.8	0.0	2.5	0.4
Median		284	90.1	9.9	7.0	2.8	0.0	2.5	0.4
Europe									
Andorra	2000	3	100.0	0.0	0.0	0.0	0.0	0.0	0.0
Austria	2000	694	95.5	4.5	3.0	1.0	0.4	1.0	0.4
Belgium	2000	562	94.0	6.0	4.5	1.2	0.3	0.4	1.2
Bosnia and Herzegovina	2000	993	97.6	2.4	2.0	0.4	0.0	0.3	0.1
Croatia	2000	780	98.2	1.8	1.5	0.3	0.0	0.1	0.1
Czech Republic	2000	616	95.6	4.4	2.6	1.1	0.6	0.6	1.1
Denmark	2000	392	88.0	12.0	7.1	4.6	0.3	4.6	0.3
Estonia	2000	410	71.5	28.5	10.7	4.4	13.4	5.6	12.2
Finland	2000	374	95.5	4.5	3.2	1.1	0.3	1.1	0.3
France	2000	947	90.7	9.3	7.3	1.5	0.5	1.2	0.8
Germany	2000	1561	93.2	6.8	4.5	1.4	0.9	1.5	0.8
Iceland	2000	8	100.0	0.0	0.0	0.0	0.0	0.0	0.0
Ireland	2000	136	97.1	2.9	2.2	0.7	0.0	0.0	0.7
Israel	2000	253	68.8	31.2	11.9	4.7	14.6	5.1	14.2
Italy	2000	688	88.7	11.3	7.0	3.3	1.0	3.2	1.2
Kazakhstan	2001	359	42.9	57.1	13.9	17.8	25.3	29.0	14.2
Latvia	2000	897	68.3	31.7	9.3	12.2	10.3	13.2	9.3
Lithuania	2002	819	70.8	29.2	10.4	8.2	10.6	9.4	9.4
Luxembourg	2000	39	92.3	7.7	7.7	0.0	0.0	0.0	0.0
Malta	2000	9	100.0	0.0	0.0	0.0	0.0	0.0	0.0
Netherlands	2000	768	89.3	10.7	7.8	2.5	0.4	2.0	0.9
Norway	2000	160	75.6	24.4	15.0	9.4	0.0	7.5	1.9
Poland	2001	3037	93.9	6.1	4.0	1.3	0.8	1.0	1.2
Russian Federation - Orel Oblast	2002	379	78.9	21.1	5.3	9.8	6.1	13.2	2.6
Russian Federation - Tomsk Oblast	2002	533	62.7	37.3	10.5	13.3	13.5	13.1	13.7
Serbia and Montenegro-Belgrade	2000	249	94.4	5.6	4.8	0.4	0.4	0.4	0.4
Slovakia	2000	465	95.9	4.1	2.4	1.3	0.4	0.6	1.1
Slovenia	2000	282	97.5	2.5	1.8	0.7	0.0	0.7	0.0
Spain - Barcelona	2001	133	89.5	10.5	7.5	2.3	0.8	2.3	0.8
Spain - Galicia	2001	360	88.3	11.7	9.7	0.6	1.4	0.6	1.4

[a] Small differences may appear between the variable "overall resistance" and "resistance to 1 drug+2 drugs+3drugs", due to rounding.

ANNEXES

COUNTRY/SETTING	Year	No. of PATIENTS TESTED	OVERALL		RESISTANCE[a] TO:			Poly-resistance	MDR
			Susceptible	Resistant	1 Drug	2 Drugs	3+Drugs		
Sweden	2000	322	88.8	11.2	7.8	2.8	0.6	2.2	1.2
Switzerland	2000	330	94.5	5.5	5.5	0.0	0.0	0.0	0.0
Turkmenistan – Dashoguz	2001	105	69.5	30.5	21.0	4.8	4.8	5.7	3.8
United Kingdom - England, Wales, Northern Ireland	2000	2312	91.6	8.4	6.4	1.3	0.6	1.1	0.9
Uzbekistan - Karakalpakstan	2001	106	51.9	48.1	15.1	13.2	19.8	19.8	13.2
Median		379	91.6	8.4	6.4	1.3	0.6	1.1	0.9
South-East Asia									
India - North Arcot	1999	282	72.3	27.7	16.7	7.1	3.9	8.2	2.8
India - Raichur District	1999	278	78.1	21.9	15.5	4.0	2.5	4.0	2.5
India - Wardha District	1999	197	80.2	19.8	15.2	4.6	0.0	4.1	0.5
Nepal	2001	755	89.0	11.0	7.0	2.8	1.2	2.6	1.3
Thailand	2001	1505	85.2	14.8	10.5	3.5	0.9	3.4	0.9
Median		282	80.2	19.8	15.2	4.0	1.2	4.0	1.3
Western Pacific									
Cambodia	2001	638	89.7	10.3	8.5	1.9	0.0	1.9	0.0
China – Henan	2001	1222	70.1	29.9	15.6	7.2	7.0	6.5	7.8
China – Hong Kong SAR	2001	3470	89.8	10.2	7.0	2.4	0.8	2.4	0.8
China – Hubei	1999	859	82.5	17.5	10.9	5.1	1.4	4.4	2.1
China – Liaoning	1999	818	57.9	42.1	21.6	10.6	9.8	10.0	10.4
Japan	1997	1374	89.7	10.3	7.6	2.1	0.6	1.8	0.9
Mongolia	1999	405	70.6	29.4	18.3	9.6	1.5	10.1	1.0
New Zealand	2001	272	88.6	11.4	9.2	2.2	0.0	2.2	0.0
Singapore	2001	823	95.0	5.0	3.2	1.2	0.6	1.3	0.5
Median		823	88.6	11.4	9.2	2.4	0.8	2.5	0.9
Overall Median		459	89.8	10.2	7.0	2.2	0.8	1.9	1.1
Overall Minimum		3	42.9	0.0	0.0	0.0	0.0	0.0	0.0
Overall Maximum		9751	100.0	57.1	21.7	17.8	25.3	29.0	14.2

[a] Small differences may appear between the variable "overall resistance" and "resistance to 1 drug+2 drugs+3drugs", due to rounding.

Annex 2: Prevalence (%) of resistance to specific drugs among new TB cases, by country/geographical setting and WHO region (1999-2002)

COUNTRY/SETTING	Year	No. of PATIENTS TESTED	INH		RMP		EMB		SM	
			MONO	ANY	MONO	ANY	MONO	ANY	MONO	ANY
Africa										
Algeria	2001	518	1.0	3.1	0.0	1.2	0.0	0.0	3.1	5.2
Botswana	2002	469	1.9	5.5	1.3	3.2	0.4	2.1	5.3	9.2
The Gambia	1999	210	1.9	2.4	0.5	1.0	0.0	0.0	1.4	1.4
South Africa - Eastern Cape	2001	506	3.8	7.1	0.2	1.2	0.0	0.7	4.0	6.7
South Africa - Free State	2001	414	3.3	6.4	0.7	2.4	0.0	0.7	1.5	4.0
South Africa - Gauteng	2001	592	1.9	4.4	0.3	1.7	0.0	0.3	1.9	3.8
South Africa - Kwazulu-Natal	2001	595	2.5	5.4	0.2	1.8	0.0	0.8	1.0	3.9
South Africa - Limpopo	2001	451	1.3	5.5	0.0	2.4	0.0	2.2	1.6	4.0
South Africa - North West	2001	631	2.2	5.9	0.5	2.7	0.0	1.3	1.7	4.4
South Africa - Western Cape	2001	427	2.6	5.2	0.0	0.9	0.0	0.0	0.5	2.3
Zambia	2000	445	3.4	6.3	0.0	1.8	0.7	2.0	4.5	5.4
**South Africa - Mpumalanga	2001	702	3.1	7.0	0.6	3.1	0.0	1.0	1.9	4.1
Median		469	2.2	5.5	0.2	1.8	0.0	0.7	1.7	4.0
Americas										
Argentina	1999	554	1.8	4.3	0.4	2.2	0.4	2.0	4.5	7.0
Canada	2000	1244	4.3	6.8	0.0	0.9	0.2	1.0	1.4	3.5
Colombia	1999	1087	3.4	9.5	0.1	1.7	0.3	0.8	5.6	11.5
Cuba	2000	377	0.3	1.1	0.0	0.8	0.0	0.0	3.4	4.5
Ecuador	2002	394	4.8	14.0	2.3	10.2	0.3	0.8	5.6	10.9
El Salvador	2001	611	0.5	1.3	0.8	1.1	0.3	0.3	3.3	3.8
Honduras	2002	169	1.2	6.5	0.0	2.4	0.0	1.2	10.1	14.8
Puerto Rico	2001	100	3.0	8.0	0.0	3.0	0.0	1.0	3.0	8.0
Uruguay	1999	315	1.3	1.6	0.0	0.3	0.0	0.0	1.6	1.6
United States of America	2001	9751	4.0	7.7	0.2	1.5	0.4	1.6	4.1	7.4
Venezuela	1998	769	1.7	3.9	0.4	1.0	0.1	1.0	2.7	4.7
**Chile	2001	867	1.5	5.0	0.1	0.9	0.0	0.2	6.56	10.0
Median		554	1.8	6.5	0.1	1.5	0.2	1.0	3.4	7.0
Eastern Mediterranean										
Egypt	2002	632	2.7	9.8	3.5	7.0	0.5	2.8	15.0	23.6

* *Not included in analysis or median calculations

ANNEXES

COUNTRY/SETTING	Year	No. of PATIENTS TESTED	INH		RMP		EMB		SM	
			MONO	ANY	MONO	ANY	MONO	ANY	MONO	ANY
Oman	2001	171	3.5	4.1	0.6	0.6	0.0	0.0	0.6	1.2
Qatar	2001	284	4.2	6.7	0.4	1.1	0.7	1.8	1.8	3.2
Median		284	3.5	6.7	0.6	1.1	0.5	1.8	1.8	3.2
Europe										
Andorra	2000	3	0.0	0.0	0.0	0.0	0.0	0.0	0.0	0.0
Austria	2000	694	1.4	2.9	0.3	0.7	0.1	0.1	1.2	2.6
Belgium	2000	562	3.7	5.3	0.4	1.6	0.4	1.1	-	-
Bosnia and Herzegovina	2000	993	0.3	0.5	0.6	0.7	0.9	1.1	0.2	0.5
Croatia	2000	780	0.8	1.0	0.0	0.1	0.0	0.0	0.8	0.9
Czech Republic	2000	616	1.6	3.4	0.0	1.1	0.2	0.8	0.8	2.0
Denmark	2000	392	2.8	7.4	0.0	0.5	0.0	0.8	4.3	8.7
Estonia	2000	410	5.1	22.9	0.0	12.2	0.0	13.2	5.6	22.4
Finland	2000	374	1.3	2.7	0.5	0.8	0.0	0.3	1.3	2.4
France	2000	947	0.5	2.5	0.0	0.8	0.8	2.1	5.9	6.4
Germany	2000	1561	1.7	3.9	0.3	1.0	0.3	1.0	2.2	4.2
Iceland	2000	8	0.0	0.0	0.0	0.0	0.0	0.0	0.0	0.0
Ireland	2000	136	2.2	2.9	0.0	0.7	0.0	0.0	0.0	0.0
Israel	2000	253	6.3	25.7	0.4	14.6	1.2	9.9	4.0	22.1
Italy	2000	688	2.0	6.4	0.4	1.6	0.6	1.5	3.9	7.8
Kazakhstan	2001	359	3.1	42.6	0.3	15.6	0.8	24.8	9.7	51.5
Latvia	2001	897	6.6	29.0	0.0	9.3	0.2	6.2	2.5	24.4
Lithuania	2002	819	6.6	25.4	0.4	9.8	0.0	7.3	3.4	21.7
Luxembourg	2000	39	5.1	5.1	0.0	0.0	0.0	0.0	2.6	2.6
Malta	2000	9	0.0	0.0	0.0	0.0	0.0	0.0	0.0	0.0
Netherlands	2000	768	2.9	5.6	0.1	0.9	0.1	0.7	5.1	6.9
Norway	2000	160	4.4	13.1	0.0	2.5	5.0	6.9	5.6	11.3
Poland	2001	3037	2.0	4.1	0.3	1.4	0.0	0.6	1.7	3.4
Russian Federation - Orel Oblast	2002	379	2.1	17.9	0.0	2.6	0.0	4.7	3.2	19.0
Russian Federation - Tomsk Oblast	2002	533	2.4	29.1	0.4	14.3	0.0	4.3	7.7	34.1
Serbia and Montenegro-Belgrade	2000	249	1.2	1.6	1.6	2.0	0.4	0.8	1.6	2.4
Slovakia	2000	465	1.7	3.2	0.2	1.5	0.0	0.2	0.4	1.3
Slovenia	2000	282	1.4	2.1	0.0	0.0	0.0	0.0	0.4	1.1
Spain - Barcelona	2001	133	3.8	6.0	0.0	1.5	0.0	0.0	3.8	6.8
Spain - Galicia	2001	360	2.5	4.4	0.0	1.4	0.6	2.2	6.7	7.2
Sweden	2000	322	7.5	10.9	0.0	1.2	0.0	0.6	0.3	2.5

COUNTRY/SETTING	Year	No. of PATIENTS TESTED	INH		RMP		EMB		SM	
			MONO	ANY	MONO	ANY	MONO	ANY	MONO	ANY
Switzerland	2000	330	5.5	5.5	0.0	0.0	0.0	0.0	–	–
Turkmenistan – Dashoguz	2001	105	5.7	15.2	0.0	3.8	0.0	1.9	15.2	24.8
United Kingdom – England, Wales, Northern Ireland	2000	2312	4.0	6.0	0.3	1.2	0.0	0.5	0.5	–
Uzbekistan – Karakalpakstan	2001	106	3.8	36.8	0.0	13.2	0.0	15.1	11.3	44.3
Median		379	2.4	5.3	0.0	1.2	0.0	0.8	2.5	4.1
South-East Asia										
India – North Arcot	1999	282	12.8	23.4	0.0	2.8	0.4	4.6	3.5	12.4
India – Raichur District	1999	278	12.2	18.7	0.0	2.5	0.0	3.2	3.2	7.2
India – Wardha District	1999	197	10.7	15.2	0.0	0.5	0.0	1.0	4.6	7.6
Nepal	2001	755	1.6	5.4	0.3	1.7	0.0	0.9	5.2	8.9
Thailand	2001	1505	5.3	9.5	0.3	1.4	0.1	1.1	4.8	8.2
Median		282	10.7	15.2	0.0	1.7	0.0	1.1	4.6	8.2
Western Pacific										
Cambodia	2001	638	4.7	6.4	0.5	0.6	0.0	0.2	3.3	5.0
China – Henan	2001	1222	3.3	17.0	1.5	9.7	0.8	4.3	10.1	22.2
China – Hong Kong SAR	2001	3470	2.3	5.5	0.2	1.0	0.0	0.5	4.5	7.5
China – Hubei	1999	859	3.7	9.7	1.2	3.8	0.1	0.6	5.9	11.4
China – Liaoning	1999	818	5.4	25.3	0.5	11.4	0.2	3.8	15.5	34.1
Japan	1997	1374	2.0	4.4	0.2	1.4	0.1	0.4	5.2	7.5
Mongolia	1999	405	4.4	15.3	0.2	1.2	0.0	1.7	13.6	24.2
New Zealand	2001	272	4.4	6.3	0.0	0.4	0.4	0.7	4.4	6.3
Singapore	2001	823	1.6	3.3	0.0	0.6	0.1	0.7	1.5	3.0
Median		823	3.7	6.4	0.3	1.2	0.1	0.7	5.2	7.5
Overall Median		459	2.6	5.9	0.2	1.4	0.0	0.8	3.3	6.3
Overall Minimum		3	0.0	0.0	0.0	0.0	0.0	0.0	0.0	0.0
Overall Maximum		9751	12.8	42.6	3.5	15.6	5.0	24.8	15.5	51.5

* *Not included in analysis or median calculations

ANNEXES

Annex 3: Prevalence (%) of drug resistance among previously treated TB cases, by country/geographical setting and WHO region (1999-2002)

COUNTRY/SETTING	Year	No. of PATIENTS TESTED	OVERALL		RESISTANCE[a] TO:			Poly-resistance	MDR
			Susceptible	Resistant	1 Drug	2 Drugs	3+Drugs		
Africa									
Botswana	2002	66	69.7	30.3	9.1	12.1	9.1	7.6	13.6
The Gambia	1999	15	100.0	0.0	0.0	0.0	0.0	0.0	0.0
South Africa - Eastern Cape	2001	283	82.3	17.7	7.4	7.4	2.8	2.8	7.8
South Africa - Free State	2001	174	90.8	9.2	6.3	2.3	.5	1.1	1.8
South Africa - Gauteng	2001	165	87.3	12.7	3.1	5.5	4.3	4.2	5.5
South Africa - Kwazulu-Natal	2001	207	81.6	18.4	8.2	4.3	5.8	2.4	7.7
South Africa - Limpopo	2001	88	83.0	17.0	9.0	4.5	3.4	1.1	7.0
South Africa - North West	2001	188	80.9	19.1	8.5	6.9	3.7	3.7	6.9
South Africa - Western Cape	2001	228	92.1	7.9	3.5	2.1	2.1	0.4	3.9
**South Africa - Mpumalanga	2001	175	76.6	23.4	6.9	5.2	11.5	2.9	13.7
Zambia	2000	44	84.1	15.9	11.4	4.5	0.0	0.0	2.3
Median		169	83.3	16.7	7.8	4.6	3.1	1.8	5.9
Americas									
Argentina	1999	149	77.2	22.8	10.1	3.4	5.4	3.4	9.4
Canada	2000	119	83.2	16.8	10.9	2.5	3.4	2.5	3.4
Cuba	2000	38	84.2	15.8	7.9	5.3	2.6	5.3	2.6
Ecuador	2002	133	52.6	47.4	16.5	18.8	12.0	6.0	24.8
El Salvador	2001	100	78.0	22.0	12.0	6.0	4.0	3.0	7.0
Honduras	2002	29	58.6	41.4	27.6	6.9	6.9	6.9	6.9
Puerto Rico	2000	4	75.0	25.0	0.0	0.0	25.0	0.0	25.0
United States	2001	537	81.2	18.8	11.0	3.9	3.9	2.6	5.2
Venezuela	1998	104	69.2	30.8	11.5	7.7	11.5	5.8	13.5
**Chile	2001	291	74.9	25.1	16.0	4.3	4.7	4.3	4.8
Median		104	75.4	24.6	11.5	5.3	6.9	3.7	7.0
Eastern Mediterranean									
Egypt	2002	217	31.8	68.2	18.4	11.1	38.7	11.5	38.2
Oman	2001	12	41.7	58.3	0.0	0.0	58.3	0.0	58.3
Median		114.5	36.7	63.3	9.2	5.5	48.5	5.8	48.3

COUNTRY/SETTING	Year	No. of PATIENTS TESTED	OVERALL		RESISTANCE[a] TO:			Poly-resistance	MDR
			Susceptible	Resistant	1 Drug	2 Drugs	3+Drugs		
Europe									
Austria	2000	67	91.0	9.0	7.5	0.0	1.5	0.0	1.5
Belgium	2000	78	85.9	14.1	7.7	2.6	3.8	1.3	5.1
Bosnia and Herzegovina	2000	153	86.9	13.1	8.5	2.6	2.0	2.6	2.0
Croatia	2000	99	93.9	6.1	5.1	0.0	1.0	0.0	1.0
Czech Republic	2000	22	86.4	13.6	4.5	4.5	4.5	0.0	9.1
Denmark	2000	33	72.7	27.3	3.0	21.2	3.0	21.2	3.0
Estonia	2000	117	41.9	58.1	10.3	4.3	43.6	2.6	45.3
Finland	2000	29	86.2	13.8	10.3	3.4	0.0	0.0	3.4
France	2000	82	72.0	28.0	13.4	9.8	4.9	6.1	8.5
Germany	2000	236	81.8	18.2	6.4	5.9	6.8	5.9	5.9
Iceland	2000	1	100.0	0.0	0.0	0.0	0.0	0.0	0.0
Ireland	2000	26	92.3	7.7	3.8	3.8	0.0	0.0	3.8
Israel	2000	24	58.3	41.7	16.7	4.2	20.8	4.2	20.8
Italy	2000	108	52.8	47.2	16.7	14.8	15.7	6.5	24.1
Kazakhstan	2001	319	17.9	82.1	8.2	11.6	62.4	17.6	56.4
Latvia	2000	247	61.9	38.1	6.5	5.7	25.9	4.5	27.1
Lithuania	2002	321	32.1	67.9	8.7	6.9	52.3	5.9	53.3
Luxembourg	2000	5	100.0	0.0	0.0	0.0	0.0	0.0	0.0
Malta	2000	1	100.0	0.0	0.0	0.0	0.0	0.0	0.0
Netherlands	2000	95	91.6	8.4	4.2	2.1	2.1	3.2	1.1
Norway	2000	10	90.0	10.0	10.0	0.0	0.0	0.0	0.0
Poland	2001	668	83.4	16.6	5.7	3.9	7.0	2.4	8.5
Russian Federation - Orel Oblast	2002	210	26.7	73.3	7.1	13.3	52.9	23.8	42.4
Russian Federation - Tomsk Oblast	2002	117	39.3	60.7	6.8	12.0	41.9	10.3	43.6
Serbia and Montenegro-Belgrade	2000	30	83.3	16.7	13.3	3.3	0.0	3.3	0.0
Slovakia	2000	110	86.4	13.6	10.0	2.7	0.9	1.8	1.8
Slovenia	2000	38	89.5	10.5	7.9	0.0	2.6	2.6	0.0
Spain-Barcelona	2001	32	68.8	31.3	12.5	9.4	9.4	6.3	12.5
Spain-Galicia	2001	40	77.5	22.5	10.0	2.5	10.0	5.0	7.5
Sweden	2000	42	92.9	7.1	4.8	2.4	0.0	0.0	2.4
Switzerland	2000	57	94.7	5.3	3.5	1.8	0.0	0.0	1.8
Turkmenistan - Dashoguz	2001	98	37.8	62.2	23.5	14.3	24.5	20.4	18.4
United Kingdom - England, Wales, Northern Ireland	2000	237	84.8	15.2	8.4	3.4	3.3	2.5	4.2
Uzbekistan - Karakalpakstan	2001	107	20.6	79.4	17.8	17.8	43.9	21.5	40.2
Median		78	84.1	15.9	7.8	3.6	3.9	2.6	4.7

[a] Small differences may appear between the variable "overall resistance" and "resistance to 1 drug+2 drugs+3drugs", due to rounding.
** Not included in analysis or median calculations

ANNEXES

ANNEXES

COUNTRY/SETTING	Year	No. of PATIENTS TESTED	OVERALL		RESISTANCE[a] TO:				Poly- resistance	MDR
			Susceptible	Resistant	1 Drug	2 Drugs	3+Drugs			
South-East Asia										
Nepal	2001	171	59.1	40.9	12.9	11.7	16.4	7.6	20.5
Thailand	2001	172	61.0	39.0	11.6	9.9	17.4	7.0	20.3
Median		171.5	60.1	39.9	12.2	10.8	16.9	7.3	20.4
Western Pacific										
Cambodia	2001	96	82.3	17.7	10.4	5.2	2.1	4.2	3.1
China - Henan	2001	265	39.2	60.8	14.3	15.5	30.9	9.8	36.6
China - Hong Kong SAR	2001	169	76.9	23.1	8.9	3.6	10.7	3.0	11.2
China - Hubei	1999	238	55.5	44.5	13.4	16.4	14.7	9.2	21.8
China - Liaoning	1999	86	44.2	55.8	15.1	20.9	19.8	16.3	24.4
Japan	1997	264	57.6	42.4	15.2	10.2	17.0	7.6	19.7
New Zealand	2001	22	90.9	9.1	4.5	4.5	0.0	4.5	0.0
Singapore	2001	126	88.1	11.9	9.5	1.6	0.8	1.6	0.8
Median		147.5	67.2	32.8	11.9	7.7	12.7	6.1	15.5
Overall Median		100	81.6	18.4	8.7	4.5	4.5	3.2	7.0
Overall Minimum		1	17.9	0.0	0.0	0.0	0.0	0.0	0.0
Overall Maximum		668	100	82.1	27.6	21.2	62.4	23.8	58.3

[a] Small differences may appear between the variable "overall resistance" and "resistance to 1 drug+2 drugs+3drugs", due to rounding.
**Not included in analysis or median calculations

Annex 4: Prevalence (%) of resistance to specific drugs among previously treated TB cases, by country/geographical setting and WHO region (1999-2002)

COUNTRY/SETTING	Year	No. of PATIENTS TESTED	INH MONO	INH ANY	RMP MONO	RMP ANY	EMB MONO	EMB ANY	SM MONO	SM ANY
Africa										
Botswana	2002	66	0.0	18.2	0.0	16.7	4.5	10.6	4.5	18.2
The Gambia	1999	15	0.0	0.0	0.0	0.0	0.0	0.0	0.0	0.0
South Africa - Eastern Cape	2001	283	3.2	13.4	0.4	7.8	0.0	1.4	3.9	8.8
South Africa - Free State	2001	174	4.0	6.9	1.1	2.9	0.0	0.6	1.1	2.9
South Africa - Gauteng	2001	165	0.6	9.7	0.0	6.1	0.0	4.8	2.4	7.9
South Africa - Kwazulu-Natal	2001	207	4.3	14.5	1.0	8.7	0.5	2.4	2.4	10.6
South Africa - Limpopo	2001	88	4.5	12.5	3.4	10.2	0.0	2.3	1.1	3.4
South Africa - North West	2001	188	0.5	11.2	2.7	9.6	0.0	1.1	5.3	12.2
South Africa - Western Cape	2001	228	2.2	6.6	0.0	3.9	0.0	1.3	1.3	3.5
Zambia	2000	44	4.5	6.8	0.0	2.3	2.3	2.3	4.5	4.5
**South Africa - Mpumalanga	2001	175	2.3	18.9	2.3	16.0	0.0	9.1	2.3	14.3
Median		168.5	2.8	10.1	0.2	7.0	0.0	1.9	2.4	6.3
Americas										
Argentina	1999	149	4.0	16.1	0.0	10.1	0.7	6.7	5.4	16.1
Canada	2000	119	6.7	12.6	0.8	4.2	0.0	3.4	3.4	6.7
Cuba	2000	38	0.0	7.9	0.0	2.6	0.0	2.6	7.9	15.8
Ecuador	2002	133	3.8	33.8	9.8	35.3	0.0	5.3	3.0	18.8
El Salvador	2001	100	3.0	12.0	5.0	13.0	1.0	3.0	3.0	9.0
Honduras	2002	29	6.9	17.2	6.9	17.2	0.0	3.4	13.8	27.6
Puerto Rico	2000	4	0.0	25.0	0.0	25.0	0.0	25.0	0.0	25.0
United States of America	2001	537	6.5	14.0	1.1	6.5	0.2	3.5	3.2	8.6
Venezuela	1998	104	5.8	23.1	2.9	18.3	0.0	7.7	2.9	15.4
**Chile	2001	291	5.2	21.6	2.6	9.5	0.0	4.3	5.1	22.5
Median		104	4.5	16.4	1.1	13.0	0.0	3.5	3.2	15.8
Eastern Mediterranean										
Egypt	2002	217	2.8	46.5	6.9	50.7	0.9	30.9	7.8	53.9
Oman	2001	12	0.0	58.3	0.0	58.3	0.0	25.0	0.0	58.3
Median		114.5	1.4	52.4	3.5	54.5	0.5	27.9	3.9	56.1

**Not included in analysis or median calculations

COUNTRY/SETTING	Year	No. of PATIENTS TESTED	INH MONO	INH ANY	RMP MONO	RMP ANY	EMB MONO	EMB ANY	SM MONO	SM ANY
Europe										
Austria	2000	67	1.5	3.0	0.0	1.5	0.0	0.0	6.0	7.5
Belgium	2000	78	6.4	12.8	1.3	6.4	0.0	5.1	-	-
Bosnia and Herzegovina	2000	153	1.3	3.3	2.6	5.9	3.3	6.5	1.3	5.2
Croatia	2000	99	3.0	4.0	2.0	3.0	0.0	1.0	0.0	1.0
Czech Republic	2000	22	0.0	9.1	4.5	13.6	0.0	4.5	0.0	4.6
Denmark	2000	33	0.0	24.2	0.0	3.0	0.0	3.0	3.0	24.2
Estonia	2000	117	6.8	54.7	0.0	45.3	0.0	41.9	3.4	48.7
Finland	2000	29	10.3	13.8	0.0	3.4	0.0	0.0	0.0	0.0
France	2000	82	4.9	18.3	1.2	11.0	1.2	2.4	6.1	15.9
Germany	2000	236	4.2	15.7	0.0	6.4	0.0	4.7	2.1	12.3
Iceland	2000	1	0.0	0.0	0.0	0.0	0.0	0.0	0.0	0.0
Ireland	2000	26	0.0	3.8	0.0	3.8	0.0	0.0	3.8	3.8
Israel	2000	24	12.5	37.5	0.0	20.8	0.0	8.3	4.2	29.2
Italy	2000	108	5.6	36.1	5.6	29.6	0.9	11.1	4.6	23.1
Kazakhstan	2001	319	0.9	67.7	0.3	61.4	1.3	54.2	5.6	77.1
Latvia	2000	247	3.6	35.2	0.0	27.1	0.0	15.0	2.8	32.8
Lithuania	2002	321	6.2	65.4	0.0	53.3	0.0	38.0	2.5	58.6
Luxembourg	2000	5	0.0	0.0	0.0	0.0	0.0	0.0	0.0	0.0
Malta	2000	1	0.0	0.0	0.0	0.0	0.0	0.0	0.0	0.0
Netherlands	2000	95	4.2	9.8	0.0	1.1	0.0	2.1	0.0	4.2
Norway	2000	10	.00	0.0	0.0	0.0	0.0	0.0	10.0	10.0
Poland	2001	668	3.4	14.4	0.4	9.0	0.0	3.3	1.8	10.0
Russian Federation - Orel Oblast	2002	210	4.8	71.0	0.0	42.4	0.5	43.8	1.9	66.2
Russian Federation - Tomsk Oblast	2002	117	0.0	51.3	1.7	47.9	5.1	13.7	5.1	57.3
Serbia and Montenegro–Belgrade	2000	30	6.7	10.0	0.0	0.0	6.7	6.7	0.0	3.3
Slovakia	2000	110	7.3	10.9	0.0	1.8	0.0	0.9	2.7	5.5
Slovenia	2000	38	5.3	7.9	0.0	0.0	0.0	2.6	2.6	5.3
Spain–Barcelona	2001	32	9.4	28.1	0.0	12.5	0.0	9.4	3.1	18.8
Spain–Galicia	2001	40	5.0	17.5	0.0	7.5	0.0	7.5	5.0	17.5
Sweden	2000	42	2.4	4.8	0.0	2.4	0.0	0.0	2.4	2.4
Switzerland	2000	57	1.8	3.5	1.8	3.5	0.0	0.0	-	-
Turkmenistan – Dashoguz	2001	98	9.2	48.0	1.0	19.4	0.0	15.3	13.3	51.0
United Kingdom - England, Wales, Northern Ireland	2000	237	3.8	10.5	1.3	5.5	0.0	2.1	-	-
Uzbekistan - Karakalpakstan	2001	107	7.5	69.2	0.0	40.2	0.0	34.6	10.3	71.0
Median		78	4.0	13.3	0.0	6.1	0.0	3.9	2.8	10.0

COUNTRY/SETTING	Year	No. of PATIENTS TESTED	INH		RMP		EMB		SM	
			MONO	ANY	MONO	ANY	MONO	ANY	MONO	ANY
South-East Asia										
Nepal	2001	171	5.3	33.3	0.0	20.5	0.0	9.9	7.6	31.0
Thailand	2001	172	4.1	30.8	1.7	22.7	0.6	15.1	5.2	24.4
Median		171.5	4.7	32.1	0.9	21.6	0.3	12.5	6.4	27.7
Western Pacific										
Cambodia	2001	96	9.4	16.7	0.0	3.1	0.0	0.0	1.0	7.3
China - Henan	2001	265	4.2	47.2	3.0	42.6	1.5	18.1	5.7	43.0
China - Hong Kong SAR	2001	169	4.7	18.9	0.0	11.2	0.0	5.9	4.1	17.8
China - Hubei	1999	238	5.5	33.2	1.7	26.9	0.0	8.8	6.3	25.6
China - Liaoning	1999	86	2.3	41.9	3.5	29.1	0.0	14.0	9.3	41.9
Japan	1997	264	6.8	33.0	0.8	21.6	0.0	15.2	7.6	24.2
New Zealand	2001	22	0.0	4.5	0.0	0.0	0.0	0.0	4.5	9.1
Singapore	2001	126	4.0	6.3	1.6	2.4	0.0	0.8	4.0	5.6
Median		147.5	4.4	25.9	1.2	16.4	0.0	7.4	5.1	21.0
Overall Median		100	4.0	14.4	0.0	8.7	0.0	3.5	3.2	11.4
Overall Minimum		1	0.0	0.0	0.0	0.0	0.0	0.0	0.0	0.0
Overall Maximum		668	12.5	71.0	9.8	61.4	6.7	54.2	13.8	77.1

ANNEXES

**Not included in analysis or median calculations

Annex 5: Prevalence (%) of resistance to specific drugs among previously treated TB cases, by country/geographical setting and WHO region (1999-2002)

COUNTRY/SETTING	Year	No. of PATIENTS TESTED	OVERALL		RESISTANCE[a] TO:				MDR
			Susceptible	Resistant	1 Drug	2 Drugs	3+Drugs	Poly-resistance	
Africa									
Botswana	2002	*	84.5	15.5	9.0	4.5	2.1	3.9	2.7
The Gambia	1999	*	95.9	4.1	3.7	0.5	0.0	0.0	0.5
Democratic Republic of Congo - Kinshasa	1999	710	61.0	39.0	18.5	11.7	8.9	14.8	5.8
South Africa - Eastern Cape	2002	*	86.6	13.4	7.7	4.3	1.3	2.5	3.1
South Africa - Free State	2001	*	91.3	8.7	5.7	1.7	1.3	1.3	1.8
South Africa - Gauteng	2001	*	92.4	7.6	3.9	2.2	1.5	1.7	2.0
South Africa - Kwazulu-Natal	2001	*	90.3	8.7	4.5	1.6	2.6	1.4	2.8
South Africa - Limpopo	2001	*	91.0	9.0	4.1	2.8	2.1	1.7	3.3
South Africa - North West	2001	*	89.1	9.9	5.1	2.7	2.0	1.8	3.0
South Africa - Western Cape	2001	*	93.6	6.4	3.2	2.3	0.9	1.2	1.9
Zambia	2000	*	88.1	11.9	9.1	2.0	0.8	1.0	1.8
**South Africa-Mpumalanga	2001	*	88.8	11.2	5.7	2.5	2.9	1.5	4.0
Median			91.0	9.0	5.1	2.3	1.4	1.7	2.7
Americas									
Argentina	1999	*	87.6	12.4	8.0	1.6	2.8	1.3	3.1
Canada	2000	1363	90.8	9.2	6.3	1.9	1.0	1.9	1.0
Cuba	2000	*	93.9	6.1	4.1	1.7	0.2	1.5	0.5
Ecuador	2002	*	73.8	26.2	13.4	9.6	3.3	4.1	8.7
El Salvador	2001	*	93.0	7.0	5.5	1.2	0.3	0.7	1.8
Honduras	2002	*	82.0	18.0	11.8	4.8	1.4	4.2	2.0
Puerto Rico	2000	139	91.4	8.6	7.2	0.7	0.7	0.7	0.7
United States	2001	10288	87.0	13.0	8.9	2.8	1.2	2.7	1.4
Venezuela	1998	*	90.4	9.6	5.5	2.7	1.4	2.4	1.7
**Chile	2001	*	86.3	13.7	9.4	2.9	1.4	2.9	1.4
Median			90.4	9.6	7.2	1.9	1.2	1.9	1.4
Eastern Mediterranean									
Egypt	2002	*	63.9	36.1	21.2	7.2	7.8	7.4	7.5
Oman	2001	183	91.3	8.7	4.4	0.5	3.8	0.5	3.8
Median			77.5	24.4	12.8	3.9	5.8	3.9	5.8

COUNTRY/SETTING	Year	No. of PATIENTS TESTED	OVERALL		RESISTANCE[a] TO:			Poly-resistance	MDR
			Susceptible	Resistant	1 Drug	2 Drugs	3+Drugs		
Europe									
Andorra	2000	3	100.0	0.0	0.0	0.0	0.0	0.0	0.0
Austria	2000	761	95.1	4.9	3.4	0.9	0.5	0.9	0.5
Belgium	2000	730	92.9	7.1	4.9	1.5	0.7	0.7	1.5
Bosnia and Herzegovina	2000	1153	96.0	4.0	2.9	0.7	0.3	0.6	0.4
Croatia	2000	879	97.7	2.3	1.9	0.2	0.1	0.1	0.2
Czech Republic	2000	584	95.3	5.0	2.7	1.4	0.9	0.7	1.5
Denmark	2000	425	86.8	13.2	6.8	5.9	0.5	5.9	0.5
Estonia	2000	527	64.9	35.1	10.6	4.4	20.1	4.9	19.5
Finland	2000	437	95.0	5.0	3.7	1.1	0.2	0.9	0.5
France	2000	1191	89.1	10.9	8.1	2.1	0.8	1.6	1.3
Germany	2000	2486	91.3	8.7	4.9	2.3	2.3	2.2	1.6
Iceland	2000	9	100.0	0.0	0.0	0.0	0.0	0.0	0.0
Ireland	2000	216	96.8	3.2	1.9	1.4	0.0	0.0	1.4
Israel	2000	281	68.0	32.0	12.5	4.6	14.9	5.0	14.6
Italy	2000	*	85.3	14.7	7.9	4.4	2.4	3.5	3.3
Kazakhstan	2001	*	36.7	63.3	12.5	16.3	34.5	26.1	24.7
Latvia	2000	1144	67.0	33.0	8.7	10.8	13.6	11.3	13.1
Lithuania	2002	1140	59.9	40.1	9.9	8.4	27.6	9.3	27.8
Luxembourg	2000	44	93.2	6.8	6.8	0.0	0.0	0.0	0.0
Malta	2000	10	100.0	0.0	0.0	0.0	0.0	0.0	0.0
Netherlands	2000	842	89.4	10.6	7.8	2.1	0.6	2.3	0.5
Norway	2000	170	76.5	23.5	14.7	8.8	0.0	7.1	1.8
Poland	2001	3705	92.0	8.0	4.3	1.8	1.9	1.2	2.5
Russian Federation - Orel Oblast	2002	589	60.3	39.7	5.9	11.0	22.8	17.0	16.8
Russian Federation - Tomsk Oblast	2002	650	58.5	41.5	9.8	13.1	18.6	12.6	19.1
Serbia and Montenegro-Belgrade	2000	279	93.2	6.8	5.7	0.7	0.4	0.7	0.4
Slovakia	2000	575	94.1	5.9	3.8	1.6	0.5	0.9	1.2
Slovenia	2000	320	96.6	3.4	2.5	0.6	0.3	0.9	0.0
Spain - Barcelona	2001	*	87.1	12.9	8.1	2.1	1.8	2.7	2.1
Spain - Galicia	2001	*	87.3	12.7	9.8	0.8	2.4	1.0	2.0
Sweden	2000	365	89.3	10.7	7.4	2.7	0.5	1.9	1.4
Switzerland	2000	492	94.9	5.1	4.7	0.4	0.0	0.0	0.4
Turkmenistan - Dashoguz	2001	*	52.5	47.5	22.3	9.9	15.3	13.6	11.6
United Kingdom - England, Wales, Northern Ireland	2000	3004	91.0	9.0	6.5	1.4	1.0	1.2	1.2

*Combined estimates were calculated through a direct standardization method
**Not included in analysis or median calculations

ANNEXES

COUNTRY/SETTING	Year	No. of PATIENTS TESTED	OVERALL		RESISTANCE[a] TO:			Poly-resistance	MDR
			Susceptible	Resistant	1 Drug	2 Drugs	3+Drugs		
United Kingdom - Scotland	2000	302	96.0	4.0	4.0	0.0	0.0	0.0	0.0
Uzbekistan - Karakalpakstan	2001	*	36.1	63.9	16.4	15.5	31.9	20.7	26.8
Median			91.2	8.8	6.2	1.7	0.6	1.2	1.3
South-East Asia									
Nepal	2001	*	84.3	15.7	7.9	4.2	3.5	3.4	4.3
Thailand	2001	*	82.7	17.3	10.6	4.1	2.6	3.8	2.9
Median			83.5	16.5	9.3	4.2	3.1	3.6	3.6
Western Pacific									
Australia	2000	766	89.7	10.3	7.7	2.1	0.5	1.6	1.0
Cambodia	2001	*	89.3	10.7	8.6	2.1	0.1	2.0	0.2
China - Hubei	1999	*	75.8	24.2	11.6	7.9	4.7	5.6	7.0
China - Liaoning	1999	*	56.4	44.6	21.4	12.5	11.6	11.2	13.0
China - Henan	2001	*	67.7	32.3	15.5	7.9	8.9	6.7	10.1
China - Hong Kong SAR	2001	3639	89.2	10.8	7.1	2.5	1.3	2.5	1.3
Japan	1997	*	87.9	12.1	7.0	2.6	2.5	2.7	2.0
New Zealand	2001	294	88.8	11.2	8.8	2.4	0.0	2.4	0.0
Singapore	2001	949	94.1	5.9	4.0	1.3	0.6	1.4	0.5
Median			88.8	11.1	8.8	2.7	1.3	2.4	1.6
Overall Median		NA	89.6	10.4	6.9	2.3	1.3	1.8	1.7
Overall Minimum		NA	31.1	0.0	0.0	0.0	0.0	0.0	0.0
Overall Maximum		NA	100.0	63.9	22.4	15.5	42.8	23.6	26.8

*Combined estimates were calculated through a direct standardization method
**Not included in analysis or median calculations

Annex 6: Prevalence (%) of resistance to specific drugs among combined TB cases, by country/geographical setting and WHO region (1999-2002)

COUNTRY/SETTING	Year	No. of PATIENTS TESTED	INH MONO	INH ANY	RMP MONO	RMP ANY	EMB MONO	EMB ANY	SM MONO	SM ANY
Africa										
Botswana	2002	*	1.7	6.6	1.1	4.7	0.9	2.7	5.2	10.2
The Gambia	1999	*	1.8	2.3	0.5	0.9	0.0	0.0	1.4	1.4
Democratic Republic of Congo – Kinshasa	1999	710	4.4	23.0	0.1	6.2	5.1	15.4	8.9	28.2
South Africa - Eastern Cape	2001	*	3.6	9.2	0.2	3.4	0.0	0.9	3.9	7.4
South Africa - Free State	2001	*	3.5	6.5	0.8	2.5	0.0	0.6	1.5	3.7
South Africa - Gauteng	2001	*	1.7	5.3	0.3	2.4	0.0	1.1	2.0	4.5
South Africa - Kwazulu-Natal	2001	*	2.9	7.0	0.3	3.1	0.1	1.1	1.3	5.1
South Africa - Limpopo	2001	*	1.9	6.9	0.6	3.9	0.0	2.2	1.5	3.9
South Africa - North West	2001	*	1.9	6.8	1.8	3.8	0.0	1.2	2.3	5.7
South Africa - Western Cape	2001	*	2.4	5.6	0.0	1.9	0.0	0.4	0.7	2.7
Zambia	2000	*	3.5	6.3	0.0	1.8	0.8	2.0	4.5	5.3
**South Africa - Mpumalanga	2001	*	3.0	8.5	0.8	4.8	0.0	2.0	1.9	5.4
Median			2.4	6.6	0.5	3.4	0.0	1.2	2.0	5.3
Americas										
Argentina	1999	*	1.8	6.0	0.1	3.4	1.0	3.1	5.1	8.9
Canada	2000	1363	4.5	7.3	0.1	1.2	0.2	1.2	1.5	3.7
Cuba	2000	*	0.2	1.7	0.0	1.0	0.0	0.2	3.9	5.5
Ecuador	2002	*	4.7	16.3	3.2	13.1	0.2	1.3	5.3	11.8
El Salvador	2001	*	0.7	2.1	1.1	2.1	0.4	0.5	3.3	4.2
Honduras	2002	*	1.4	6.9	1.2	2.9	0.0	1.3	10.2	15.2
Puerto Rico	2000	139	2.9	4.3	0.7	1.4	0.7	1.4	2.9	4.3
United States	2001	10288	4.1	8.0	0.3	1.7	0.4	1.7	4.1	7.4
Venezuela	1998	*	2.1	5.6	0.6	2.6	0.1	1.6	2.7	5.6
**Chile	2001	*	2.1	7.5	0.5	2.2	0.0	0.9	6.8	11.9
Median			2.0	6.5	0.2	2.4	0.2	1.3	4.0	6.5
Eastern Mediterranean										
Egypt	2002	*	2.7	15.2	4.0	13.4	0.5	7.0	14.0	28.1
Oman	2001	183	3.3	7.7	0.5	4.4	0.0	1.6	0.5	4.9
Median			3.0	11.6	2.3	8.9	0.3	4.3	7.3	16.5

*Combined estimates were calculated through a direct standardization method
**Not included in analysis or median calculations

ANNEXES

COUNTRY/SETTING	Year	No. of PATIENTS TESTED	INH		RMP		EMB		SM	
			MONO	ANY	MONO	ANY	MONO	ANY	MONO	ANY
Europe										
Andorra	2000	3	0.0	0.0	0.0	0.0	0.0	0.0	0.0	0.0
Austria	2000	761	1.4	2.9	0.3	0.8	0.1	0.1	1.6	3.0
Belgium	2000	730	4.2	6.4	0.4	1.9	0.3	1.6	-	-
Bosnia and Herzegovina	2000	1153	0.4	1.0	0.9	1.5	1.2	1.8	0.4	1.3
Croatia	2000	879	1.0	1.4	0.2	0.5	0.0	0.1	0.7	.9
Czech Republic	2000	584	1.5	3.8	0.2	1.7	0.2	1.0	0.9	2.2
Denmark	2000	425	2.6	8.7	0.0	0.7	0.0	0.9	4.2	9.9
Estonia	2000	527	5.5	30.0	0.0	19.5	0.0	19.5	5.1	28.3
Finland	2000	437	2.1	3.4	0.5	0.9	0.0	0.2	1.1	2.1
France	2000	1191	1.0	3.8	0.2	1.5	0.8	1.9	6.0	7.4
Germany	2000	2486	2.3	6.1	0.2	1.8	0.2	1.4	2.2	5.5
Iceland	2000	9	0.0	0.0	0.0	0.0	0.0	0.0	0.0	0.0
Ireland	2000	216	1.4	2.8	0.0	1.4	0.0	0.0	0.5	0.5
Israel	2000	281	6.8	26.3	0.4	14.9	1.4	10.0	3.9	22.4
Italy	2000	*	2.4	9.2	0.9	4.3	0.6	2.4	4.0	9.3
Kazakhstan	2001	*	2.5	58.8	0.3	27.0	0.9	32.1	8.7	57.9
Latvia	2000	1144	5.9	30.3	0.0	13.1	0.2	8.1	2.5	26.2
Lithuania	2002	1140	6.5	36.7	0.3	22.0	0.0	16.0	3.2	32.1
Luxembourg	2000	44	4.5	4.5	0.0	0.0	0.0	0.0	2.3	2.3
Malta	2000	10	0.0	0.0	0.0	0.0	0.0	0.0	0.0	0.0
Netherlands	2000	842	3.1	5.8	0.1	0.6	0.1	0.8	4.5	6.9
Norway	2000	170	4.1	12.4	0.0	2.4	4.7	6.5	5.9	11.2
Poland	2001	3705	2.3	6.0	0.3	2.8	0.0	1.1	1.7	4.6
Russian Federation - Orel Oblast	2002	589	3.1	36.8	0.0	16.8	0.2	18.7	2.7	35.8
Russian Federation - Tomsk Oblast	2002	650	2.0	33.1	0.6	20.3	0.0	6.0	7.2	38.3
Serbia and Montenegro- Belgrade	2000	279	1.8	2.5	1.4	1.8	1.1	1.4	1.4	2.5
Slovakia	2000	575	2.8	4.7	0.2	1.6	0.3	0.3	0.9	2.1
Slovenia	2000	320	1.9	2.8	0.0	0.0	0.0	0.3	0.6	1.6
Spain - Barcelona	2001	*	4.4	8.5	0.0	2.8	0.0	1.1	3.7	8.1
Spain - Galicia	2001	*	2.8	5.8	0.0	2.0	0.5	2.8	6.5	8.3
Sweden	2000	365	6.8	10.1	0.0	1.4	0.0	0.5	0.5	2.5
Switzerland	2000	492	4.5	4.9	0.2	0.6	0.0	0.0	-	-
Turkmenistan – Dashoguz	2001	*	7.6	32.8	0.5	12.2	0.0	9.1	14.2	38.9
United Kingdom - Scotland	2000	302	3.6	3.6	0.0	0.0	0.0	0.0	0.3	0.3

COUNTRY/SETTING	Year	No. of PATIENTS TESTED	INH		RMP		EMB		SM	
			MONO	ANY	MONO	ANY	MONO	ANY	MONO	ANY
United Kingdom - England, Wales, Northern Ireland	2000	3004	4.0	6.4	0.4	1.6	0.0	0.6	-	-
Uzbekistan - Karakalpakstan	2001	*	5.6	53.1	0.0	26.8	0.0	24.9	10.8	57.8
Median			2.7	6.0	0.2	1.6	0.0	1.1	2.3	5.0
South-East Asia										
Nepal	2001	*	2.2	9.8	0.2	4.7	0.0	2.3	5.5	12.4
Thailand	2001	*	5.2	11.7	0.5	3.6	0.1	2.6	4.8	9.9
Median			3.7	10.8	0.4	4.2	0.1	2.5	5.2	11.2
Western Pacific										
Australia	2000	766	7.4	10.1	0.3	1.3	0.0	0.9	0.0	1.2
Cambodia	2001	*	5.0	7.0	0.4	0.8	0.0	0.1	3.2	5.1
China - Hubei	1999	*	4.2	15.5	1.3	9.6	0.1	2.6	6.0	14.9
China - Liaoning	1999	*	4.8	28.3	0.1	14.6	0.2	5.7	14.4	35.5
China - Henan	2001	*	3.3	19.4	1.6	12.3	0.9	5.4	9.7	23.8
China - Hong Kong	2001	3639	2.4	6.1	0.2	1.4	0.0	0.8	4.5	8.0
Japan	1997	*	2.3	6.0	0.1	2.6	0.1	1.3	5.6	8.5
New Zealand	2001	294	4.1	6.1	0.0	0.3	0.3	0.7	4.4	6.5
Singapore	2001	949	1.9	3.7	0.2	0.8	0.1	0.7	1.8	3.4
Median			4.1	8.6	0.3	1.7	0.1	0.8	4.5	8.0
Overall Median		NA	2.7	6.6	0.2	2.2	0.1	1.3	3.1	5.8
Overall Minimum		NA	0.0	0.0	0.0	0.0	0.0	0.0	0.0	0.0
Overall Maximum		NA	7.7	58.8	4.4	27.0	5.1	32.1	14.9	57.9

*Combined estimates were calculated through a direct standardization method

**Not included in analysis or median calculations

ANNEXES

Annex 7: Trends of resistance (%) against any TB drug among new TB cases in 26 countries/settings (1994–2002)

Country/Setting	Years of observation									P-Value
	1994	1995	1996	1997	1998	1999	2000	2001	2002	
Botswana	.	3.7	.	.	.	6.3	.	.	10.4	<0.0001
Canada	.	.	.	9.8	9.4	9.5	8.5	.	.	ns
China, Hong Kong SAR	.	.	12.2	11.8	12.0	12.8	11.5	10.2	.	0.023
Cuba	.	8.3	.	.	4.6	.	5.0	.	.	0.017
Czech Republic	.	2.0	.	.	.	2.7	4.4	.	.	ns
Denmark	.	.	.	.	13.1	15.3	12.0	.	.	ns
Estonia	28.2	.	.	.	36.9	33.4	28.5	.	.	ns
Finland	.	.	.	4.9	.	2.2	4.5	.	.	ns
France	.	8.2	.	9.3	.	9.2	9.3	.	.	ns
Germany	.	.	.	5.8	9.0	6.8	6.8	.	.	ns
Lithuania	.	.	.	.	.	28.1	27.7	.	29.2	ns
Latvia	.	.	34.0	.	29.9	30.8	31.7	.	.	ns
Nepal	.	.	9.8	.	.	13.3	.	11.0	.	ns
Netherlands	.	.	10.3	.	.	8.8	10.7	.	.	ns
New Zealand	.	5.6	4.4	13.0	12.9	8.3	13.4	11.4	.	0.015
Norway	.	.	10.9	.	.	16.0	24.4	.	.	0.006
Oman	.	.	.	.	4.5	.	8.7	5.3	.	ns
Puerto Rico	10.0	.	.	11.3	9.5	7.2	8.1	12.0	.	ns
Russian Fed., Tomsk Oblast	.	.	.	.	29.0	.	35.3	36.8	37.3	0.005
Slovakia	.	.	.	.	2.7	2.9	4.1	.	.	ns
Slovenia	.	.	.	2.4	.	3.0	2.5	.	.	ns
Spain, Barcelona	.	9.6	.	3.5	.	6.3	8.9	10.5	.	ns
Sweden	.	.	.	7.9	.	11.7	11.2	.	.	ns
Switzerland	.	.	.	3.1	.	6.1	5.5	.	.	ns
United Kingdom - England, Wales, Northern Ireland[a]	.	6.8	.	7.1	.	8.7	8.4	.	.	----
United States	.	12.3	.	12.0	12.3	11.6	12.7	12.7	.	ns

[a] Data from England, Wales and Northern Ireland reported before 1999 cannot be compared with data reported after 1999, because of changes in surveillance methodologies.

ANNEXES

Annex 8: Trends of MDR (%) among new TB cases in 26 countries/ settings (1994-2002)

Country/Setting	Years of observation									P-Value
	1994	1995	1996	1997	1998	1999	2000	2001	2002	
Botswana	.	0.2	.	.	.	0.5	.	.	0.8	ns
Canada	.	.	.	0.8	0.6	0.6	0.7	.	.	ns
China, Hong Kong SAR	.	.	1.4	1.1	1.3	1.0	1.1	0.8	.	0.01
Cuba	.	0.7	.	.	0.0	.	0.3	.	.	-
Czech Republic	.	1.0	.	.	.	0.3	1.1	.	.	ns
Denmark	.	.	.	.	0.5	0.0	0.3	.	.	-
Estonia	10.2	.	.	.	14.1	17.5	12.2	.	.	ns
Finland	.	.	.	0.0	.	0.0	0.3	.	.	-
France	.	0.5	.	0.0	.	.	0.8	.	.	-
Germany	.	.	.	0.5	1.0	0.8	0.8	.	.	ns
Latvia	.	.	14.4	.	9.0	10.4	9.3	.	.	0.032
Lithuania	.	.	.	.	.	7.8	8.7	.	9.4	ns
Nepal	.	.	1.1	.	.	3.7	.	1.3	.	ns
Netherlands	.	.	0.6	.	.	0.4	0.9	.	.	ns
New Zealand	.	1.4	0.0	0.8	1.3	0.9	0.4	0.0	.	-
Norway	.	.	2.2	.	.	2.1	1.9	.	.	ns
Oman	.	.	.	.	0.8	.	3.5	0.0	.	-
Puerto Rico	1.9	.	.	2.5	1.6	0.0	0.0	2.0	.	-
Russian Fed., Tomsk Oblast	.	.	.	.	6.5	.	8.6	10.7	13.7	0.0001
Spain, Barcelona	.	0.5	.	0.3	.	0.0	2.2	0.8	.	-
Slovakia	.	.	.	.	0.3	0.7	1.1	.	.	ns
Slovenia	.	.	.	0.7	.	0.0	0.0	.	.	-
Sweden	.	.	.	0.6	.	0.8	1.2	.	.	ns
Switzerland	.	.	.	0.0	.	0.7	0.0	.	.	-
United Kingdom - England, Wales, Northern Ireland[a]	.	1.1	.	0.8	.	0.5	0.9	.	.	----
United States	.	1.6	.	1.2	1.1	1.1	1.2	1.1	.	0.0002

[a] Data from England, Wales and Northern Ireland reported before 1999 cannot be compared with data reported after 1999, because of changes in surveillance methodologies.

Annex 9: Trends of any INH resistance (%) among new TB cases in 26 countries/settings (1994-2002)

Country/Setting	Years of observation									P-Value
	1994	1995	1996	1997	1998	1999	2000	2001	2002	
Botswana	.	1.5	.	.	.	4.4	.	.	4.5	0.012
Canada	.	.	.	7.2	7.2	7.7	6.8	.	.	ns
China, Hong Kong SAR	.	.	6.1	5.8	6.9	5.9	6.2	5.5	.	ns
Cuba	.	2.0	.	.	0.7	.	1.1	.	.	ns
Czech Republic	.	2.0	.	.	.	1.6	3.4	.	.	ns
Denmark	.	.	.	.	6.1	7.4	7.4	.	.	ns
Estonia	21.1	.	.	.	26.0	27.3	22.9	.	.	ns
Finland	.	.	.	4.6	.	0.5	2.7	.	.	0.02
France	.	3.4	.	3.6	.	3.4	2.5	.	.	ns
Germany	.	.	.	4.0	5.5	4.2	3.9	.	.	ns
Latvia	.	.	31.7	.	28.1	27.8	29.0	.	.	ns
Lithuania	.	.	.	.	.	21.7	21.8	.	25.4	ns
Nepal	.	.	5.6	.	.	7.6	.	5.4	.	ns
Netherlands	.	.	6.2	.	.	5.8	5.6	.	.	ns
New Zealand	.	4.2	4.4	10.6	11.6	5.7	8.7	6.3	.	ns
Norway	.	.	8.0	.	.	7.6	13.1	.	.	ns
Oman	.	.	.	.	3.0	.	5.8	4.1	.	ns
Puerto Rico	6.8	.	.	6.9	8.7	1.2	3.7	8.0	.	ns
Russian Fed., Tomsk Oblast	.	.	.	.	19.4	.	24.4	28.2	29.1	0.0002
Slovakia	.	.	.	.	2.0	1.8	3.2	.	.	ns
Slovenia	.	.	.	1.0	.	2.3	2.1	.	.	ns
Spain, Barcelona	.	3.2	.	2.2	.	3.9	5.9	.	.	ns
Sweden	.	.	.	5.6	.	9.3	10.9	.	.	0.02
Switzerland	.	.	.	2.8	.	5.6	5.5	.	.	ns
United Kingdom - England, Wales, Northern Ireland[a]	.	5.5	.	5.0	.	6.2	6.0	.	.	---
United States	.	7.8	.	8.0	8.3	7.6	8.1	7.7	.	ns

[a] Data from England, Wales and Northern Ireland reported before 1999 cannot be compared with data reported after 1999, because of changes in surveillance methodologies.

ANNEXES

Annex 10: Trends of any rifampicin resistance (%) among new TB cases in 26 countries/settings (1994-2002)

Country/Setting	Years of observation									P-Value
	1994	1995	1996	1997	1998	1999	2000	2001	2002	
Botswana	.	1.0	.	.	.	0.6	.	.	2.0	ns
Canada	.	.	.	0.9	0.6	0.8	0.8	.	.	ns
China, Hong Kong SAR	.	.	1.6	1.4	1.4	1.3	1.2	1.0	.	0.01
Cuba	.	0.9	.	.	0.0	.	0.8	.	.	-
Czech Republic	.	1.0	.	.	.	0.8	1.1	.	.	ns
Denmark	.	.	.	.	0.5	0.3	0.5	.	.	ns
Estonia	10.2	.	.	.	14.3	17.8	12.2	.	.	ns
Finland	.	.	.	0.0	.	0.0	0.8	.	.	-
France	.	0.7	.	0.3	.	0.8	0.8	.	.	ns
Germany	.	.	.	0.8	1.7	1.1	1.0	.	.	ns
Latvia	.	.	14.7	.	9.0	10.4	9.3	.	.	0.02
Lithuania	.	.	.	.	.	10.1	9.6	.	9.8	ns
Nepal	.	.	1.7	.	.	3.7	.	1.7	.	ns
Netherlands	.	.	1.1	.	.	0.8	0.9	.	.	ns
New Zealand	.	1.4	0.0	0.8	1.3	1.3	0.4	0.4	.	-
Norway	.	.	2.2	.	.	2.1	2.5	.	.	ns
Oman	.	.	.	.	1.5	.	3.5	0.6	.	ns
Puerto Rico	2.7	.	.	3.1	1.6	0.6	0.7	3.0	.	ns
Russian Fed., Tomsk Oblast	.	.	.	.	7.9	.	10.3	11.8	14.3	0.001
Slovakia	.	.	.	.	0.3	1.1	1.5	.	.	0.04
Slovenia	.	.	.	0.7	.	0.0	0.0	.	.	-
Spain, Barcelona	.	0.9	.	0.3	.	0.8	2.2	1.5	.	ns
Sweden	.	.	.	0.6	.	1.3	1.2	.	.	ns
Switzerland	.	.	.	0.0	.	0.9	0.0	.	.	-
United Kingdom - England, Wales, Northern Ireland[a]	.	1.2	.	0.8	.	0.5	1.2	.	.	---
United States	.	2.4	.	1.7	1.5	1.3	1.5	1.5	.	0.0001

ANNEXES

[a] Data from England, Wales and Northern Ireland reported before 1999 cannot be compared with data reported after 1999, because of changes in surveillance methodologies.

Annex 11: Trends of resistance (%) to any TB drug among previously treated TB cases in 24 countries/settings (1994-2002)

Country/Setting	Years of observation									P-Value
	1994	1995	1996	1997	1998	1999	2000	2001	2002	
Botswana	.	14.9	.	.	.	22.8	.	.	21.7	ns
Canada	.	.	.	16.0	11.1	13.7	16.8	.	.	ns
China, Hong Kong SAR	.	.	26.9	27.1	25.6	26.4	23.7	23.1	.	ns
Cuba	.	91.3	.	.	32.6	.	15.8	.	.	0.0001
Czech Republic	.	12.5	.	.	.	8.6	13.6	.	.	ns
Denmark	.	.	.	.	12.5	16.7	27.3	.	.	ns
Estonia	46.2	.	.	.	59.8	55.1	58.1	.	.	ns
Finland	.	.	.	0.0	.	3.7	13.8	.	.	-
France	.	21.5	.	20.0	.	16.0	28.0	.	.	ns
Germany	.	.	.	21.0	19.8	19.8	18.2	.	.	ns
Latvia	.	.	73.7	.	30.8	33.7	38.1	.	.	<0.0001
Lithuania	.	.	.	.	.	61.7	61.8	.	67.9	ns
Netherlands	.	.	15.7	.	.	9.5	8.4	.	.	ns
New Zealand	.	0.0	6.7	21.4	27.3	17.4	29.4	9.1	.	-
Norway	.	.	16.7	.	.	2.5	10.0	.	.	ns
Puerto Rico	27.3	.	.	58.3	7.1	14.3	25.0	.	.	ns
Russian Fed. Tomsk Oblast	.	.	.	.	57.8	.	62.0	67.6	60.7	ns
Slovakia	.	.	.	.	15.9	6.6	13.6	.	.	ns
Slovenia	.	.	.	8.3	.	5.7	10.5	.	.	ns
Spain-Barcelona	.	29.5	.	23.2	.	34.1	22.2	31.3	.	ns
Sweden	.	.	.	16.7	.	25.8	7.1	.	.	ns
Switzerland	.	.	.	27.5	.	21.1	5.3	.	.	0.006
United Kingdom - England, Wales, Northern Ireland[a]	.	32.4	.	22.2	.	5.9	15.2	.	.	---
United States	.	23.6	.	20.9	17.0	17.7	18.2	18.8	.	<0.0001

[a] Data from England, Wales and Northern Ireland reported before 1999 cannot be compared with data reported after 1999, because of changes in surveillance methodologies.

Annex 12: MDR trends among previously treated TB cases in 24 countries/settings (1994-2002)

Country/Setting	Years of observation									P-Value
	1994	1995	1996	1997	1998	1999	2000	2001	2002	
Botswana	.	6.1	.	.	.	9.0	.	.	10.4	ns
Canada	.	.	.	3.2	3.7	3.2	3.4	.	.	ns
China, Hong Kong SAR	.	.	9.6	7.6	11.3	7.7	9.2	11.2	.	ns
Cuba	.	13.0	.	.	7.0	.	2.6	.	.	ns
Czech Republic	.	6.3	.	.	.	2.9	9.1	.	.	ns
Denmark	.	.	.	.	3.1	0.0	3.0	.	.	-
Estonia	19.2	.	.	.	37.8	48.3	45.3	.	.	<0.0001
Finland	.	.	.	0.0	.	0.0	3.4	.	.	-
France	.	4.1	.	3.1	.	8.5	8.5	.	.	ns
Germany	.	.	.	9.6	7.2	6.9	5.9	.	.	ns
Latvia	.	.	54.4	.	23.7	26.8	27.1	.	.	<0.0001
Lithuania	.	.	.	.	.	42.5	43.2	.	53.3	0.007
Netherlands	.	.	0.6	.	.	0.0	1.1	.	.	-
New Zealand	.	0.0	0.0	0.0	9.1	0.0	0.0	0.0	.	-
Norway	.	16.7	.	.	.	0.0	0.0	.	.	ns
Puerto Rico	13.6	.	.	16.7	0.0	14.3	25.0	.	.	-
Russian Fed. Tomsk Oblast	.	.	.	.	26.7	.	32.2	42.4	43.6	0.0002
Slovakia	.	.	.	.	8.3	2.5	1.8	.	.	0.009
Slovenia	.	.	.	2.8	.	5.7	0.0	.	.	-
Spain-Barcelona	.	20.5	.	11.6	.	20.5	11.1	12.5	.	ns
Sweden	.	.	.	8.3	.	12.9	2.4	.	.	ns
Switzerland	.	.	.	12.5	.	10.5	1.8	.	.	ns
United Kingdom - England, Wales, Northern Ireland[a]	.	16.9	.	13.2	.	2.7	4.2	.	.	---
United States	.	7.1	.	5.6	3.4	4.0	3.9	5.2	.	0.01

ANNEXES

[a] Data from England, Wales and Northern Ireland reported before 1999 cannot be compared with data reported after 1999, because of changes in surveillance methodologies.

Annex 13: Trends of RMP resistance among previously treated TB cases in 24 countries/settings (1994-2002)

Country/Setting	Years of observation									P-Value
	1994	1995	1996	1997	1998	1999	2000	2001	2002	
Botswana	.	7.9	.	.	.	13.1	.	.	12.3	ns
Canada	.	.	.	3.2	3.7	3.2	4.2	.	.	ns
China, Hong Kong SAR	.	.	11.6	9.2	12.8	7.7	9.2	11.2	.	ns
Cuba	.	17.4	.	.	7.0	.	2.6	.	.	0.03
Czech Republic	.	6.3	.	.	.	4.3	2.6	.	.	ns
Denmark	.	.	.	.	3.1	0.0	3.0	.	.	ns
Estonia	19.2	.	.	.	39.0	48.3	45.3	.	.	0.01
Finland	.	.	.	0.0	.	0.0	3.4	.	.	ns
France	.	6.7	.	6.2	.	9.4	11.0	.	.	ns
Germany	.	.	.	10.3	7.2	8.9	6.4	.	.	ns
Latvia	.	.	57.9	.	25.0	27.9	27.1	.	.	0.0003
Lithuania	.	.	.	.	.	46.1	45.0	.	53.3	ns
Netherlands	.	.	0.6	.	.	2.4	1.1	.	.	ns
New Zealand	.	0.0	0.0	14.3	9.1	0.0	0.0	0.0	.	ns
Norway	.	.	16.7	.	.	0.0	0.0	.	.	ns
Puerto Rico	18.2	.	.	25.0	0.0	14.3	25.0	.	.	ns
Russian Fed. Tomsk Oblast	.	.	.	.	31.0	.	38.0	46.0	47.9	0.0004
Slovakia	.	.	.	.	10.2	4.1	1.8	.	.	0.003
Slovenia	.	.	.	2.8	.	5.7	0.0	.	.	ns
Spain-Barcelona	.	20.5	.	11.6	.	22.7	11.1	12.5	.	ns
Sweden	.	.	.	8.3	.	12.9	2.4	.	.	ns
Switzerland	.	.	.	15.0	.	10.5	3.5	.	.	ns
United Kingdom - England, Wales, Northern Ireland[a]	.	17.6	.	13.2	.	3.6	5.5	.	.	---
United States	.	8.4	.	8.0	3.6	5.3	4.8	6.5	.	0.007

[a] Data from England, Wales and Northern Ireland reported before 1999 cannot be compared with data reported after 1999, because of changes in surveillance methodologies.

ANNEXES

Annex 14: Trends of resistance (%) to any TB drug among combined cases in 26 countries/settings (1994-2002)

Country/Setting	Years of observation									P-Value
	1994	1995	1996	1997	1998	1999	2000	2001	2002	
Australia	.	9.5	10.5	.	13.0	10.7	10.3	.	.	ns
Botswana	.	4.8	.	.	.	7.7	.	.	15.5	S
Canada	.	.	.	10.4	9.5	9.8	9.2	.	.	ns
China-Hong Kong SAR	.	.	14.4	13.1	12.9	13.6	12.2	10.8		<0.0001
Cuba	.	10.7	.	.	8.3	.	6.1	.	.	S
Czech Republic	.	2.8	.	.	.	3.3	5.0	.	.	S
Denmark	.	.	.	.	13.1	15.4	13.2	.	.	ns
Estonia	29.8	.	.	.	41.0	37.1	35.1	.	.	S
Finland	.	.	.	4.9	.	2.0	5.0	.	.	ns
France	.	9.6	.	11.1	.	10.4	10.9	.	.	S
Germany	.	.	.	7.7	9.3	8.3	8.7	.	.	ns
Israel	.	.	.	.	19.2	16.6	32.0	.	.	0.002
Latvia	.	.	49.7	.	30.1	31.3	33.0	.	.	S
Lithuania	.	.	.	.	.	44.5	44.3	.	48.1	0.002
Netherlands	.	14.1	11.0	.	.	8.8	10.6	.	.	0.002
New Zealand	.	5.3	4.6	13.9	13.9	9.2	14.5	11.2	.	0.01
Norway	.	.	11.1	13.0	23.5	.	.	.	.	0.01
Puerto Rico	11.0	.	.	14.5	9.3	7.5	8.6	.	.	ns
Russian Fed. -Tomsk Oblast	.	.	.	.	39.3	.	40.0	43.2	41.5	ns
Slovakia	.	.	.	.	5.5	3.6	5.9	.	.	ns
Slovenia	.	.	.	3.1	.	3.2	3.4	.	.	ns
Spain-Barcelona	.	12.9	.	5.4	.	9.4	10.2	12.9	.	S
Sweden	.	.	.	8.4	.	12.7	10.7	.	.	ns
Switzerland	.	.	.	5.8	.	7.0	5.1	.	.	ns
United Kingdom - England, Wales, Northern Ireland[a]	.	8.2	.	8.1	.	8.4	9.0	.	.	---
United States	.	12.9	.	12.4	12.5	11.9	12.9	13.0	.	ns

[a] Data from England, Wales and Northern Ireland reported before 1999 cannot be compared with data reported after 1999, because of changes in surveillance methodologies.

S: Given the adjustment of the combined rates, due to the survey particularities, no P-values can be determined

Annex 15: Trends of MDR resistance (%) among combined cases in 26 countries/settings (1994-2002)

Country/Setting	Years of observation									P-Value
	1994	1995	1996	1997	1998	1999	2000	2001	2002	
Australia	.	0.7	2.0	.	0.9	0.5	1.0	.	.	ns
Botswana	.	0.8	.	.	.	1.2	.	.	2.7	S
Canada	.	.	.	1.1	0.9	0.8	1.0	.	.	ns
China-Hong Kong SAR	.	.	2.6	1.7	2.0	1.4	1.5	1.3	.	<0.0001
Cuba	.	1.0	.	.	0.9	.	0.5	.	.	S
Czech Republic	.	1.4	.	.	.	0.6	1.5	.	.	S
Denmark	.	.	.	.	0.7	0.0	0..5	.	.	ns
Estonia	11.0	.	.	.	18.3	22.8	19.5	.	.	S
Finland	.	.	.	0.0	.	0.0	0..5	.	.	ns
France	.	0..9	.	0.4	.	1.4	1.3	.	.	S
Germany	.	.	.	1.4	1.4	1.4	1.6	.	.	ns
Israel	.	.	.	.	8.1	7.9	14.6	.	.	0.009
Latvia	.	.	30.3	.	12.2	13.5	13.1	.	.	S
Lithuania	.	.	.	.	.	24.7	25.5	.	30.8	<0.0001
Netherlands	.	1.1	0.6	.	.	0.4	0.9	.	.	ns
New Zealand	.	1.3	0.0	0.7	1.8	0.8	0.4	0.0	.	ns
Norway	.	.	2.8	.	.	1.6	1.8	.	.	ns
Puerto Rico	2.6	.	.	3.5	1.4	0.6	0.7	.	.	ns
Russian Fed. Tomsk Oblast	.	.	.	.	13.7	.	12.8	17.3	19.1	0.003
Slovakia	.	.	.	.	2.0	1.0	1.2	.	.	ns
Slovenia	.	.	.	0.9	.	0.6	0.0	.	.	ns
Spain-Barcelona	.	2.0	.	1.4	.	2.2	3.7	3.7	.	S
Sweden	.	.	.	1.1	.	1.7	1.4	.	.	ns
Switzerland	.	.	.	1.4	.	1.8	0.4	.	.	ns
United Kingdom - England, Wales, Northern Ireland[a]	.	1.9	.	1.5	.	0.6	1.2	.	.	0.0008
United States	.	2.0	.	1.4	1.2	1.3	1.3	1.4	.	<0.0001

[a] Data from England, Wales and Northern Ireland reported before 1999 cannot be compared with data reported after 1999, because of changes in surveillance methodologies.

S: Given the adjustment of the combined rates, due to the survey particularities, no P-values can be determined

ANNEXES

Annex 16: Trends of any INH resistance (%) among combined cases in 26 countries/settings (1994-2002)

Country/Setting	Year sof observation									P-Value
	1994	1995	1996	1997	1998	1999	2000	2001	2002	
Australia	.	7.5	9.7	.	9.0	6.8	10.1	.	.	ns
Botswana	.	2.4	.	.	.	5.4	.	6.6		S
Canada	.	.	.	7.8	7.4	8.0	7.3	.	.	0.003
China-Hong Kong SAR	.	.	7.8	6.9	7.6	6.5	6.9	6.1	.	ns
Cuba	.	2.8	.	.	3.1	.	1.7	.	.	S
Czech Republic	.	2.8	.	.	.	2.1	3.6	.	.	S
Denmark	.	.	.	.	6.5	7.5	8.7	.	.	ns
Estonia	23.3	.	.	.	31.2	31.9	30.0	.	.	S
Finland	.	.	.	4.6	.	0.7	3.4	.	.	ns
France	.	4.5	.	4.0	.	4.7	3.8	.	.	S
Germany	.	.	.	5.8	6.5	5.5	6.1	.	.	ns
Israel	.	.	.	.	15.6	13.3	26.3	.	.	0.001
Latvia	.	.	46.8	.	28.3	28.5	30.3	.	.	S
Lithuania	.	.	.	.	.	37.4	38.7	.	44.9	<0.0001
Netherlands	.	8.6	6.8	.	.	5.8	5.9	.	.	0.01
New Zealand	.	4.0	4.6	10.2	12.0	6.4	10.1	6.1	.	ns
Norway	.	.	8.3	.	.	6.0	12.4	.	.	ns
Puerto Rico	7.7	.	.	9.9	8.6	1.7	4.3	.	.	S
Russian Fed. Tomsk Oblast	.	.	.	.	27.7	.	29.0	34.6	33.1	0.008
Slovakia	.	.	.	.	4.6	2.4	4.7	.	.	ns
Slovenia	.	.	.	1.5	.	2.7	2.8	.	.	ns
Spain-Barcelona	.	8.4	.	4.1	.	6.3	7.5	8.5	.	S
Sweden	.	.	.	6.3	.	10.3	10.1	.	.	0.04
Switzerland	.	.	.	5.2	.	6.5	4.9	.	.	ns
United Kingdom - England, Wales, Northern Ireland[a]	.	6.8	.	5.9	.	5.9	6.4	.	.	---
United States	.	8.4	.	8.34	8.6	7.9	8.3	8.0	.	ns

[a] Data from England, Wales and Northern Ireland reported before 1999 cannot be compared with data reported after 1999, because of changes in surveillance methodologies.

S: Given the adjustment of the combined rates, due to the survey particularities, no P-values can be determined

Annex 17: Trends of any RMP resistance (%) among combined cases in 26 countries/settings (1994-2002)

Country/Setting	Years of observation									P-Value
	1994	1995	1996	1997	1998	1999	2000	2001	2002	
Australia	.	1.1	2.1	.	1.1	0.8	1.3	.	.	ns
Botswana	.	1.7	.	.	.	1.7	.	.	4.7	S
Canada	.	.	.	1.1	0.9	1.0	1.2	.	.	ns
China-Hong Kong SAR	.	.	3.1	2.1	2.2	1.7	1.6	1.4	.	<0.0001
Cuba	.	1.4	.	.	0.9	.	1.0	.	.	S
Czech Republic	.	1.4	.	.	.	1.1	1.6	.	.	S
Denmark	.	.	.	.	0.7	0.2	0.7	.	.	ns
Estonia	11.0	.	.	.	18.7	23.0	19.5	.	.	S
Finland	.	.	.	0.0	.	0.0	0.9	.	.	-
France	.	1.3	.	0.8	.	1.5	1.5	.	.	S
Germany	.	.	.	1.7	1.8	1.8	1.8	.	.	ns
Israel	.	.	.	.	8.5	8.5	14.9	.	.	0.01
Latvia	.	.	31.8	.	12.5	13.7	13.1	.	.	S
Lithuania	.	.	.	.	.	27.6	26.9	.	31.0	0.0004
Netherlands	.	0.2	1.0	.	.	0.9	0.9	.	.	ns
New Zealand	.	1.3	0.0	2.2	1.8	1.2	0.4	0.3	.	ns
Norway	.	.	2.8	.	.	1.6	2.4	.	.	ns
Puerto Rico	3.6	.	.	4.7	1.4	1.2	1.4	.	.	ns
Russian Fed. Tomsk Oblast	.	.	.	.	16.2	.	15.2	18.9	20.3	0.031
Slovakia	.	.	.	.	2.4	1.7	1.6	.	.	ns
Slovenia	.	.	.	0.9	.	0.6	0.0	.	.	ns
Spain-Barcelona	.	2.7	.	1.4	.	3.3	3.1	2.8	.	S
Sweden	.	.	.	1.1	.	2.2	1.4	.	.	ns
Switzerland	.	.	.	1.7	.	2.1	.	0.6	.	ns
United Kingdom - England, Wales, Northern Ireland[a]	.	2.1	.	1.6	.	0.7	.	1.6	.	---
United States	.	2.7	.	2.0	1.6	1.5	1.7	1.7	.	<0.0001

[a] Data from England, Wales and Northern Ireland reported before 1999 cannot be compared with data reported after 1999, because of changes in surveillance methodologies.
S: Given the adjustment of the combined rates, due to the survey particularities, no P-values can be determined

Annex 18: Ecological bivariate analysis among new TB cases in all countries/settings

All countries/settings (n=60)	Any resistance rate rs (P-value)	MDR rate rs (P-value)
Out-of-pocket health expenditure	0.297 (0.021)	0.257 (0.047)
Human Development Index	0.253 (0.051)	- 0.259 (0.046)
GDP	- 0.284 (0.028)	- 0.314 (0.015)
GINI	0.294 (0.023)	0.306 (0.017)
Responsiveness level		
- level index	- 0.150 (0.252)	- 0.257 (0.047)
- distribution index	- 0.191 (0.151)	- 0.265 (0.045)
Fairness index	- 0.293 (0.023)	- 0.343 (0.007)
Performance index	- 0.411 (0.001)	- 0.393 (0.002)
Notified TB incidence rate (new cases)	0.353 (0.006)	0.401 (0.001)
% Re-treatment cases	0.224 (0.085)	0.337 (0.006)
Human Poverty Index	0.313 (0.015)	0.358 (0.005)
Duration of introduction of RIF	0.214 (0.122)	0.301 (0.047)

Annex 19: Selective ecological bivariate analysis among new TB cases in medium- and low- income

Medium- and low-income countries/settings (n=36)	Any resistance rate rs (P-value)	MDR rate rs (P-value)
Out-of-pocket health expenditure	0.327 (0.045)	0.182 (0.289)
GDP	- 0.348 (0.038)	- 0.145 (0.397)
GINI	0.338 (0.044)	0.317 (0.060)
Health expenditure	- 0.374 (0.025)	- 0.311 (0.065)
Fairness index	- 0.437 (0.008)	- 0.367 (0.028)
Performance index	- 0.500 (0.002)	- 0.475 (0.003)
Notified TB incidence rate (new cases)	0.449 (0.006)	- 0.342 (0.041)
% Re-treatment cases	0.402 (0.015)	0.591 (0.001)

ANNEXES

Annex 20: Ecological bivariate analysis among combined TB cases in all countries/settings

All countries/settings (n=56)	Any resistance rate rs (P-value)	MDR rate rs (P-value)
Out of pocket health expenditure	0.303 (0.024)	0.244 (0.070)
Human Development Index	0.296 (0.024)	- 0.376 (0.004)
GDP	- 0.353 (0.008)	- 0.403 (0.002)
GINI	0.310 (0.020)	0.299 (0.025)
Human Poverty Index	0.362 (0.006)	0.467 (0.001)
Education index	0.148 (0.277)	0.270 (0.044)
Responsiveness		
- level index	- 0.235 (0.082)	- 0.331 (0.013)
- distribution index	- 0.266 (0.052)	- 0.341 (0.012)
Fairness index	- 0.407 (0.002)	- 0.447 (0.001)
Performance index	- 0.412 (0.002)	- 0.371 (0.005)
Health expenditure	- 0.324 (0.015)	- 0.404 (0.002)
Notified TB incidence rate (new cases)	0.401 (0.002)	0.462 (0.001)
% Re-treatment cases	0.227 (0.067)	0.309 (0.021)
HIV rate in adults	0.275 (0.040)	0.251 (0.062)

Annex 21: Selective ecological bivariate analysis among combined TB cases in medium- and low-income

Medium- and low-income countries/settings (n=32)	Any resistance rate rs (P-value)	MDR rate rs (P-value)
GINI	0.355 (0.046)	0.247 (0.174)
Health expenditure	- 0.476 (0.006)	- 0.491 (0.004)
Fairness index	- 0.468 (0.007)	- 0.338 (0.058)
Performance index	- 0.471 (0.007)	- 0.410 (0.020)
Notified TB incidence rate (new cases)	0.416 (0.018)	- 0.308 (0.086)
% Re-treatment cases	0.457 (0.009)	0.537 (0.002)

Annex 22: **Ecological multivariate analysis among new TB cases in all countries/settings**

All countries/settings (n=60)

OUTCOME VARIABLE: PREVALENCE OF ANY RESISTANCE
Model = 0.189 + 0.0065 Re-treatment – 0.0035 HPI

Re-treatment: p<0.001	HPI: p= 0.054	R^2=25%[a]

OUTCOME VARIABLE: PREVALENCE OF MDR
Model = 0.094 + 0.0039 Re-treatment – 0.00002 GDP

Re-treatment: p<0.0001	GDP: p= 0.068	R^2=28%

Low- and middle-income countries (n=36)

OUTCOME VARIABLE: PREVALENCE OF ANY RESISTANCE
Model = 0.38 + 0.0067 Re-treatment – 0.00001 GDP

Re-treatment: p=0.001	GDP: p= 0.006	R^2=40%

OUTCOME VARIABLE: PREVALENCE OF MDR
Model = -0.326 + 0.003 Re-treatment – 0.0001 GDP + 0.004 HPI - 0,571 HDI

Re-treatment: p=0.006	GDP: p= 0.025	HPI: p=0.065	HDI :p=0.0044	R^2=42%

ANNEXES

[a] The R^2, called also "coefficient of determination" is a measure of the goodness of fit of the linear regression model to the data. It expresses the percentage of the variation in the outcome variable that has been explained by the regression on the explanatory variables. In the example, R^2 = 25% implies that 25% of the variation of any resistance rate over the 60 countries is explained by the variables "re-treatment cases" and "HPI".

Annex 23: Ecological multivariate analysis among combined TB cases in all countries/settings

All countries/settings (n=56)

OUTCOME VARIABLE: PREVALENCE OF ANY RESISTANCE
Model = 0.327 + 0.009 Re-treatment − 0.00005 GDP
Re-treatment: $p<0.0001$ GDP: $p= 0.068$ $R^2=28\%$

OUTCOME VARIABLE: PREVALENCE OF MDR
Model = 0.129 + 0.0076 Re-treatment − 0.0000037 GDP
Re-treatment: $p<0.0001$ GDP: $p= 0.010$ $R^2=45\%$

Low- and median-income countries (n=32)

OUTCOME VARIABLE: PREVALENCE OF ANY RESISTANCE
Model = 0.382 + 0.010 Re-treatment − 0.00002 GDP
Re-treatment: $p< 0.001$ GDP: $p= 0.006$ $R^2=50\%$

OUTCOME VARIABLE: PREVALENCE OF MDR
Model = 0.096 + 0.0076 Re-treatment
Re-treatment: $p<0.0001$ $R^2=40\%$

ANNEXES

Annex 24: Forecast of the number of MDR cases (with 95% CI) 1999-2002

COUNTRY/SETTING	TOTAL NO. OF CASES	% MDR	LOWER 95% CI	UPPER 95% CI	LOWER ESTIMATE OF NO. OF MDR CASES	ESTIMATE OF NO. OF MDR CASES	HIGHER ESTIMATE OF NO. OF MDR CASES
South Africa*	103626	2.9	2.8	3.0	2902	2957	3109
Kazakhstan*	11980	24.4	23.7	25.2	2839	2926	3019
China, Hubei Province*	23633	7.0	6.7	7.3	1583	1653	1725
China, Henan Province*	15125	10.1	9.6	10.6	1452	1527	1603
China, Liaoning Province	8002	13.0	12.2	13.7	976	1037	1096
Nepal*	15727	3.8	3.5	4.1	550	600	645
Thailand*	29768	1.8	1.7	2.0	506	541	595
Egypt*	5470	8.5	7.8	9.3	427	467	509
Ecuador*	5029	8.7	8.0	9.6	402	439	483
Uzbekistan, Karakalpakstan	1294	26.8	24.4	29.3	316	347	379
Zambia*	14546	1.8	1.6	2.1	233	269	305
Lithuania	1140	21.8	19.4	24.3	221	248	277
Japan, sentinel*	12013	1.8	1.6	2.1	192	222	252
Argentina*	6602	3.0	2.6	3.4	172	196	224
Latvia	1144	13.1	11.2	15.2	128	150	174
United States	10288	1.4	1.1	1.6	113	140	165
Russian Federation, Tomsk Oblast	650	19.1	16.2	22.4	105	124	146
Colombia*	8022	1.5	1.3	1.8	104	121	144
Estonia	527	19.5	16.3	23.2	86	103	122
Russian Federation, Orel Oblast	589	16.8	13.9	20.1	82	99	118
Botswana*	3452	2.7	2.2	3.3	76	94	114
Poland	3705	2.5	2.0	3.1	74	92	115
Turkmenistan, Dashoguz	791	11.6	9.5	14.1	75	92	112
Algeria*#	7953	1.1	.9	1.4	72	88	111
Venezuela*	3812	1.7	1.3	2.1	50	63	80
Honduras*	2983	2.0	1.6	2.6	48	61	78
Germany	2780	1.7	1.3	2.3	36	47	64
China, Hong Kong SAR	3639	1.3	.9	1.7	33	46	62
Israel	281	14.6	10.8	19.4	30	41	55
United Kingdom - England, Wales and Northern Ireland	3004	1.2	.9	1.7	27	37	51
India, Raichur District	1241	2.6	1.8	3.7	22	32	46
Cambodia*	15188	.2	.1	.3	15	26	46
Italy (half of the country)	1387	1.7	1.1	2.5	15	23	35

* Survey methodology applied. For countries conducting surveys on a sample of the population, estimates were generated by applying prevalences determined in surveys to reported notification figures for the corresponding population and thus are dependent upon the level of case-finding in the country and quality of recording and reporting of the national programme.
# New cases only.

ANNEXES

COUNTRY/SETTING	TOTAL NO. OF CASES	% MDR	LOWER 95% CI	UPPER 95% CI	LOWER ESTIMATE OF NO. OF MDR CASES	ESTIMATE OF NO. OF MDR CASES	HIGHER ESTIMATE OF NO. OF MDR CASES
Chile*	1505	1.4	.9	2.2	14	21	33
France, sentinel sites*	2398	.8	.5	1.3	12	20	31
El Salvador*	1184	1.4	.9	2.3	11	17	27
Mongolia*#	1631	1.0	.6	1.7	10	17	28
Canada	1363	1.0	.5	1.7	7	13	23
Belgium	730	1.5	.8	2.8	6	11	20
Spain, Galicia State*	493	2.2	1.2	4.1	6	11	20
Czech Republic	638	1.4	.7	2.8	4	9	18
Netherlands	863	.9	.4	1.9	3	8	16
Oman	183	3.8	1.7	8.0	3	7	15
Slovakia	575	1.2	.5	2.6	3	7	15
Spain, Barcelona City*	240	2.5	1.0	5.6	2	6	13
The Gambia*	876	.6	.2	1.4	2	5	12
Bosnia and Herzegovina	1153	.4	.2	1.1	2	5	13
Sweden	365	1.4	.5	3.4	2	5	12
Singapore	949	.5	.2	1.3	2	5	12
Cuba, sentinel*	620	.6	.2	1.8	1	4	11
Austria	761	.5	.2	1.4	2	4	11
India, Wardha District,	800	.5	.2	1.4	2	4	11
Ireland	225	1.3	.3	4.2	1	3	9
Norway	170	1.8	.5	5.5	1	3	9
Croatia	879	.2	.1	.9	1	2	8
Uruguay*#	392	.5	.1	2.0	0	2	8
Denmark	425	.5	.1	1.9	0	2	8
Finland	437	.5	.1	1.8	0	2	8
Switzerland	492	.4	.1	1.6	0	2	8
Puerto Rico	139	.7	.1	4.5	0	1	6
Qatar#	284	.4	.1	2.3	0	1	7
Serbia and Montenegro	279	.4	.0	2.3	0	1	6
Luxembourg	44	.0	.0	10.0	0	0	4
Andorra	3	.0	.0	69.0	0	0	2
Malta	10	.0	.0	34.5	0	0	3
Iceland	9	.0	.0	37.1	0	0	3
Slovenia	320	.0	.0	1.5	0	0	5
New Zealand	294	.0	.0	1.6	0	0	5
Scotland	302	.0	.0	1.6	0	0	5

ANNEXES

* Survey methodology applied. For countries conducting surveys on a sample of the population, estimates were generated by applying prevalences determined in surveys to reported notification figures for the corresponding population and thus are dependent upon the level of case-finding in the country and quality of recording and reporting of the national programme.
# New cases only.

Annex 25: GLC operations June 2000-November 2004

Countries with DOTS-Plus approved projects	Countries with projects under review	Pipeline
Peru	Azerbaijan	Kosovo
Estonia	Dominican Republic	Tadjikistan
Latvia	Moldova	Ecuador
Russia (Tomsk)	Kenya	Viet Nam
Russia (Orel)	India (Delhi)	Morocco
Russia (Arkhangelsk)	Tunisia	Paraguay
Russia (Ivanovo)		Mongolia
Philippines		South Africa
Mexico		India
Malawi		Iran
Bolivia		
Haiti		
Costa Rica		
Uzbekistan		
Nepal		
Lebanon		
El Salvador		
Egypt		
Nicaragua		
Romania		
Honduras		
Kyrgyzstan		
Abkhazia		
Syria		
Jordan		
Kenya		
Georgia		

REFERENCES

1   Stýblo K, Daňková D, Drápela J, Calliová J, Jezek Z, Krivánek J, et al. Epidemiological and clinical study of tuberculosis in the district of Kolín, Czechoslovakia. *Bulletin of the World Health Organization,* 1967, 37:819-74.

2   Dye C, Zhao F, Scheele S, Williams B. Evaluating the impact of tuberculosis control: number of deaths prevented by short-course chemotherapy in China. *International Journal of Epidemiology,* 2000, 29:558-564.

3   Chaulet P, Boulahbal F, Grosset J. Surveillance of drug resistance for tuberculosis control: why and how? *Tubercle and Lung Disease,* 1995, 76:487-492.

4   World Health Organization. *WHO Global Strategy for Containment of Antimicrobial Resistance.* Geneva, 2001 (WHO/CDS/CSR/DRS/2001.2).

5   Crofton J, Mitchison DA. Streptomycin resistance in pulmonary tuberculosis. *British Medical Journal,* 1948, **2**:1009-1015.

6   Mitchison DA. Development of streptomycin resistant isolates of tubercle bacilli in pulmonary tuberculosis. *Thorax,* 1950, **4**:144.

7   Canetti G. Present aspects of bacterial resistance in tuberculosis. *American Review of Respiratory Diseases,* 1965, **92**:687-703.

8   Hong Kong Government Tuberculosis Services / British Medical Research Council Cooperative Investigation. Drug resistance in patients with pulmonary tuberculosis presenting at chest clinics in Hong Kong. *Tubercle,* 1964, **45**:77-95.

9   Public Health Service Cooperative Investigation. Prevalence of drug resistance in previously untreated patients. *American Review of Respiratory Diseases,* 1964, **89**:327-336.

10 Pyle MM. Relative numbers of resistant tubercle bacilli in sputa of patients before and during treatment with streptomycin. *Proceedings of the Mayo Clinic,* 1947, **22**: 465.

11 Mahmoudi A, Iseman MD. Pitfalls in care of patients with tuberculosis. *Journal of the American Medical Association,* 1993, **270**:65-68.

12   Kochi A, Vareldzis B, Styblo K. Multi-drug resistant tuberculosis and its control. *Research in Microbiology*, 1993, **73**:219-224.

13   Mitchison DA. Natural sensitivity of *M. tuberculosis* to thiacetazone. *Tubercle*, 1968, 49:38.

14   Konno K, Feldmann FM, McDermott W. Pyrazinamide susceptibility and amidase activity of tubercle bacilli. *American Review of Respiratory Diseases*, 1967, **95**:461.

15   Stewart SM, Hall E, Riddell RW, Somner AR. Bacteriological aspects of the use of ethionamide, pyrazinamide and cycloserine in the treatment of chronic pulmonary tuberculosis. *Tubercle*, 1962, 43:417-31.

16   World Health Organization. *Anti-tuberculosis drug resistance in the world: The WHO/ IUATLD Global Project on Anti-Tuberculosis Dug Resistance Surveillance. Report 2: Prevalence and trends.* Geneva, 2000 (WHO/CDS/TB/2000.278).

17   Espinal MA, Laszlo A, Simonsen L, Boulahbal F, Kim SJ, Reniero A, et al. Global trends in resistance to antituberculosis drugs. *New England Journal of Medicine,* 2001, 344:1294-1302.

18   World Health Organization. *Guidelines for surveillance of drug resistance in tuberculosis.* Geneva, 2003 (WHO/CDS/CSR/RMD/2003.3).

19   Laserson KF, Kenyon AS, Kenyon TA, Layloff T, Binkin NJ. Substandard tuberculosis drugs on the global market and their simple detection. *International Journal of Tuberculosis and Lung Disease,* 2001, 5(5):448-454.

20   World Health Organization. *Involving private practitioners in tuberculosis control: issues, interventions, and emerging policy framework.* Geneva, 2001 (WHO/CDS/ TB/2001.285).

21   Lansang MA, Lucas-Aquino R, Tupasi TE, Minaus Salazare LS, Juban N, Limjoco TT, et al. Purchase of antibiotics without prescription in Manila, the Philippines: inappropriate choices and doses. *Journal of Clinical Epidemiology,* 1990, 43(1):61-67

22   Greenhalgh T. Drug prescription and self-medication in India. *Social Science and Medicine,* 1987, 25(3):307-318.

23   Lonnroth K, Lambregts K, Nhien DTT, Quy HT, Diwan VK. Private pharmacies and TB control – a survey of case detection skills and reported anti-TB dispensing in private pharmacies in Ho Chi Minh City, Vietnam. *International Journal of Tuberculosis and Lung Disease,* 2000, 4: 1052-1059.

24   Hurtig AK, Pande SB, Baral SC, Porter JDH, Bam DS. Anti-tuberculosis treatment in private pharmacies, Kathmandu Valley, Nepal. *International Journal of Tuberculosis and Lung Disease,* 2000, 4(8):730-736.

25   Aluoch JA, Edwards EA, Stott H, Fox W, Sutherland I. A fourth study of case-finding methods for pulmonary tuberculosis in Kenya. *Transactions of the Royal Society of Tropical Medicine and Hygiene,* 1982, 79:679-691.

26   Ollé-Goig JE, Cullity JE, Vargas R. A survey of prescribing patterns for tuberculosis treatment amongst doctors in a Bolivian city. *International Journal of Tuberculosis and Lung Disease,* 1999, **3**:74-78.

27   Sumartojo EM, Geiter LJ, Miller B, Hale BE. Can physicians treat tuberculosis? Report on a national survey of physician practice. *American Journal of Public Health,* 1997, **87**:2008-2011.

28   Liu Z, Shilkret KL, Finelli L. Initial drug regimens for the treatment of tuberculosis: evaluation of physician prescribing practice in New Jersey, 1994-1995. *Chest,* 1998, **113**:1446-1451.

29   Corbett LE, Watt CJ, Walker N, Maher D, Williams BG, Raviglione MC, Dye C. The growing burden of tuberculosis. *Archives of Internal Medicine,* 2003, **163**:1009-1021.

30   World Health Organization. *Forty-fourth World Health Assembly.* Geneva, 1991 (WHA44/1991/REC/1).

31   World Health Organization. *An expanded DOTS framework for effective tuberculosis control.* Geneva, 2002 (WHO/CDS/TB/2002.297).

32   World Bank. *World Development Report 1993: investing in health.* New York, Oxford University Press, 1993.

33   World Health Organization. *Anti-tuberculosis drug resistance in the world: the WHO/ IUATLD Global Project on Anti-Tuberculosis Drug Resistance Surveillance.* Geneva, 1997 (WHO/TB/97.229).

34   Pablos-Méndez A, Raviglione MC, Laszlo A, Binkin N, Rieder HL, Bustreo F, et al. Global surveillance for antituberculosis-drug resistance, 1994–1997. *New England Journal of Medicine,* 1998, **338**:1641-1649.

35   Espinal MA, Kim SJ, Suarez PG, Kam KM, Khomenko AG, Migliori GB, et al. Standard short-course chemotherapy for drug-resistant tuberculosis: Treatment Outcomes in 6 Countries. *Journal of the American Medical Association,* 2000, **283**(19): 2537-2545.

36   World Health Organization. *Guidelines for establishing DOTS- PLUS pilot projects for the management of multi-drug resistant tuberculosis (MDR-TB).* Geneva, 2000 (WHO/CDS/ TB/2000.279).

37   Cohn DL, Bustreo F, Raviglione MC. Drug-resistant tuberculosis: review of the worldwide situation and the WHO/IUATLD Global Surveillance Project. *Clinicallinfectious Diseases,* 1997, 24(Suppl 1):S121-30.

38   Smith I, Arnold V, Kumaresan J. Global Drug Facility: improving access to TB drugs. *WHO Essential Drugs Monitor*, 2003, 32.

39   Kumaresan J, Smith I, Arnold V, Evans P. The Global TB Drug Facility: innovative global procurement. *International Journal of Tuberculosis and Lung Disease*, 2004, 8(1):130-138.

40   Gupta R, Cegielski JP, Espinal MA, Henkens M, Kim JY, Lambregts-Van Weezenbeek CS, et al. Increasing transparency in partnerships for health: introducing the Green Light Committee. *Tropical Medicine and International Health*, 2002, 7(11):970-976.

41   Gupta R, Kim JK, Espinal MA. Responding to market failures in tuberculosis control. *Science*, **293**:1049-1051.

42   Gordin FM, Nelson ET, Matts JP, et al. The impact of human immunodeficiency virus infection on drug resistant tuberculosis. *American Journal of Respiratory and Critical Care Medicine*, 1996, 154:1478-1483.

43   Espinal MA, Laserson K, Camacho M, Fusheng Z, Kim SJ, Tlali RE, et al. Determinants of drug-resistant tuberculosis: analysis of 11 countries. *International Journal of Tuberculosis and Lung Disease,* 2001, **5**(10): 887-893.

44   Dupon M, Texier-Maugein J, Leroy V, et al. Tuberculosis and HIV infection: a cohort study of incidence and susceptibility to antituberculosis drugs, Bordeaux, 1985-1993. AIDS, 1995, 9:577-578.

45   Dooley SW, Jarvis WR, Marlone WJ, Snider DE. Multi-drug resistant tuberculosis. *Annals of Internal Medicine*, 1992, **117**:257-259.

46   Edlin BR, Tokars JL, Grieco MH, et al. An outbreak of multi-drug resistant tuberculosis among hospitalized patients with the acquired immunodeficiency syndrome. *New England Journal of Medicine*, 1992, **326**:1514-1521.

47   Coronado VG, Beck-Sague CM, Hutton MD, et al. Transmission of multi-drug resistant *Mycobacterium tuberculosis* among persons with human immunodeficiency virus infection in an urban hospital: epidemiologic and restriction fragment length polymorphism analysis. *Journal of Infectious Diseases,* 1993, **168**:1052-1055.

48   Centers for Disease Control and Prevention. Nosocomial transmission of multidrug-resistant tuberculosis among HIV-infected persons – Florida and New York, 1988-1991. *Morbidity and Mortality Weekly Report*, 1991, **40**:585-591.

49   Ritacco V, DiLonardo M, Reniero A, Ambroggi M, Barrera, Dambrosi A, et al. Nosocomial spread of HIV-related multidrug resistant tuberculosis in Buenos Aires. *Journal of Infectious Diseases,* 1997, 176:637-642.

50   Monno L, Angarano G, Carbonara S, et al. Emergence of drug resistant *Mycobacterium tuberculosis* in HIV-infected patients. *Lancet*, 1991, **337**:852.

51   Bouvet E. Transmission nosocomiale de tuberculose multirésistante parmi les patients infectés par le VIH: en France, à Paris. *Bulletin epidémiologique hebdomadaire*, 1991, **45**:196-197.

52   Coronodo VG, Beck-Sague CM, Hutton MD, Davis BJ, Nicholas P, Villareal C, et al. Transmission of drug-resistant *Mycobacterium tuberculosis* among persons with human immunodeficiency virus infection in urban hospital: epidemiologic and restriction fragment length polymorphism analysis. *Journal of Infectious Diseases*, 1993, 168:1052-1055.

53   Rajeswari R, Balasubramanian R, Bose MSC, Sekar L, Rahman F. Private pharmacies in tuberculosis control- a neglected link *International Journal of Tuberculosis and Lung Disease*, 2002, **6**(2):171-173.

54   Uplekar MW, Rangan S. Private doctors and tuberculosis control in India. *Tubercle and Lung Disease*, 1993, 74:332-337.

55   Uplekar MW, Juvekar SK, Parande DB, et al. Tuberculosis management in private practice and its implications. *Indian Journal of Tuberculosis*, 1996, 43:19-22.

56   Singla N, Sharma PP, Singla R, Jain RC. Survey of knowledge, attitudes and practices for tuberculosis among general practitioners in Delhi, India. *International Journal of Tuberculosis and Lung Disease*, 1998, 2:384-389.

57   Uplekar M, Juvekar S, Morankar S, Rangan S, Nunn P. Tuberculosis patients and practitioners in private clinics in India. *International Journal of Tuberculosis and Lung Disease,* 1998, 2:324-329.

58   World Health Organization. *Laboratory services in tuberculosis control. Part III: Culture.* Geneva, 1998 (WHO/TB/98.258).

59   Vestal AL, Kubica GP. Differential identification of mycobacteria III. Use of thiacetazone, thiophen-2-carboxylic acid hydrazide and triphenyltetrazolium chloride. *Scandinavian Journal of Respiratory Diseases,* 1967, **48**:142-148.

60   Canetti G, Froman S, Grosset J, Hauduroy P, Langerova M, Mahler HT, et al. Mycobacteria: laboratory methods for testing drug sensitivity and resistance. *Bulletin of the World Health Organization*, 1963, **29**:565-578.

61   Canetti G, Fox W, Khomenko A, Mahler HT, Menon NK, Mitchison DA, et al. Advances in techniques of testing mycobacterial drug sensitivity, and the use of sensitivity tests in tuberculosis control programmes. *Bulletin of the World Health Organization*. 1969; 41(1):21-43.

62   Siddiqi SH. *BACTEC 460TB system. Product and procedure manual,* 1996. Becton Dickinson and Company, 1996.

63   Brenner E. *Surveillance of drug resistance in tuberculosis software: SDRTB3.* Geneva, World Health Organization Geneva. 2000.

64   World Health Organization. *Global tuberculosis control; surveillance, planning, financing.* Geneva, 2003 (WHO/CDS/TB/2003.316).

65   Ford BL. An overview of hot-deck procedures. In: Madow WG, Olkin I, Rubin DB, eds., *Incomplete data in sample surveys.* New York, Academic Press, 1983:185-207.

66   Laszlo A, Rahman M, Espinal M, Raviglione M. Quality assurance programme for drug susceptibility testing of *Mycobacterium tuberculosis* in the WHO/IUATLD Supranational Reference Laboratory Network: five rounds of proficiency testing, 1994–1998. *The International Journal of Tuberculosis and Lung Disease*, 2002, 6(9):748-756.

67   United Nations Development Programme. *Human Development Report 2002: Deepening democracy in a fragmented world.* New York, 2002.

68   World Health Organization. *Global tuberculosis control; surveillance, planning, financing.* Geneva, 2002 (WHO/CDS/TB/2002.295).

69   Joint United Nations Programme on HIV/AIDS (UNAIDS). *Report on the global HIV/AIDS epidemic.* Geneva, 2002 (UNAIDS/02.26E).

70   United Nations Development Programme. *Human Development Report 2003: Millennium Development Goals: A compact among nations to end human poverty.* New York, 2003.

71   World Health Organization. *The World Health Report 2002: changing history.* Geneva, 2002.

72   World Health Organization. *The World Health Report 2000: Health systems: improving performance.* Geneva, 2000.

73   Watterson S, Wilson SM, Yates MD, Drobniewski F. A comparison of three molecular assays for rapid detection of rifampin resistance in *Mycobacterium tuberculosis*. *Journal of clinical microbiology*, 1998, **36**:1969-1973.

74   Gamboa F, Cardona PJ, Mandeerola JM, et al. Evaluation of a commercial probe assay for detection of rifampin resistance in *Mycobacterium tuberculosis* directly from respiratory and non respiratory clinical specimens. *European Journal of Clinical Microbiology and Infectious Diseases*, 1998, **17**:189-192.

75   Traore H, Fissette K, Bastian I, Devleeschhouver F, Portaels F. Detection of rifampicin resistance in *Mycobacterium tuberculosis* isolates from diverse countries by a commercial line probe assay as an initial indicator of multidrug resistance. *International Journal of Tuberculosis and Lung Disease*, 2000, **4**(5):481-484.

76   Drobniewski F, Balabanova Y, Ruddy M, Weldon L, Jeltkova K, Brown T, et al. Rifampin-
      and multidrug-resistant tuberculosis in Russian civilians and prison inmates:
      dominance of the beijing strain family. *Emerging Infectious Disease*, 2002, **8**(11):1320-
      1326.

77   Kenyon TA, Mwasekaga MJ, Huebner R, Rumisha D, Binkin N, Maganu E. Low levels of
      drug resistance amidst rapidly increasing tuberculosis and human immunodeficiency
      virus: co-epidemics in Botswana. *International Journal of Tuberculosis and Lung
      Disease,* 1999, 3: 4-11.

78   Weyer K, Groenwald P, Zwarenstein M, Lombard CJ. Tuberculosis drug resistance in
      the Western Cape. *South African Medical Journal*, 1995, **85**(6):499-504.

79   Chemtob D, Epstein L, Slater P, Weiler-Ravell D. Epidemiological analysis of
      tuberculosis treatment outcome as a tool for changing tuberculosis control policy in
      Israel. *Israel Medical Association Journal*, 2001, 3:479-483.

80   Sosna J, Shulimzon T, Roznman J, Lidgi M, Lavy A, Ben-Dov IZ, Ben-Dov I. Drug-
      resistant pulmnonary tuberculosis in Israel, a society of immigrants: 1985-1994.
      International Journal of Tuberculosis and Lung Disease, 1999, **3**(8):689-694.

81   Chemtob D, Leventhal A, Weiler-Ravell D. Screening and management of tuberculosis
      in immigrants: the challenge beyond professional competence. *Interational Journal
      of Tuberculosis and Lung Disease,* 2003, **7**(10):959-966.

82   Chemtob D, Leventhal A, Berlowitz Y, Weiler-Ravell D.The new National Tuberculosis
      Control Programme in Israel, a country of high immigration. *International Journal of
      Tuberculosis and Lung Disease,* 2003, **7**(8):828-836.

83   Augustynowicz-Kopec E, Zwolska Z, Jaworski A, Kostrzewa E, Klatt M. Drug-resistant
      tuberculosis in Poland in 2000: second national survey and comparison with the
      1997 survey. *International Journal of Tuberculosis and Lung Disease,* 2003, **4**(7):645-
      651.

84   Yoshiyama T, Supawitkul S, Kunyanone N, Riengthong D, Yanai H, Abe C, et al.
      Prevalence of drug-resistant tuberculosis in an HIV endemic area in northern
      Thailand. *International Journal of Tuberculosis and Lung Disease,* 2001, 5(1):32-39.

85   Kai Man Kam, Chi Wai Yip, Lai Wa Tse, Oi Chi Leung, Lai Ping Sin, Mei Yuk Chan, Wai
      Sum Wong, Trends in multidrug-resistant Mycobacterium tuberculosis in relation to
      sputum smear positivity in Hong Kong, 1989-1999. *Clinical Infectious Disease* 2002:34.

86   Quy HTW, Lan NTN, Borgdorff MW, Grosset J, Linh PD, Tung LB, et al. Drug resistance
      among failure and relapse cases of tuberculosis: is the standard re-treatment
      regimen adequate? *International Journal of Tuberculosis and Lung Disease,* 2003,
      7(7):631-636.

REFERENCES

COUNTRY PROFILES

ALGERIA

Countrywide: 2001

PROFILE OF THE COUNTRY AND ITS CONTROL PROGRAMME

Population in year of survey	**30,350,007**		Year N.T.P was established	**1969**		
Notification all cases (rate)	**60.4**	**/100,000**	Year of Rifampicin introduction	**1980**		
Estimated incidence (all cases)	**65.2**	**/100,000**	Year of Isoniazid introduction	**1952**		
Notification new sputum smear +	**7998**		Use of Standardized Regimens	**Yes**		
Notification new sputum smear + (rate)	**26.3**	**/100,000**	% Use of Short Course Chemotherapy	**Yes**	**100**	**%**
Treatment Success	**87.3**	**%**	Use of Directly Observed Therapy	**Yes**	**100**	**%**
Retreatment cases	**635**		During continuation phase	**No**		
Retreatment as % of NTP	**7.9**	**%**	Use of Fixed Dose Combination	**Yes**	**100**	**%**
Estimated HIV positive TB cases	**.30**	**%**	Treatment in private sector	**Cat 1**		

Category 1: virtually all TB patients public sector
Category 2: <15% in private sector
Category 3: 15% or more in private sector

TB drugs available on the private market	**No**

CHARACTERISTICS OF THE SURVEY/SURVEILLANCE PROGRAMME

Study Duration	**12 Months**
Target Area	**Countrywide**
Sampling Method	**Cluster**
Culture Media	**Löwenstein-Jensen**
DST Method	**Proportion**
Supranational Reference Laboratory	**Institut Pasteur, Centre National de Référence des Mycobacteries, Paris, France**

*Notations to accompany profile: Estimated HIV positive TB cases is a WHO estimate
Retreatment indicates sputum smear positive pulmonary cases only.

*For survey settings where less than 100% of cases are sampled, combined estimates are based on the rates of new and previously treated cases obtained in the survey, but weighted by the absolute number of new and previously treated sputum positive TB cases, as published by the national authorities.

COUNTRY PROFILES

PREVALENCE OF DRUG RESISTANCE

Countrywide: 2001

	New		Previous		Combined	
	N	%	N	%	N	%
Total number of strains tested	518	100.00				
SUSCEPTIBLE TO ALL 4 DRUGS	**486**	**93.6**				
ANY RESISTANCE	**32**	**6.2**				
- Isoniazid (INH)	16	3.2				
- Rifampicin (RMP)	6	1.2				
- Ethambutol (EMB)	0	0.0				
- Streptomycin (SM)	27	5.2				
MONORESISTANCE	**21**	**4.1**				
- Isoniazid (INH)	5	1.0				
- Rifampicin (RMP)	0	0.0				
- Ethambutol (EMB)	0	0.0				
- Streptomycin (SM)	16	3.1				
MULTIDRUG RESISTANCE	**6**	**1.1**				
- INH + RMP	0	0.0				
- INH + RMP + EMB	0	0.0				
- INH + RMP + SM	6	1.1				
- INH + RMP + EMB + SM	0	0.0				
OTHER PATTERNS	**5**	**1.0**				
- INH + EMB	0	0.0				
- INH + SM	5	5.0				
- INH + EMB + SM	0	0.0				
- RMP + EMB	0	0.0				
- RMP + SM	0	0.0				
- RMP + EMB + SM	0	0.0				
- EMB + SM	0	0.0				
NUMBER OF DRUGS RESISTANT TO:						
susceptible to 4 drugs	486	93.6				
resistant to 1 drug	21	4.1				
resistant to 2 drugs	5	1.0				
resistant to 3 drugs	6	1.1				
resistant to 4 drugs	0	0.0				

COUNTRY PROFILES

ANDORRA

Countrywide: 2000

PROFILE OF THE COUNTRY AND ITS CONTROL PROGRAMME

Population in year of survey	**66,000**	Year N.T.P was established	
Notification all cases (rate)	**/100,000**	Year of Rifampicin introduction	
Estimated incidence (all cases)	**/100,000**	Year of Isoniazid introduction	
Notification new sputum smear +	**1**	Use of Standardized Regimens	
Notification new sputum smear + (rate)	**/100,000**	% Use of Short Course Chemotherapy	**%**
Treatment Success	**%**	Use of Directly Observed Therapy	**%**
Retreatment cases	**0**	During continuation phase	
Retreatment as % of NTP	**%**	Use of Fixed Dose Combination	**%**
Estimated HIV positive TB cases	**.34 %**	Treatment in private sector Category 1: virtually all TB patients public sector Category 2: <15% in private sector Category 3: 15% or more in private sector	
		TB drugs available on the private market	

CHARACTERISTICS OF THE SURVEY/SURVEILLANCE PROGRAMME

Study Duration	**12 Months**
Target Area	**Countrywide**
Sampling Method	**All cases**
Culture Media	
DST Method	
Supranational Reference Laboratory	**Servicio de Microbiologia, Hospital Universitaris Vall d'Hebron, Barcelona, Spain**

*Notations to accompany profile: Estimated HIV positive TB cases is a WHO estimate

*For survey settings where less than 100% of cases are sampled, combined estimates are based on the rates of new and previously treated cases obtained in the survey, but weighted by the absolute number of new and previously treated sputum positive TB cases, as published by the national authorities.

PREVALENCE OF DRUG RESISTANCE

Countrywide: 2000

	New		Previous		Combined	
	N	%	N	%	N	%
Total number of strains tested	3	100.0	0	0.0	3	100.0
SUSCEPTIBLE TO ALL 4 DRUGS	3	100.0	0	0.0	3	100.0
ANY RESISTANCE	0	0.0	0	0.0	0	0.0
- Isoniazid (INH)	0	0.0	0	0.0	0	0.0
- Rifampicin (RMP)	0	0.0	0	0.0	0	0.0
- Ethambutol (EMB)	0	0.0	0	0.0	0	0.0
- Streptomycin (SM)	0	0.0	0	0.0	0	0.0
MONORESISTANCE	0	0.0	0	0.0	0	0.0
- Isoniazid (INH)	0	0.0	0	0.0	0	0.0
- Rifampicin (RMP)	0	0.0	0	0.0	0	0.0
- Ethambutol (EMB)	0	0.0	0	0.0	0	0.0
- Streptomycin (SM)	0	0.0	0	0.0	0	0.0
MULTIDRUG RESISTANCE	0	0.0	0	0.0	0	0.0
- INH + RMP	0	0.0	0	0.0	0	0.0
- INH + RMP + EMB	0	0.0	0	0.0	0	0.0
- INH + RMP + SM	0	0.0	0	0.0	0	0.0
- INH + RMP + EMB + SM	0	0.0	0	0.0	0	0.0
OTHER PATTERNS	0	0.0	0	0.0	0	0.0
- INH + EMB	0	0.0	0	0.0	0	0.0
- INH + SM	0	0.0	0	0.0	0	0.0
- INH + EMB + SM	0	0.0	0	0.0	0	0.0
- RMP + EMB	0	0.0	0	0.0	0	0.0
- RMP + SM	0	0.0	0	0.0	0	0.0
- RMP + EMB + SM	0	0.0	0	0.0	0	0.0
- EMB + SM	0	0.0	0	0.0	0	0.0
NUMBER OF DRUGS RESISTANT TO:						
susceptible to 4 drugs	3	100.0	0	0.0	3	100.0
resistant to 1 drug	0	0.0	0	0.0	0	0.0
resistant to 2 drugs	0	0.0	0	0.0	0	0.0
resistant to 3 drugs	0	0.0	0	0.0	0	0.0
resistant to 4 drugs	0	0.0	0	0.0	0	0.0

COUNTRY PROFILES

ARGENTINA

Countrywide: 1999

PROFILE OF THE COUNTRY AND ITS CONTROL PROGRAMME

Population in year of survey	**36,577,000**		Year N.T.P was established	**1960**		
Notification all cases (rate)	**32.5**	**/100,000**	Year of Rifampicin introduction	**1974**		
Estimated incidence (all cases)		**/100,000**	Year of Isoniazid introduction	**1960**		
Notification new sputum smear +	**5234**		Use of Standardized Regimens	**Yes**		
Notification new sputum smear + (rate)	**14.3**	**/100,000**	% Use of Short Course Chemotherapy	**Yes**	**100**	**%**
Treatment Success	**74.3**	**%**	Use of Directly Observed Therapy	**Yes**	**51.6**	**%**
Retreatment cases	**NA**		During continuation phase	**Yes**		
Retreatment as % of NTP	**18**	**%**	Use of Fixed Dose Combination	**Yes**	**90**	**%**
Estimated HIV positive TB cases	**8.0**	**%**	Treatment in private sector	**Cat 2**		

Category 1: virtually all TB patients public sector
Category 2: <15% in private sector
Category 3: 15% or more in private sector

TB drugs available on the private market	**Yes**

CHARACTERISTICS OF THE SURVEY/SURVEILLANCE PROGRAMME

Study Duration	**12 Months**
Target Area	**Countrywide**
Sampling Method	**Cluster**
Culture Media	**Löwenstein-Jensen and BACTEC**
DST Method	**Proportion and BACTEC**
Supranational Reference Laboratory	**Instituto Panamericano de Proteccion de Alimentos y Zoonosis (INPPAZ) Buenos Aires, Argentina**

*Notations to accompany profile:

*For survey settings where less than 100% of cases are sampled, combined estimates are based on the rates of new and previously treated cases obtained in the survey, but weighted by the absolute number of new and previously treated sputum positive TB cases, as published by the national authorities.

COUNTRY PROFILES

PREVALENCE OF DRUG RESISTANCE

Countrywide: 1999

	New		Previous		Combined	
	N	%	N	%	N	%
Total number of strains tested	679	100.0	149	100.0		100.0
SUSCEPTIBLE TO ALL 4 DRUGS	610	89.8	115	77.2		87.6
ANY RESISTANCE	69	10.2	34	22.8		12.4
- Isoniazid (INH)	26	3.8	24	16.1		6.0
- Rifampicin (RMP)	13	1.9	15	10.1		3.4
- Ethambutol (EMB)	16	2.4	10	6.7		3.1
- Streptomycin (SM)	50	7.4	24	16.1		8.9
MONORESISTANCE	51	7.5	15	10.1		8.0
- Isoniazid (INH)	9	1.3	6	4.0		1.8
- Rifampicin (RMP)	1	0.1	0	0.0		0.1
- Ethambutol (EMB)	7	1.0	1	0.7		1.0
- Streptomycin (SM)	34	5.0	8	5.4		5.1
MULTIDRUG RESISTANCE	12	1.8	14	9.4		3.1
- INH + RMP	2	0.3	1	0.7		0.4
- INH + RMP + EMB	0	0.0	2	1.3		0.2
- INH + RMP + SM	2	0.3	5	3.4		0.8
- INH + RMP + EMB + SM	8	1.2	6	4.0		1.7
OTHER PATTERNS	6	0.9	5	3.4		1.3
- INH + EMB	0	0.0	0	0.0		0.0
- INH + SM	5	0.7	3	2.0		1.0
- INH + EMB + SM	0	0.0	1	0.7		0.1
- RMP + EMB	0	0.0	0	0.0		0.0
- RMP + SM	0	0.0	1	0.7		0.1
- RMP + EMB + SM	0	0.0	0	0.0		0.0
- EMB + SM	1	0.1	0	0.0		0.2
NUMBER OF DRUGS RESISTANT TO:						
susceptible to 4 drugs	610	89.8	115	77.2		87.6
resistant to 1 drug	51	7.5	15	10.1		8.0
resistant to 2 drugs	8	1.2	5	3.4		1.6
resistant to 3 drugs	2	0.3	8	5.4		1.1
resistant to 4 drugs	8	1.2	6	4.0		1.7

COUNTRY PROFILES

AUSTRALIA

Countrywide: 2001

PROFILE OF THE COUNTRY AND ITS CONTROL PROGRAMME

Population in year of survey	**19,383,424**		Year N.T.P was established	**1948**		
Notification all cases (rate)		**/100,000**	Year of Rifampicin introduction	**early 1970s**		
Estimated incidence (all cases)	**5.1**	**/100,000**	Year of Isoniazid introduction	**early 1950s**		
Notification new sputum smear +	**261**		Use of Standardized Regimens	**Yes**		
Notification new sputum smear + (rate)	**1.3**	**/100,000**	% Use of Short Course Chemotherapy	**Yes**	**>95**	**%**
Treatment Success		**%**	Use of Directly Observed Therapy	**Yes**	**>95**	**%**
Retreatment cases			During continuation phase	**50%**		
Retreatment as % of NTP		**%**	Use of Fixed Dose Combination	**No**		**%**
Estimated HIV positive TB cases	**2.56**	**%**	Treatment in private sector	**Cat 2**		
			Category 1: virtually all TB patients public sector			
			Category 2: <15% in private sector			
			Category 3: 15% or more in private sector			
			TB drugs available on the private market	**No**		

CHARACTERISTICS OF THE SURVEY/SURVEILLANCE PROGRAMME

Study Duration	**12 Months**
Target Area	**Countrywide**
Sampling Method	**All cases**
Culture Media	**Various**
DST Method	**Radiometric**
Supranational Reference Laboratory	**Queensland Mycobacterium Reference Laboratory, Australia**

*Notations to accompany profile: Estimated HIV positive TB cases is a WHO estimate

Only 29.6% of isolates tested for SM.

*For survey settings where less than 100% of cases are sampled, combined estimates are based on the rates of new and previously treated cases obtained in the survey, but weighted by the absolute number of new and previously treated sputum positive TB cases, as published by the national authorities.

COUNTRY PROFILES

PREVALENCE OF DRUG RESISTANCE

Countrywide: 2001

	New		Previous		Combined	
	N	%	N	%	N	%
Total number of strains tested					770	100.0
SUSCEPTIBLE TO ALL 4 DRUGS					**694**	**90.1**
ANY RESISTANCE					**76**	**9.9**
- Isoniazid (INH)					66	8.6
- Rifampicin (RMP)					13	1.7
- Ethambutol (EMB)					2	0.3
- Streptomycin (SM)					21	2.7
MONORESISTANCE					**53**	**6.9**
- Isoniazid (INH)					43	5.6
- Rifampicin (RMP)					1	0.1
- Ethambutol (EMB)					1	0.1
- Streptomycin (SM)					8	1.0
MULTIDRUG RESISTANCE					**12**	**1.6**
- INH + RMP					10	1.3
- INH + RMP + EMB					0	0.0
- INH + RMP + SM					1	0.1
- INH + RMP + EMB + SM					1	0.1
OTHER PATTERNS					**11**	**1.4**
- INH + EMB					0	0.0
- INH + SM					11	1.4
- INH + EMB + SM					0	0.0
- RMP + EMB					0	0.0
- RMP + SM					0	0.0
- RMP + EMB + SM					0	0.0
- EMB + SM					0	0.0
NUMBER OF DRUGS RESISTANT TO:						
susceptible to 4 drugs					694	90.1
resistant to 1 drug					53	6.9
resistant to 2 drugs					21	2.7
resistant to 3 drugs					1	0.1
resistant to 4 drugs					1	0.1

COUNTRY PROFILES

AUSTRIA

Countrywide: 2000

PROFILE OF THE COUNTRY AND ITS CONTROL PROGRAMME

Population in year of survey	**8,080,000**		Year N.T.P was established	
Notification all cases (rate)	**15**	**/100,000**	Year of Rifampicin introduction	
Estimated incidence (all cases)		**/100,000**	Year of Isoniazid introduction	
Notification new sputum smear +	**324**		Use of Standardized Regimens	
Notification new sputum smear + (rate)	**4**	**/100,000**	% Use of Short Course Chemotherapy	**%**
Treatment Success		**%**	Use of Directly Observed Therapy	**%**
Retreatment cases	**25**		During continuation phase	
Retreatment as % of NTP		**%**	Use of Fixed Dose Combination	**%**
Estimated HIV positive TB cases	**6.92**	**%**	Treatment in private sector	

Category 1: virtually all TB patients public sector
Category 2: <15% in private sector
Category 3: 15% or more in private sector

TB drugs available on the private market

CHARACTERISTICS OF THE SURVEY/SURVEILLANCE PROGRAMME

Study Duration	**12 Months**
Target Area	**Countrywide**
Sampling Method	**All cases**
Culture Media	
DST Method	
Supranational Reference Laboratory	

*Notations to accompany profile: Estimated HIV positive TB cases is a WHO estimate

*For survey settings where less than 100% of cases are sampled, combined estimates are based on the rates of new and previously treated cases obtained in the survey, but weighted by the absolute number of new and previously treated sputum positive TB cases, as published by the national authorities.

PREVALENCE OF DRUG RESISTANCE

Countrywide: 2000

	New		Previous		Combined	
	N	%	N	%	N	%
Total number of strains tested	694	100.0	67	100.0	761	100.0
SUSCEPTIBLE TO ALL 4 DRUGS	**663**	**95.5**	**61**	**91.0**	**724**	**95.1**
ANY RESISTANCE	**31**	**4.5**	**6**	**9.0**	**37**	**4.9**
- Isoniazid (INH)	20	2.9	2	3.0	22	2.9
- Rifampicin (RMP)	5	0.7	1	1.5	6	0.8
- Ethambutol (EMB)	1	0.1	0	0.0	1	0.1
- Streptomycin (SM)	18	2.6	5	7.5	23	3.0
MONORESISTANCE	**21**	**3.0**	**5**	**7.5**	**26**	**3.4**
- Isoniazid (INH)	10	1.4	1	1.5	11	1.4
- Rifampicin (RMP)	2	0.3	0	0.0	2	0.3
- Ethambutol (EMB)	1	0.1	0	0.0	1	0.1
- Streptomycin (SM)	8	1.2	4	6.0	12	1.6
MULTIDRUG RESISTANCE	**3**	**0.4**	**1**	**1.5**	**4**	**0.5**
- INH + RMP	0	0.0	0	0.0	0	0.0
- INH + RMP + EMB	0	0.0	0	0.0	0	0.0
- INH + RMP + SM	3	0.4	1	1.5	4	0.5
- INH + RMP + EMB + SM	0	0.0	0	0.0	0	0.0
OTHER PATTERNS	**7**	**1.0**	**0**	**0.0**	**7**	**0.9**
- INH + EMB	0	0.0	0	0.0	0	0.0
- INH + SM	7	1.0	0	0.0	7	0.9
- INH + EMB + SM	0	0.0	0	0.0	0	0.0
- RMP + EMB	0	0.0	0	0.0	0	0.0
- RMP + SM	0	0.0	0	0.0	0	0.0
- RMP + EMB + SM	0	0.0	0	0.0	0	0.0
- EMB + SM	0	0.0	0	0.0	0	0.0
NUMBER OF DRUGS RESISTANT TO:						
susceptible to 4 drugs	663	95.5	61	91.0	724	95.1
resistant to 1 drug	21	3.0	5	7.5	26	3.4
resistant to 2 drugs	7	1.0	0	0.0	7	0.9
resistant to 3 drugs	3	0.4	1	1.5	4	0.5
resistant to 4 drugs	0	0.0	0	0.0	0	0.0

COUNTRY PROFILES

BELGIUM

Countrywide: 2000

PROFILE OF THE COUNTRY AND ITS CONTROL PROGRAMME

Population in year of survey	**10,239,085**		Year N.T.P was established			
Notification all cases (rate)	**12.8**	**/100,000**	Year of Rifampicin introduction	**1967**		
Estimated incidence (all cases)	**12.8**	**/100,000**	Year of Isoniazid introduction			
Notification new sputum smear +	**361**		Use of Standardized Regimens	**Yes**		
Notification new sputum smear + (rate)	**3.5**	**/100,000**	% Use of Short Course Chemotherapy			**%**
Treatment Success	**75.5**	**%**	Use of Directly Observed Therapy	**Yes**	**2**	**%**
Retreatment cases	**124**		During continuation phase	**Yes**		
Retreatment as % of NTP		**%**	Use of Fixed Dose Combination	**Yes**	**4**	**%**
Estimated HIV positive TB cases	**4.89**	**%**	Treatment in private sector	**Cat 3**		

Category 1: virtually all TB patients public sector
Category 2: <15% in private sector
Category 3: 15% or more in private sector

TB drugs available on the private market	**Rx required**

CHARACTERISTICS OF THE SURVEY/SURVEILLANCE PROGRAMME

Study Duration	**12 Months**
Target Area	**Countrywide**
Sampling Method	**All cases**
Culture Media	**Löwenstein-Jensen and BACTEC**
DST Method	**Proportion**
Supranational Reference Laboratory	**Prince Leopold Institute of Tropical Medicine, Antwerp, Belgium**

*Notations to accompany profile: Estimated HIV positive TB cases is a WHO estimate
The combined column includes patients with unknown treatment history
Streptomycin is not routinely tested

*For survey settings where less than 100% of cases are sampled, combined estimates are based on the rates of new and previously treated cases obtained in the survey, but weighted by the absolute number of new and previously treated sputum positive TB cases, as published by the national authorities.

COUNTRY PROFILES

PREVALENCE OF DRUG RESISTANCE

Countrywide: 2000

	New		Previous		Combined	
	N	%	N	%	N	%
Total number of strains tested	562	100.0	78	100.0	730	100.0
SUSCEPTIBLE TO ALL 4 DRUGS	**528**	**94.0**	**67**	**85.9**	**678**	**92.9**
ANY RESISTANCE	**34**	**6.0**	**11**	**14.1**	**52**	**7.1**
- Isoniazid (INH)	30	5.3	10	12.8	47	6.4
- Rifampicin (RMP)	9	1.6	5	6.4	14	1.9
- Ethambutol (EMB)	6	1.1	4	5.1	12	1.6
- Streptomycin (SM)	-	-	-	-	-	-
MONORESISTANCE	**25**	**4.4**	**6**	**7.7**	**36**	**4.9**
- Isoniazid (INH)	21	3.7	5	6.4	31	4.2
- Rifampicin (RMP)	2	0.4	1	1.3	3	0.4
- Ethambutol (EMB)	2	0.4	0	0.0	2	0.3
- Streptomycin (SM)	-	-	-	-	-	-
MULTIDRUG RESISTANCE	**7**	**1.2**	**4**	**5.1**	**11**	**1.5**
- INH + RMP	5	0.9	1	1.3	6	0.8
- INH + RMP + EMB	2	0.4	3	3.8	5	0.7
- INH + RMP + SM	-	-	-	-	-	-
- INH + RMP + EMB + SM	-	-	-	-	-	-
OTHER PATTERNS	**2**	**0.4**	**1**	**1.3**	**5**	**0.7**
- INH + EMB	2	0.4	1	1.3	5	0.7
- INH + SM	-	-	-	-	-	-
- INH + EMB + SM	-	-	-	-	-	-
- RMP + EMB	0	0.0	0	0.0	0	0.0
- RMP + SM	-	-	-	-	-	-
- RMP + EMB + SM	-	-	-	-	-	-
- EMB + SM	-	-	-	-	-	-
NUMBER OF DRUGS RESISTANT TO:						
susceptible to 4 drugs	528	94.0	67	85.9	678	92.9
resistant to 1 drug	25	4.4	6	7.7	36	4.9
resistant to 2 drugs	7	1.2	2	2.6	11	1.5
resistant to 3 drugs	2	0.4	3	3.8	5	0.7
resistant to 4 drugs	-	-	-	-	-	-

COUNTRY PROFILES

BOSNIA AND HERZEGOVINA

Countrywide: 2000

PROFILE OF THE COUNTRY AND ITS CONTROL PROGRAMME

Population in year of survey	**3,977,000**		Year N.T.P was established	**1998**		
Notification all cases (rate)	**60**	**/100,000**	Year of Rifampicin introduction	**1974**		
Estimated incidence (all cases)	**61**	**/100,000**	Year of Isoniazid introduction	**1957**		
Notification new sputum smear +	**759**		Use of Standardized Regimens	**Yes**		
Notification new sputum smear + (rate)	**16**	**/100,000**	% Use of Short Course Chemotherapy	**Yes**	**90**	**%**
Treatment Success	**84**	**%**	Use of Directly Observed Therapy	**Yes**	**90**	**%**
Retreatment cases	**145**		During continuation phase	**Yes**		
Retreatment as % of NTP	**12**	**%**	Use of Fixed Dose Combination	**No**		**%**
Estimated HIV positive TB cases	**0.14**	**%**	Treatment in private sector Category 1: virtually all TB patients public sector Category 2: <15% in private sector Category 3: 15% or more in private sector	**Cat 1**		
			TB drugs available on the private market	**1st line infrequently**		

CHARACTERISTICS OF THE SURVEY/SURVEILLANCE PROGRAMME

Study Duration	**12 Months**
Target Area	**Countrywide**
Sampling Method	**All cases**
Culture Media	**Löwenstein-Jensen**
DST Method	**Proportion**
Supranational Reference Laboratory	**National Reference Center for Mycobacteria, Borstel, Germany**

*Notations to accompany profile: Estimated HIV positive TB cases is a WHO estimate
The combined column includes patients with unknown treatment history

*For survey settings where less than 100% of cases are sampled, combined estimates are based on the rates of new and previously treated cases obtained in the survey, but weighted by the absolute number of new and previously treated sputum positive TB cases, as published by the national authorities.

COUNTRY PROFILES

PREVALENCE OF DRUG RESISTANCE

Countrywide: 2000

	New		Previous		Combined	
	N	%	N	%	N	%
Total number of strains tested	993	100.0	153	100.0	1,153	100.0
SUSCEPTIBLE TO ALL 4 DRUGS	**969**	**97.6**	**133**	**86.9**	**1,107**	**96.0**
ANY RESISTANCE	**24**	**2.4**	**20**	**13.1**	**46**	**4.0**
- Isoniazid (INH)	5	0.5	5	3.3	11	1.0
- Rifampicin (RMP)	7	0.7	9	5.9	17	1.5
- Ethambutol (EMB)	11	1.1	10	6.5	21	1.8
- Streptomycin (SM)	5	0.5	8	5.2	15	1.3
MONORESISTANCE	**20**	**2.0**	**13**	**8.5**	**34**	**2.9**
- Isoniazid (INH)	3	0.3	2	1.3	5	0.4
- Rifampicin (RMP)	6	0.6	4	2.6	10	0.9
- Ethambutol (EMB)	9	0.9	5	3.3	14	1.2
- Streptomycin (SM)	2	0.2	2	1.3	5	0.4
MULTIDRUG RESISTANCE	**1**	**0.1**	**3**	**2.0**	**5**	**0.4**
- INH + RMP	1	0.1	0	0.0	1	0.1
- INH + RMP + EMB	0	0.0	0	0.0	0	0.0
- INH + RMP + SM	0	0.0	1	0.7	2	0.2
- INH + RMP + EMB + SM	0	0.0	2	1.3	2	0.2
OTHER PATTERNS	**3**	**0.3**	**4**	**2.6**	**7**	**0.6**
- INH + EMB	0	0.0	0	0.0	0	0.0
- INH + SM	1	0.1	0	0.0	1	0.1
- INH + EMB + SM	0	0.0	0	0.0	0	0.0
- RMP + EMB	0	0.0	1	0.7	1	0.1
- RMP + SM	0	0.0	1	0.7	1	0.1
- RMP + EMB + SM	0	0.0	0	0.0	0	0.0
- EMB + SM	2	0.2	2	1.3	4	0.3
NUMBER OF DRUGS RESISTANT TO:						
susceptible to 4 drugs	969	97.6	133	86.9	1,107	96.0
resistant to 1 drug	20	2.0	13	8.5	34	2.9
resistant to 2 drugs	4	0.4	4	2.6	8	0.7
resistant to 3 drugs	6	0.0	1	0.7	2	0.2
resistant to 4 drugs	0	0.0	2	1.3	2	0.2

COUNTRY PROFILES

BOTSWANA

Countrywide: 2002

PROFILE OF THE COUNTRY AND ITS CONTROL PROGRAMME

Population in year of survey	1,680,863		Year N.T.P was established	1975		
Notification all cases (rate)	442	/100,000	Year of Rifampicin introduction	1986		
Estimated incidence (all cases)	620	/100,000	Year of Isoniazid introduction	NA		
Notification new sputum smear +	3128		Use of Standardized Regimens	Yes		
Notification new sputum smear + (rate)	186	/100,000	% Use of Short Course Chemotherapy	Yes	100	%
Treatment Success	71	%	Use of Directly Observed Therapy	Yes	100	%
Retreatment cases	306		During continuation phase	Yes		
Retreatment as % of NTP	7.2	%	Use of Fixed Dose Combination	No		%
Estimated HIV positive TB cases	60.0	%	Treatment in private sector	Cat 1		

Category 1: virtually all TB patients public sector
Category 2: <15% in private sector
Category 3: 15% or more in private sector

TB drugs available on the private market   **No**

CHARACTERISTICS OF THE SURVEY/SURVEILLANCE PROGRAMME

Study Duration	**8 Months**
Target Area	**Countrywide**
Sampling Method	**All diagnostic centers**
Culture Media	**BACTEC MGIT and Löwenstein-Jensen**
DST Method	**Resistance ratio method**
Supranational Reference Laboratory	**Centers for Disease Control and Prevention (CDC), Atlanta, United States of America**

*Notations to accompany profile: Estimated HIV positive TB cases is a WHO estimate
Retreatment indicates sputum smear positive pulmonary cases only

*For survey settings where less than 100% of cases are sampled, combined estimates are based on the rates of new and previously treated cases obtained in the survey, but weighted by the absolute number of new and previously treated sputum positive TB cases, as published by the national authorities.

COUNTRY PROFILES

PREVALENCE OF DRUG RESISTANCE

Countrywide: 2002

	New		Previous		Combined	
	N	%	N	%	N	%
Total number of strains tested	1,182	100.0	106	100.0		100.0
SUSCEPTIBLE TO ALL 4 DRUGS	**1,059**	**89,6**	**82**	**77.3**		**88.5**
ANY RESISTANCE	**123**	**10.4**	**23**	**21.7**		**11.4**
- Isoniazid (INH)	53	4.5	15	14.2		5.3
- Rifampicin (RMP)	24	2.0	13	12.3		2.9
- Ethambutol (EMB)	15	1.3	9	8.5		1.9
- Streptomycin (SM)	82	6.9	17	16.0		7.7
MONORESISTANCE	**86**	**7.3**	**7**	**6.6**		**7.2**
- Isoniazid (INH)	22	1.9	0	0.0		1.7
- Rifampicin (RMP)	10	0.8	0	0.0		0.8
- Ethambutol (EMB)	2	0.2	2	1.9		0.3
- Streptomycin (SM)	52	4.4	5	4.7		4.4
MULTIDRUG RESISTANCE	**10**	**0.8**	**11**	**10.4**		**1.7**
- INH + RMP	3	0.3	3	2.8		0.5
- INH + RMP + EMB	2	0.2	2	1.9		0.3
- INH + RMP + SM	3	0.3	1	0.9		0.3
- INH + RMP + EMB + SM	2	0.2	5	4.7		0.6
OTHER PATTERNS	**27**	**2.3**	**6**	**5.7**		**2.6**
- INH + EMB	2	0.2	0	0.0		0.2
- INH + SM	15	1.3	4	3.8		1.5
- INH + EMB + SM	4	0.3	0	0.0		0.3
- RMP + EMB	0	0.0	0	0.0		0.0
- RMP + SM	3	0.3	2	1.9		0.4
- RMP + EMB + SM	1	0.1	0	0.0		0.1
- EMB + SM	2	0.2	0	0.0		0.2
NUMBER OF DRUGS RESISTANT TO:						
susceptible to 4 drugs	1,059	89.6	82	77.3		88.5
resistant to 1 drug	86	7.3	7	6.6		7.2
resistant to 2 drugs	25	2.1	9	8.5		2.7
resistant to 3 drugs	10	0.8	3	2.8		1.0
resistant to 4 drugs	2	0.2	5	4.7		0.6

CAMBODIA

Countrywide: 2001

PROFILE OF THE COUNTRY AND ITS CONTROL PROGRAMME

Population in year of survey	**11,739,999**		Year N.T.P was established	**1980**		
Notification all cases (rate)	**164**	**/100,000**	Year of Rifampicin introduction	**1994**		
Estimated incidence (all cases)	**573**	**/100,000**	Year of Isoniazid introduction	**1980**		
Notification new sputum smear +	**14361**		Use of Standardized Regimens	**Yes**		
Notification new sputum smear + (rate)	**122**	**/100,000**	% Use of Short Course Chemotherapy	**Yes**	**100**	**%**
Treatment Success	**91**	**%**	Use of Directly Observed Therapy	**Yes**	**>90**	**%**
Retreatment cases	**833**		During continuation phase	**No**		
Retreatment as % of NTP		**%**	Use of Fixed Dose Combination	**Yes**	**100**	**%**
Estimated HIV positive TB cases	**12.24**	**%**	Treatment in private sector	**Cat 3**		

Category 1: virtually all TB patients public sector
Category 2: <15% in private sector
Category 3: 15% or more in private sector

TB drugs available on the private market	**All drugs**

CHARACTERISTICS OF THE SURVEY/SURVEILLANCE PROGRAMME

Study Duration	**7 Months**
Target Area	**Countrywide**
Sampling Method	**Proportionate Cluster**
Culture Media	**Ogawa and Löwenstein-Jensen**
DST Method	**Proportion**
Supranational Reference Laboratory	**Research Institute of Tuberculosis (RIT), Tokyo, Japan**

*Notations to accompany profile: Estimated HIV positive TB cases is a WHO estimate
Retreatment indicates sputum smear positive pulmonary cases only

*For survey settings where less than 100% of cases are sampled, combined estimates are based on the rates of new and previously treated cases obtained in the survey, but weighted by the absolute number of new and previously treated sputum positive TB cases, as published by the national authorities.

COUNTRY PROFILES

PREVALENCE OF DRUG RESISTANCE

Countrywide: 2001

	New		Previous		Combined	
	N	%	N	%	N	%
Total number of strains tested	638	100.0	96	100.0		100.0
SUSCEPTIBLE TO ALL 4 DRUGS	**572**	**89.7**	**79**	**82.3**		**89.3**
ANY RESISTANCE	**66**	**10.3**	**17**	**17.7**		**10.7**
- Isoniazid (INH)	41	6.4	16	16.7		7.0
- Rifampicin (RMP)	4	0.6	3	3.1		0.8
- Ethambutol (EMB)	1	0.1	0	0.0		0.1
- Streptomycin (SM)	32	5.0	7	7.3		5.1
MONORESISTANCE	**54**	**8.4**	**10**	**10.4**		**8.6**
- Isoniazid (INH)	30	4.7	9	9.3		5.0
- Rifampicin (RMP)	3	0.5	0	0.0		0.4
- Ethambutol (EMB)	0	0.0	0	0.0		0.0
- Streptomycin (SM)	21	3.3	1	1.0		3.2
MULTIDRUG RESISTANCE	**0**	**0.0**	**3**	**3.1**		**0.2**
- INH + RMP	0	0.0	1	1.0		0.3
- INH + RMP + EMB	0	0.0	0	0.0		0.0
- INH + RMP + SM	0	0.0	2	2.0		0.1
- INH + RMP + EMB + SM	0	0.0	0	0.0		0.0
OTHER PATTERNS	**12**	**1.9**	**4**	**4.2**		**2.0**
- INH + EMB	1	0.1	0	0.0		0.1
- INH + SM	10	1.6	4	4.2		1.7
- INH + EMB + SM	0	0.0	0	0.0		0.0
- RMP + EMB	0	0.0	0	0.0		0.0
- RMP + SM	1	0.1	0	0.0		0.1
- RMP + EMB + SM	0	0.0	0	0.0		0.0
- EMB + SM	0	0.0	0	0.0		0.0
NUMBER OF DRUGS RESISTANT TO:						
susceptible to 4 drugs	572	89.7	79	82.3		89.3
resistant to 1 drug	54	8.4	10	10.4		8.6
resistant to 2 drugs	12	1.9	5	5.2		2.1
resistant to 3 drugs	0	0.0	2	2.0		0.1
resistant to 4 drugs	0	0.0	0	0.0		0.0

COUNTRY PROFILES

CANADA

Countrywide: 2000

PROFILE OF THE COUNTRY AND ITS CONTROL PROGRAMME

Population in year of survey	**30,941,252**		Year N.T.P was established	**1994**		
Notification all cases (rate)	**4.0**	**/100,000**	Year of Rifampicin introduction	**1969**		
Estimated incidence (all cases)	**5.5**	**/100,000**	Year of Isoniazid introduction	**1952**		
Notification new sputum smear +	**506**		Use of Standardized Regimens	**Yes, recommended**		
Notification new sputum smear + (rate)	**1.6**	**/100,000**	% Use of Short Course Chemotherapy	**NA**		**%**
Treatment Success		**%**	Use of Directly Observed Therapy	**Yes**	**20**	**%**
Retreatment cases	**47**		During continuation phase	**Yes**		
Retreatment as % of NTP		**%**	Use of Fixed Dose Combination	**Yes**		**%**
Estimated HIV positive TB cases	**9.06**	**%**	Treatment in private sector	**Cat 1**		

Category 1: virtually all TB patients public sector
Category 2: <15% in private sector
Category 3: 15% or more in private sector

TB drugs available on the private market	**No**	

CHARACTERISTICS OF THE SURVEY/SURVEILLANCE PROGRAMME

Study Duration	**12 Months**
Target Area	**Countrywide**
Sampling Method	**All cases**
Culture Media	**Various**
DST Method	**Indirect proportion using radiometric method**
Supranational Reference Laboratory	

*Notations to accompany profile: Estimated HIV positive TB cases is a WHO estimate
Retreatment indicates sputum smear positive pulmonary cases only

*For survey settings where less than 100% of cases are sampled, combined estimates are based on the rates of new and previously treated cases obtained in the survey, but weighted by the absolute number of new and previously treated sputum positive TB cases, as published by the national authorities.

COUNTRY PROFILES

PREVALENCE OF DRUG RESISTANCE

Countrywide: 2000

	New		Previous		Combined	
	N	%	N	%	N	%
Total number of strains tested	1,244	100.0	119	100.0	1,363	100.0
SUSCEPTIBLE TO ALL 4 DRUGS	**1,138**	**91.5**	**99**	**83.2**	**1,237**	**90.8**
ANY RESISTANCE	**106**	**8.5**	**20**	**16.8**	**126**	**9.2**
- Isoniazid (INH)	84	6.8	15	12.6	99	7.3
- Rifampicin (RMP)	11	0.9	5	4.2	16	1.2
- Ethambutol (EMB)	13	1.0	4	3.4	17	1.2
- Streptomycin (SM)	43	3.4	8	6.7	51	3.7
MONORESISTANCE	**73**	**5.8**	**13**	**10.9**	**86**	**6.3**
- Isoniazid (INH)	53	4.3	8	6.7	61	4.5
- Rifampicin (RMP)	0	0.0	1	0.8	1	0.0
- Ethambutol (EMB)	3	0.2	0	0.0	3	0.2
- Streptomycin (SM)	17	1.4	4	3.4	21	1.5
MULTIDRUG RESISTANCE	**9**	**0.7**	**4**	**3.4**	**13**	**0.9**
- INH + RMP	2	0.1	1	0.8	3	0.2
- INH + RMP + EMB	2	0.1	1	0.8	3	0.2
- INH + RMP + SM	3	0.2	1	0.8	4	0.3
- INH + RMP + EMB + SM	2	0.1	1	0.8	3	0.2
OTHER PATTERNS	**24**	**1.9**	**3**	**2.5**	**27**	**1.9**
- INH + EMB	1	0.0	1	0.8	2	0.1
- INH + SM	18	1.4	1	0.8	19	1.4
- INH + EMB + SM	3	0.2	1	0.8	4	0.2
- RMP + EMB	2	0.1	0	0.0	2	0.1
- RMP + SM	0	0.0	0	0.0	0	0.0
- RMP + EMB + SM	0	0.0	0	0.0	0	0.0
- EMB + SM	0	0.0	0	0.0	0	0.0
NUMBER OF DRUGS RESISTANT TO:						
susceptible to 4 drugs	1,138	91.5	99	83.2	1,237	90.8
resistant to 1 drug	73	5.8	13	10.9	86	6.3
resistant to 2 drugs	23	1.8	3	2.5	26	1.9
resistant to 3 drugs	8	0.6	3	2.5	11	0.8
resistant to 4 drugs	2	0.1	1	0.8	3	0.2

COUNTRY PROFILES

CHILE

Countrywide: 2001

PROFILE OF THE COUNTRY AND ITS CONTROL PROGRAMME

Population in year of survey	**15,401,952**		Year N.T.P was established	**1973**		
Notification all cases (rate)	**19.7**	**/100,000**	Year of Rifampicin introduction	**1970**		
Estimated incidence (all cases)	**20.3**	**/100,000**	Year of Isoniazid introduction	**1955**		
Notification new sputum smear +	**1355**		Use of Standardized Regimens	**Yes**		
Notification new sputum smear + (rate)	**8.8**	**/100,000**	% Use of Short Course Chemotherapy	**Yes**	**100**	**%**
Treatment Success	**82**	**%**	Use of Directly Observed Therapy	**Yes**	**>95**	**%**
Retreatment cases	**234**		During continuation phase	**Yes**		
Retreatment as % of NTP	**14.7**	**%**	Use of Fixed Dose Combination	**No**		**%**
Estimated HIV positive TB cases	**0.63**	**%**	Treatment in private sector	**Cat 2**		

Category 1: virtually all TB patients public sector
Category 2: <15% in private sector
Category 3: 15% or more in private sector

TB drugs available on the private market — **No**

CHARACTERISTICS OF THE SURVEY/SURVEILLANCE PROGRAMME

Study Duration	**6 Months**
Target Area	**Countrywide**
Sampling Method	**Cluster**
Culture Media	**Löwenstein-Jensen**
DST Method	**Proportion method and MGIT 960**
Supranational Reference Laboratory	**Instituto de Salud Pública de Chile, Santiago, Chile**

*Notations to accompany profile: Estimated HIV positive TB cases is a WHO estimate
Retreatment indicates sputum smear positive pulmonary cases only

*For survey settings where less than 100% of cases are sampled, combined estimates are based on the rates of new and previously treated cases obtained in the survey, but weighted by the absolute number of new and previously treated sputum positive TB cases, as published by the national authorities.

COUNTRY PROFILES

PREVALENCE OF DRUG RESISTANCE

Countrywide: 2001

	New		Previous		Combined	
	N	%	N	%	N	%
Total number of strains tested	867	100.0	291	100.0		100.0
SUSCEPTIBLE TO ALL 4 DRUGS	**776**	**89.5**	**231**	**74.9**		**86.3**
ANY RESISTANCE	**91**	**11.7**	**60**	**25.1**		**13.7**
- Isoniazid (INH)	39	5.0	50	21.6		7.5
- Rifampicin (RMP)	7	0.9	17	5.8		2.2
- Ethambutol (EMB)	2	0.2	10	4.3		0.9
- Streptomycin (SM)	78	10.0	52	22.5		11.9
MONORESISTANCE	**64**	**8.2**	**37**	**16.0**		**9.4**
- Isoniazid (INH)	12	1.5	12	5.2		2.1
- Rifampicin (RMP)	1	0.1	6	2.6		0.5
- Ethambutol (EMB)	0	0.0	0	0.0		0.0
- Streptomycin (SM)	51	6.5	19	5.1		6.8
MULTIDRUG RESISTANCE	**6**	**0.7**	**11**	**4.8**		**1.4**
- INH + RMP	0	0.0	0	0.0		0.0
- INH + RMP + EMB	0	0.0	3	1.3		0.2
- INH + RMP + SM	4	0.5	1	0.4		0.5
- INH + RMP + EMB + SM	2	0.2	7	3.0		0.7
OTHER PATTERNS	**21**	**2.7**	**10**	**4.3**		**2.9**
- INH + EMB	0	0.0	0	0.0		0.0
- INH + SM	21	2.7	10	4.3		2.9
- INH + EMB + SM	0	0.0	0	0.0		0.0
- RMP + EMB	0	0.0	0	0.0		0.0
- RMP + SM	0	0.0	0	0.0		0.0
- RMP + EMB + SM	0	0.0	0	0.0		0.0
- EMB + SM	0	0.0	0	0.0		0.0
NUMBER OF DRUGS RESISTANT TO:						
susceptible to 4 drugs	776	89.5	231	74.9		86.3
resistant to 1 drug	64	8.2	37	16.0		9.4
resistant to 2 drugs	21	2.7	10	4.3		2.9
resistant to 3 drugs	4	0.5	4	1.7		0.7
resistant to 4 drugs	2	0.3	7	3.0		0.7

COUNTRY PROFILES

CHINA

Henan: 2001

PROFILE OF THE COUNTRY AND ITS CONTROL PROGRAMME

Population in year of survey	**94,350,000**		Year N.T.P was established	**1991**	
Notification all cases (rate)	**38.5**	**/100,000**	Year of Rifampicin introduction	**1972**	
Estimated incidence (all cases)		**/100,000**	Year of Isoniazid introduction	**1951**	
Notification new sputum smear +	**13942**		Use of Standardized Regimens	**Yes**	
Notification new sputum smear + (rate)	**14.8**	**/100,000**	% Use of Short Course Chemotherapy	**Yes**	**%**
Treatment Success		**%**	Use of Directly Observed Therapy	**Yes**	**%**
Retreatment cases	**1201**		During continuation phase	**Yes**	
Retreatment as % of NTP		**%**	Use of Fixed Dose Combination	**Yes 42**	**%**
Estimated HIV positive TB cases	**NA**	**%**	Treatment in private sector	**Cat 3**	

Category 1: virtually all TB patients public sector
Category 2: <15% in private sector
Category 3: 15% or more in private sector

TB drugs available on the private market	**All 1st line drugs including PZA**

CHARACTERISTICS OF THE SURVEY/SURVEILLANCE PROGRAMME

Study Duration	**12 Months**
Target Area	**Province**
Sampling Method	**Proportionate cluster**
Culture Media	**Ogawa and Löwenstein-Jensen**
DST Method	**Proportion**
Supranational Reference Laboratory	**Korean Institute of Tuberculosis (KIT), Seoul, Republic of Korea**

*Notations to accompany profile: Retreatment indicates sputum smear positive pulmonary cases only

*For survey settings where less than 100% of cases are sampled, combined estimates are based on the rates of new and previously treated cases obtained in the survey, but weighted by the absolute number of new and previously treated sputum positive TB cases, as published by the national authorities.

PREVALENCE OF DRUG RESISTANCE

Henan: 2001

	New		Previous		Combined	
	N	%	N	%	N	%
Total number of strains tested	1,222	100.0	265	100.0		100.0
SUSCEPTIBLE TO ALL 4 DRUGS	**858**	**70.2**	**104**	**39.2**		**67.7**
ANY RESISTANCE	**364**	**29.8**	**161**	**60.8**		**32.3**
- Isoniazid (INH)	208	17.0	125	47.2		19.4
- Rifampicin (RMP)	117	9.6	113	42.6		12.3
- Ethambutol (EMB)	53	4.3	48	18.1		5.4
- Streptomycin (SM)	271	22.2	114	43.0		23.8
MONORESISTANCE	**190**	**15.6**	**38**	**14.3**		**15.5**
- Isoniazid (INH)	40	3.3	11	4.2		3.3
- Rifampicin (RMP)	17	1.4	8	3.0		1.6
- Ethambutol (EMB)	10	0.8	4	1.5		0.9
- Streptomycin (SM)	123	10.1	15	5.7		9.7
MULTIDRUG RESISTANCE	**95**	**7.8**	**97**	**36.6**		**10.1**
- INH + RMP	18	1.5	20	7.5		5.5
- INH + RMP + EMB	5	0.4	2	0.8		0.4
- INH + RMP + SM	47	3.9	41	15.5		4.8
- INH + RMP + EMB + SM	25	2.0	34	12.8		2.9
OTHER PATTERNS	**79**	**6.5**	**26**	**9.8**		**6.7**
- INH + EMB	2	0.2	0	0.0		0.2
- INH + SM	62	5.1	13	4.9		5.1
- INH + EMB + SM	9	0.7	4	1.5		0.8
- RMP + EMB	1	0.1	2	0.8		0.1
- RMP + SM	4	0.3	5	1.9		0.5
- RMP + EMB + SM	0	0.0	1	0.4		0.0
- EMB + SM	1	0.1	1	0.4		0.1
NUMBER OF DRUGS RESISTANT TO:						
susceptible to 4 drugs	858	70.2	104	39.2		67.7
resistant to 1 drug	190	15.6	38	14.3		15.5
resistant to 2 drugs	88	7.1	41	15.5		7.9
resistant to 3 drugs	61	5.0	48	18.1		6.0
resistant to 4 drugs	25	2.0	34	12.9		2.9

CHINA

Hubei: 1999

PROFILE OF THE COUNTRY AND ITS CONTROL PROGRAMME

Population in year of survey	**59,165,000**		Year N.T.P was established	**1990**		
Notification all cases (rate)	**55.7**	**/100,000**	Year of Rifampicin introduction	**1997**		
Estimated incidence (all cases)	**440**	**/100,000**	Year of Isoniazid introduction	**1951**		
Notification new sputum smear +	**17765**		Use of Standardized Regimens	**Yes**		
Notification new sputum smear + (rate)	**30.02**	**/100,000**	% Use of Short Course Chemotherapy	**Yes**	**100**	**%**
Treatment Success		**%**	Use of Directly Observed Therapy	**Yes**	**95**	**%**
Retreatment cases	**5868**		During continuation phase	**Yes**		
Retreatment as % of NTP	**20**	**%**	Use of Fixed Dose Combination	**Yes**	**100**	**%**
Estimated HIV positive TB cases	**NA**	**%**	Treatment in private sector	**Cat 2**		

Category 1: virtually all TB patients public sector
Category 2: <15% in private sector
Category 3: 15% or more in private sector

TB drugs available on the private market	**All**

CHARACTERISTICS OF THE SURVEY/SURVEILLANCE PROGRAMME

Study Duration	**10 Months**
Target Area	**Province**
Sampling Method	**Cluster**
Culture Media	**Löwenstein-Jensen**
DST Method	**Proportion**
Supranational Reference Laboratory	**Korean Institute of Tuberculosis (KIT), Seoul, Republic of Korea**

*Notations to accompany profile: Retreatment indicates sputum smear positive pulmonary cases only

*For survey settings where less than 100% of cases are sampled, combined estimates are based on the rates of new and previously treated cases obtained in the survey, but weighted by the absolute number of new and previously treated sputum positive TB cases, as published by the national authorities.

PREVALENCE OF DRUG RESISTANCE

Hubei: 1999

	New		Previous		Combined	
	N	%	N	%	N	%
Total number of strains tested	859	100.0	238	100.0		100.0
SUSCEPTIBLE TO ALL 4 DRUGS	**709**	**82.5**	**132**	**55.5**		**75.8**
ANY RESISTANCE	**150**	**17.5**	**106**	**44.5**		**24.2**
- Isoniazid (INH)	83	9.7	79	33.2		15.5
- Rifampicin (RMP)	33	3.8	64	26.9		9.6
- Ethambutol (EMB)	5	0.6	21	8.8		2.6
- Streptomycin (SM)	98	11.4	61	25.6		14.9
MONORESISTANCE	**94**	**10.9**	**32**	**13.4**		**11.6**
- Isoniazid (INH)	32	3.7	13	5.5		4.2
- Rifampicin (RMP)	10	1.2	4	1.7		1.3
- Ethambutol (EMB)	1	0.1	0	0.0		0.1
- Streptomycin (SM)	51	5.9	15	6.3		6.0
MULTIDRUG RESISTANCE	**18**	**2.1**	**52**	**21.8**		**7.0**
- INH + RMP	6	0.7	19	8.0		7.5
- INH + RMP + EMB	2	0.2	5	2.1		0.7
- INH + RMP + SM	9	1.0	18	7.6		2.7
- INH + RMP + EMB + SM	1	0.1	10	4.2		1.1
OTHER PATTERNS	**38**	**4.4**	**22**	**9.2**		**5.6**
- INH + EMB	1	0.1	1	0.4		0.2
- INH + SM	32	3.7	11	4.6		3.9
- INH + EMB + SM	0	0.0	2	0.8		0.2
- RMP + EMB	0	0.0	3	1.3		0.3
- RMP + SM	5	0.6	5	2.1		1.0
- RMP + EMB + SM	0	0.0	0	0.0		0.0
- EMB + SM	0	0.0	0	0.0		0.0
NUMBER OF DRUGS RESISTANT TO:						
susceptible to 4 drugs	709	82.5	132	55.5		75.8
resistant to 1 drug	94	10.9	32	13.4		11.6
resistant to 2 drugs	44	5.1	39	16.4		7.9
resistant to 3 drugs	11	1.2	25	10.5		3.6
resistant to 4 drugs	1	0.1	10	4.2		1.1

COUNTRY PROFILES

CHINA

Hong Kong: 2001

PROFILE OF THE COUNTRY AND ITS CONTROL PROGRAMME

Population in year of survey	**6,665,000**		Year N.T.P was established	**1979**		
Notification all cases (rate)	**112.5**	**/100,000**	Year of Rifampicin introduction	**1970s**		
Estimated incidence (all cases)	**113.7**	**/100,000**	Year of Isoniazid introduction	**1950s-1960s**		
Notification new sputum smear +	**1926**		Use of Standardized Regimens	**Yes**		
Notification new sputum smear + (rate)	**28.9**	**/100,000**	% Use of Short Course Chemotherapy	**Yes**	**100**	**%**
Treatment Success	**89**	**%**	Use of Directly Observed Therapy	**Yes**	**85**	**%**
Retreatment cases	**207**		During continuation phase	**Yes**		
Retreatment as % of NTP	**3.11**	**%**	Use of Fixed Dose Combination	**Yes**		**%**
Estimated HIV positive TB cases	**0.49**	**%**	Treatment in private sector	**Cat 1**		

Category 1: virtually all TB patients public sector
Category 2: <15% in private sector
Category 3: 15% or more in private sector

TB drugs available on the private market	**All 1st and 2nd line drugs**

CHARACTERISTICS OF THE SURVEY/SURVEILLANCE PROGRAMME

Study Duration	**12 Months**
Target Area	**Countrywide**
Sampling Method	**All culture positive cases**
Culture Media	**Löwenstein-Jensen and BACTEC**
DST Method	**Absolute concentration**
Supranational Reference Laboratory	**Korean Institute of Tuberculosis (KIT), Seoul, Republic of Korea**

*Notations to accompany profile: Retreatment indicates sputum smear positive pulmonary cases only

*For survey settings where less than 100% of cases are sampled, combined estimates are based on the rates of new and previously treated cases obtained in the survey, but weighted by the absolute number of new and previously treated sputum positive TB cases, as published by the national authorities.

PREVALENCE OF DRUG RESISTANCE

Hong Kong: 2001

	New		Previous		Combined	
	N	%	N	%	N	%
Total number of strains tested	3,470	100.0	169	100.0	3,639	100.0
SUSCEPTIBLE TO ALL 4 DRUGS	**3,115**	**89.8**	**130**	**76.9**	**3,245**	**89.2**
ANY RESISTANCE	**355**	**10.2**	**39**	**23.1**	**394**	**10.8**
- Isoniazid (INH)	191	5.5	32	18.9	223	6.1
- Rifampicin (RMP)	33	1.0	19	11.2	52	1.4
- Ethambutol (EMB)	19	0.5	10	5.9	29	0.8
- Streptomycin (SM)	260	7.5	30	17.8	290	8.0
MONORESISTANCE	**243**	**7.1**	**15**	**8.8**	**258**	**7.1**
- Isoniazid (INH)	80	2.3	8	4.7	88	2.4
- Rifampicin (RMP)	6	0.2	0	0.0	6	0.2
- Ethambutol (EMB)	1	0.1	0	0.0	1	0.1
- Streptomycin (SM)	156	4.1	7	4.1	163	4.5
MULTIDRUG RESISTANCE	**27**	**0.8**	**19**	**11.2**	**46**	**1.3**
- INH + RMP	6	0.2	1	0.6	7	0.2
- INH + RMP + EMB	0	0.0	0	0.0	0	0.0
- INH + RMP + SM	13	0.4	8	4.7	21	0.6
- INH + RMP + EMB + SM	8	0.2	10	5.9	18	0.5
OTHER PATTERNS	**85**	**2.5**	**5**	**3.0**	**90**	**2.4**
- INH + EMB	2	0.1	0	0.0	2	0.1
- INH + SM	75	2.2	5	3.0	80	2.2
- INH + EMB + SM	7	0.2	0	0.0	7	0.2
- RMP + EMB	0	0.0	0	0.0	0	0.0
- RMP + SM	0	0.0	0	0.0	0	0.0
- RMP + EMB + SM	0	0.0	0	0.0	0	0.0
- EMB + SM	1	0.1	0	0.0	1	0.1
NUMBER OF DRUGS RESISTANT TO:						
susceptible to 4 drugs	3,115	89.8	130	76.9	3,245	89.2
resistant to 1 drug	243	7.0	15	8.9	258	7.1
resistant to 2 drugs	84	2.4	6	3.6	90	2.5
resistant to 3 drugs	20	0.6	8	4.7	28	0.8
resistant to 4 drugs	8	0.2	10	5.9	18	0.5

COUNTRY PROFILES

CHINA

Liaoning: 1999

PROFILE OF THE COUNTRY AND ITS CONTROL PROGRAMME

Population in year of survey	**40,900,000**		Year N.T.P was established	**1992**		
Notification all cases (rate)	**37.2**	**/100,000**	Year of Rifampicin introduction	**1970**		
Estimated incidence (all cases)	**80**	**/100,000**	Year of Isoniazid introduction	**1952**		
Notification new sputum smear +	**6537**		Use of Standardized Regimens	**Yes**		
Notification new sputum smear + (rate)	**15.98**	**/100,000**	% Use of Short Course Chemotherapy	**Yes**	**95**	**%**
Treatment Success		**%**	Use of Directly Observed Therapy	**Yes**	**95**	**%**
Retreatment cases	**1465**		During continuation phase	**Yes**		
Retreatment as % of NTP		**%**	Use of Fixed Dose Combination			**%**
Estimated HIV positive TB cases	**NA**	**%**	Treatment in private sector	**Cat 2**		
			Category 1: virtually all TB patients public sector Category 2: <15% in private sector Category 3: 15% or more in private sector			
			TB drugs available on the private market	**All drugs**		

CHARACTERISTICS OF THE SURVEY/SURVEILLANCE PROGRAMME

Study Duration	**12 Months**
Target Area	**Province**
Sampling Method	**Cluster**
Culture Media	**Ogawa and Löwenstein-Jensen**
DST Method	**Proportion**
Supranational Reference Laboratory	**Korean Institute of Tuberculosis (KIT), Seoul, Republic of Korea**

*Notations to accompany profile: Retreatment indicates sputum smear positive pulmonary cases only Based on some patient re-interviews 25-30% of new drug resistant cases are suspected to have been misclassified. Therefore, MDR among new cases could be reduced from 10% to 8%. The reduction would be less if susceptible patients were also misclassified.

*For survey settings where less than 100% of cases are sampled, combined estimates are based on the rates of new and previously treated cases obtained in the survey, but weighted by the absolute number of new and previously treated sputum positive TB cases, as published by the national authorities.

COUNTRY PROFILES

PREVALENCE OF DRUG RESISTANCE

Liaoning: 1999

	New		Previous		Combined	
	N	%	N	%	N	%
Total number of strains tested	818	100.0	86	100.0		100.0
SUSCEPTIBLE TO ALL 4 DRUGS	**474**	**57.9**	**38**	**44.2**		**55.4**
ANY RESISTANCE	**344**	**42.1**	**48**	**55.8**		**44.6**
- Isoniazid (INH)	207	25.3	36	41.9		28.3
- Rifampicin (RMP)	93	11.4	25	29.0		14.6
- Ethambutol (EMB)	31	3.8	12	14.0		5.7
- Streptomycin (SM)	279	34.1	36	41.9		35.5
MONORESISTANCE	**177**	**21.6**	**13**	**15.1**		**20.4**
- Isoniazid (INH)	44	5.4	2	2.3		4.8
- Rifampicin (RMP)	4	0.5	3	3.5		1.0
- Ethambutol (EMB)	2	0.2	0	0.0		0.2
- Streptomycin (SM)	127	15.5	8	9.3		14.4
MULTIDRUG RESISTANCE	**85**	**10.4**	**21**	**24.4**		**13.0**
- INH + RMP	10	1.2	6	7.0		4.7
- INH + RMP + EMB	2	0.2	0	0.0		0.2
- INH + RMP + SM	54	6.6	6	7.0		6.7
- INH + RMP + EMB + SM	19	2.3	9	10.5		3.8
OTHER PATTERNS	**82**	**10.0**	**14**	**16.3**		**11.2**
- INH + EMB	2	0.2	1	1.2		0.4
- INH + SM	71	8.7	11	12.8		9.4
- INH + EMB + SM	5	0.6	1	1.2		0.7
- RMP + EMB	1	0.1	0	0.0		0.1
- RMP + SM	3	0.4	0	0.0		0.3
- RMP + EMB + SM	0	0.0	1	1.2		0.2
- EMB + SM	0	0.0	0	0.0		0.0
NUMBER OF DRUGS RESISTANT TO:						
susceptible to 4 drugs	474	57.9	38	44.2		55.4
resistant to 1 drug	177	21.6	13	15.1		20.4
resistant to 2 drugs	87	10.6	18	20.9		12.5
resistant to 3 drugs	61	7.4	8	9.3		7.8
resistant to 4 drugs	19	2.3	9	10.5		3.8

COUNTRY PROFILES

COLOMBIA

Countrywide: 1999-2000

PROFILE OF THE COUNTRY AND ITS CONTROL PROGRAMME

Population in year of survey	**40,772,994**		Year N.T.P was established	**1960**		
Notification all cases (rate)	**21.1**	**/100,000**	Year of Rifampicin introduction	**1981**		
Estimated incidence (all cases)	**55**	**/100,000**	Year of Isoniazid introduction			
Notification new sputum smear +	**8329**		Use of Standardized Regimens	**Yes**		
Notification new sputum smear + (rate)	**20.0**	**/100,000**	% Use of Short Course Chemotherapy	**Yes**	**90**	**%**
Treatment Success	**NA**	**%**	Use of Directly Observed Therapy	**NA**		**%**
Retreatment cases	**NA**		During continuation phase			
Retreatment as % of NTP	**20**	**%**	Use of Fixed Dose Combination	**Yes**	**100**	**%**
Estimated HIV positive TB cases	**1.05**	**%**	Treatment in private sector			

Category 1: virtually all TB patients public sector
Category 2: <15% in private sector
Category 3: 15% or more in private sector

TB drugs available on the private market

CHARACTERISTICS OF THE SURVEY/SURVEILLANCE PROGRAMME

Study Duration	**12 Months**
Target Area	**Countrywide**
Sampling Method	**Cluster**
Culture Media	**Ogawa**
DST Method	**Proportion**
Supranational Reference Laboratory	**Instituto de Salud Pública de Chile, Santiago, Chile**

*Notations to accompany profile: Estimated HIV positive TB cases is a WHO estimate

*For survey settings where less than 100% of cases are sampled, combined estimates are based on the rates of new and previously treated cases obtained in the survey, but weighted by the absolute number of new and previously treated sputum positive TB cases, as published by the national authorities.

COUNTRY PROFILES

PREVALENCE OF DRUG RESISTANCE

Countrywide: 1999-2000

	New		Previous		Combined	
	N	%	N	%	N	%
Total number of strains tested	1,087	100.0				
SUSCEPTIBLE TO ALL 4 DRUGS	**918**	**84.5**				
ANY RESISTANCE	**169**	**15.5**				
- Isoniazid (INH)	103	9.5				
- Rifampicin (RMP)	18	1.7				
- Ethambutol (EMB)	9	0.8				
- Streptomycin (SM)	125	11.5				
MONORESISTANCE	**102**	**9.4**				
- Isoniazid (INH)	37	3.4				
- Rifampicin (RMP)	1	0.1				
- Ethambutol (EMB)	3	0.3				
- Streptomycin (SM)	61	5.6				
MULTIDRUG RESISTANCE	**16**	**1.5**				
- INH + RMP	1	0.1				
- INH + RMP + EMB	2	0.2				
- INH + RMP + SM	11	1.0				
- INH + RMP + EMB + SM	2	0.2				
OTHER PATTERNS	**51**	**4.7**				
- INH + EMB	0	0.0				
- INH + SM	48	4.4				
- INH + EMB + SM	2	0.2				
- RMP + EMB	0	0.0				
- RMP + SM	1	0.1				
- RMP + EMB + SM	0	0.0				
- EMB + SM	0	0.0				
NUMBER OF DRUGS RESISTANT TO:						
susceptible to 4 drugs	918	84.5				
resistant to 1 drug	102	9.4				
resistant to 2 drugs	50	4.6				
resistant to 3 drugs	15	1.4				
resistant to 4 drugs	2	0.2				

CROATIA

Countrywide: 2000

PROFILE OF THE COUNTRY AND ITS CONTROL PROGRAMME

Population in year of survey	**4,446,000**	Year N.T.P was established	
Notification all cases (rate)	**/100,000**	Year of Rifampicin introduction	
Estimated incidence (all cases)	**/100,000**	Year of Isoniazid introduction	
Notification new sputum smear +	**866**	Use of Standardized Regimens	
Notification new sputum smear + (rate)	**/100,000**	% Use of Short Course Chemotherapy	**%**
Treatment Success	**%**	Use of Directly Observed Therapy	**%**
Retreatment cases		During continuation phase	
Retreatment as % of NTP	**%**	Use of Fixed Dose Combination	**%**
Estimated HIV positive TB cases	**0.06 %**	Treatment in private sector	

Category 1: virtually all TB patients public sector
Category 2: <15% in private sector
Category 3: 15% or more in private sector

TB drugs available on the private market

CHARACTERISTICS OF THE SURVEY/SURVEILLANCE PROGRAMME

Study Duration	**Months**
Target Area	**Countrywide**
Sampling Method	**All cases**
Culture Media	
DST Method	
Supranational Reference Laboratory	**National Reference Center for Mycobacteria, Borstel, Germany**

*Notations to accompany profile: Estimated HIV positive TB cases is a WHO estimate

*For survey settings where less than 100% of cases are sampled, combined estimates are based on the rates of new and previously treated cases obtained in the survey, but weighted by the absolute number of new and previously treated sputum positive TB cases, as published by the national authorities.

COUNTRY PROFILES

PREVALENCE OF DRUG RESISTANCE

Countrywide: 2000

	New		Previous		Combined	
	N	%	N	%	N	%
Total number of strains tested	780	100.0	99	100.0	879	100.0
SUSCEPTIBLE TO ALL 4 DRUGS	**766**	**98.2**	**93**	**93.9**	**859**	**98.0**
ANY RESISTANCE	**14**	**1.8**	**6**	**6.1**	**20**	**2.0**
- Isoniazid (INH)	8	1.0	4	4.0	12	1.4
- Rifampicin (RMP)	1	0.1	3	3.0	4	0.5
- Ethambutol (EMB)	0	0.0	1	1.0	1	0.1
- Streptomycin (SM)	7	0.9	1	1.0	8	0.9
MONORESISTANCE	**12**	**1.5**	**5**	**5.1**	**17**	**1.9**
- Isoniazid (INH)	6	0.8	3	3.0	9	1.0
- Rifampicin (RMP)	0	0.0	2	2.0	2	0.2
- Ethambutol (EMB)	0	0.0	0	0.0	0	0.0
- Streptomycin (SM)	6	0.8	1	1.0	6	0.7
MULTIDRUG RESISTANCE	**1**	**0.1**	**1**	**1.0**	**2**	**0.2**
- INH + RMP	1	0.1	0	0.0	1	0.1
- INH + RMP + EMB	0	0.0	0	0.0	0	0.0
- INH + RMP + SM	0	0.0	0	0.0	0	0.0
- INH + RMP + EMB + SM	0	0.0	1	0.1	1	0.1
OTHER PATTERNS	**1**	**0.1**	**0**	**0.0**	**1**	**0.1**
- INH + EMB	0	0.0	0	0.0	0	0.0
- INH + SM	1	0.1	0	0.0	1	0.1
- INH + EMB + SM	0	0.0	0	0.0	0	0.0
- RMP + EMB	0	0.0	0	0.0	0	0.0
- RMP + SM	0	0.0	0	0.0	0	0.0
- RMP + EMB + SM	0	0.0	0	0.0	0	0.0
- EMB + SM	0	0.0	0	0.0	0	0.0
NUMBER OF DRUGS RESISTANT TO:						
susceptible to 4 drugs	766	98.2	93	93.9	859	98.0
resistant to 1 drug	12	1.5	5	5.1	17	1.9
resistant to 2 drugs	2	0.2	0	0.0	2	0.2
resistant to 3 drugs	0	0.0	0	0.0	0	0.0
resistant to 4 drugs	0	0.0	1	1.0	1	0.1

COUNTRY PROFILES

CUBA

Countrywide: 2000

PROFILE OF THE COUNTRY AND ITS CONTROL PROGRAMME

Population in year of survey	**11,187,673**		Year N.T.P was established	**1963**		
Notification all cases (rate)	**10**	**/100,000**	Year of Rifampicin introduction	**1982**		
Estimated incidence (all cases)	**10.1**	**/100,000**	Year of Isoniazid introduction	**1950**		
Notification new sputum smear +	**677**		Use of Standardized Regimens	**Yes**		
Notification new sputum smear + (rate)	**6.0**	**/100,000**	% Use of Short Course Chemotherapy	**Yes**	**100**	**%**
Treatment Success	**93**	**%**	Use of Directly Observed Therapy	**Yes**	**100**	**%**
Retreatment cases	**71**		During continuation phase	**Yes**		
Retreatment as % of NTP		**%**	Use of Fixed Dose Combination	**No**		**%**
Estimated HIV positive TB cases	**0.11**	**%**	Treatment in private sector	**Cat 1**		

Category 1: virtually all TB patients public sector
Category 2: <15% in private sector
Category 3: 15% or more in private sector

TB drugs available on the private market	**No**

CHARACTERISTICS OF THE SURVEY/SURVEILLANCE PROGRAMME

Study Duration	**12 Months**
Target Area	**Countrywide**
Sampling Method	**Proportionate cluster**
Culture Media	**Löwenstein-Jensen**
DST Method	**Proportion**
Supranational Reference Laboratory	**Instituto de Salud Pública de Chile, Santiago, Chile**

*Notations to accompany profile: Estimated HIV positive TB cases is a WHO estimate

*For survey settings where less than 100% of cases are sampled, combined estimates are based on the rates of new and previously treated cases obtained in the survey, but weighted by the absolute number of new and previously treated sputum positive TB cases, as published by the national authorities.

COUNTRY PROFILES

PREVALENCE OF DRUG RESISTANCE

Countrywide: 2000

	New		Previous		Combined	
	N	%	N	%	N	%
Total number of strains tested	377	100.0	38	100.0		100.0
SUSCEPTIBLE TO ALL 4 DRUGS	358	95.0	32	84.2		93.9
ANY RESISTANCE	19	5.0	6	15.8		6.1
- Isoniazid (INH)	4	1.0	3	7.9		1.7
- Rifampicin (RMP)	3	0.8	1	2.6		1.0
- Ethambutol (EMB)	0	0.0	1	2.6		0.2
- Streptomycin (SM)	17	4.5	6	15.8		5.5
MONORESISTANCE	14	3.7	3	7.9		4.1
- Isoniazid (INH)	1	0.3	0	0.0		0.2
- Rifampicin (RMP)	0	0.0	0	0.0		0.0
- Ethambutol (EMB)	0	0.0	0	0.0		0.0
- Streptomycin (SM)	13	3.5	3	7.9		3.9
MULTIDRUG RESISTANCE	1	0.3	1	2.6		0.5
- INH + RMP	1	0.3	0	0.0		0.2
- INH + RMP + EMB	0	0.0	0	0.0		0.0
- INH + RMP + SM	0	0.0	0	0.0		0.0
- INH + RMP + EMB + SM	0	0.0	1	2.6		0.2
OTHER PATTERNS	4	1.0	2	5.2		1.5
- INH + EMB	0	0.0	0	0.0		0.0
- INH + SM	2	0.5	2	5.2		1.0
- INH + EMB + SM	0	0.0	0	0.0		0.0
- RMP + EMB	0	0.0	0	0.0		0.0
- RMP + SM	2	0.5	0	0.0		0.5
- RMP + EMB + SM	0	0.0	0	0.0		0.0
- EMB + SM	0	0.0	0	0.0		0.0
NUMBER OF DRUGS RESISTANT TO:						
susceptible to 4 drugs	358	95.0	32	84.2		93.9
resistant to 1 drug	14	3.7	3	7.9		4.1
resistant to 2 drugs	5	1.3	2	5.2		1.7
resistant to 3 drugs	0	0.0	0	0.0		0.0
resistant to 4 drugs	0	0.0	1	2.6		0.2

COUNTRY PROFILES

CZECH REPUBLIC

Countrywide: 2000

PROFILE OF THE COUNTRY AND ITS CONTROL PROGRAMME

Population in year of survey	10,269,000		Year N.T.P was established	1982	
Notification all cases (rate)		/100,000	Year of Rifampicin introduction	1980	
Estimated incidence (all cases)		/100,000	Year of Isoniazid introduction		
Notification new sputum smear +	420		Use of Standardized Regimens	Yes	
Notification new sputum smear + (rate)		/100,000	% Use of Short Course Chemotherapy	Yes	80 %
Treatment Success		%	Use of Directly Observed Therapy	Yes	90 %
Retreatment cases	26		During continuation phase	Yes	
Retreatment as % of NTP		%	Use of Fixed Dose Combination	Yes	100 %
Estimated HIV positive TB cases	1.46	%	Treatment in private sector	Cat 3	

Category 1: virtually all TB patients public sector
Category 2: <15% in private sector
Category 3: 15% or more in private sector

TB drugs available on the private market	NA

CHARACTERISTICS OF THE SURVEY/SURVEILLANCE PROGRAMME

Study Duration	**12 Months**
Target Area	**Countrywide**
Sampling Method	**All cases**
Culture Media	**Löwenstein-Jensen and others**
DST Method	**Proportion**
Supranational Reference Laboratory	**National Institute of Public Health, Prague, Czech Republic**

*Notations to accompany profile: Estimated HIV positive TB cases is a WHO estimate

*For survey settings where less than 100% of cases are sampled, combined estimates are based on the rates of new and previously treated cases obtained in the survey, but weighted by the absolute number of new and previously treated sputum positive TB cases, as published by the national authorities.

COUNTRY PROFILES

PREVALENCE OF DRUG RESISTANCE

Countrywide: 2000

	New		Previous		Combined	
	N	%	N	%	N	%
Total number of strains tested	616	100.0	22	100.0	638	100.0
SUSCEPTIBLE TO ALL 4 DRUGS	**589**	**95.6**	**19**	**86.4**	**608**	**95.3**
ANY RESISTANCE	**27**	**4.4**	**3**	**13.6**	**30**	**4.7**
- Isoniazid (INH)	21	3.4	2	9.1	23	3.6
- Rifampicin (RMP)	7	1.1	3	13.6	10	1.6
- Ethambutol (EMB)	5	0.8	1	4.5	6	0.9
- Streptomycin (SM)	12	1.9	1	4.5	13	2.0
MONORESISTANCE	**16**	**2.6**	**1**	**4.5**	**17**	**2.7**
- Isoniazid (INH)	10	1.6	0	0.0	10	1.6
- Rifampicin (RMP)	0	0.0	1	4.5	1	0.2
- Ethambutol (EMB)	1	0.2	0	0.0	1	0.2
- Streptomycin (SM)	5	0.8	0	0.0	5	0.8
MULTIDRUG RESISTANCE	**7**	**1.1**	**2**	**9.1**	**9**	**1.4**
- INH + RMP	3	0.5	1	4.5	4	0.6
- INH + RMP + EMB	1	0.2	0	0.0	1	0.2
- INH + RMP + SM	0	0.0	0	0.0	0	0.0
- INH + RMP + EMB + SM	3	0.5	1	4.5	4	0.6
OTHER PATTERNS	**4**	**0.6**	**0**	**0.0**	**4**	**0.6**
- INH + EMB	0	0.0	0	0.0	0	0.0
- INH + SM	4	0.6	0	0.0	4	0.6
- INH + EMB + SM	0	0.0	0	0.0	0	0.0
- RMP + EMB	0	0.0	0	0.0	0	0.0
- RMP + SM	0	0.0	0	0.0	0	0.0
- RMP + EMB + SM	0	0.0	0	0.0	0	0.0
- EMB + SM	0	0.0	0	0.0	0	0.0
NUMBER OF DRUGS RESISTANT TO:						
susceptible to 4 drugs	589	95.6	19	86.4	608	95.3
resistant to 1 drug	16	2.6	1	4.5	17	2.7
resistant to 2 drugs	7	1.1	1	4.5	8	1.3
resistant to 3 drugs	1	0.2	0	0.0	1	0.1
resistant to 4 drugs	3	0.5	1	4.5	4	0.6

COUNTRY PROFILES

DEMOCRATIC REPUBLIC OF THE CONGO

Kinshasa: 1999

PROFILE OF THE COUNTRY AND ITS CONTROL PROGRAMME

Population in year of survey		Year N.T.P was established	
Notification all cases (rate)	/100,000	Year of Rifampicin introduction	
Estimated incidence (all cases)	/100,000	Year of Isoniazid introduction	
Notification new sputum smear +	10710	Use of Standardized Regimens	
Notification new sputum smear + (rate)	/100,000	% Use of Short Course Chemotherapy	%
Treatment Success	%	Use of Directly Observed Therapy	%
Retreatment cases	1338	During continuation phase	
Retreatment as % of NTP	%	Use of Fixed Dose Combination	%
Estimated HIV positive TB cases	NA %	Treatment in private sector	

Category 1: virtually all TB patients public sector
Category 2: <15% in private sector
Category 3: 15% or more in private sector

TB drugs available on the private market

CHARACTERISTICS OF THE SURVEY/SURVEILLANCE PROGRAMME

Study Duration	Months
Target Area	
Sampling Method	Cluster
Culture Media	
DST Method	
Supranational Reference Laboratory	Prince Leopold Institute of Tropical Medicine, Antwerp, Belgium

*Notations to accompany profile: Retreatment indicates sputum smear positive pulmonary cases only

*For survey settings where less than 100% of cases are sampled, combined estimates are based on the rates of new and previously treated cases obtained in the survey, but weighted by the absolute number of new and previously treated sputum positive TB cases, as published by the national authorities.

PREVALENCE OF DRUG RESISTANCE

Kinshasa: 1999

	New		Previous		Combined	
	N	%	N	%	N	%
Total number of strains tested					710	100.0
SUSCEPTIBLE TO ALL 4 DRUGS					433	61.0
ANY RESISTANCE					277	39.0
- Isoniazid (INH)					163	23.0
- Rifampicin (RMP)					44	6.2
- Ethambutol (EMB)					109	15.4
- Streptomycin (SM)					200	28.2
MONORESISTANCE					131	18.4
- Isoniazid (INH)					31	4.4
- Rifampicin (RMP)					1	0.1
- Ethambutol (EMB)					36	5.1
- Streptomycin (SM)					63	8.9
MULTIDRUG RESISTANCE					41	5.8
- INH + RMP					2	0.3
- INH + RMP + EMB					4	0.6
- INH + RMP + SM					5	0.7
- INH + RMP + EMB + SM					30	4.2
OTHER PATTERNS					105	14.8
- INH + EMB					3	0.4
- INH + SM					66	9.3
- INH + EMB + SM					22	3.1
- RMP + EMB					0	0.0
- RMP + SM					0	0.0
- RMP + EMB + SM					2	0.3
- EMB + SM					12	1.7
NUMBER OF DRUGS RESISTANT TO:						
susceptible to 4 drugs					433	61.0
resistant to 1 drug					131	18.4
resistant to 2 drugs					83	11.7
resistant to 3 drugs					33	4.6
resistant to 4 drugs					30	4.2

DENMARK

Countrywide: 2000

PROFILE OF THE COUNTRY AND ITS CONTROL PROGRAMME

Population in year of survey	**5,330,020**		Year N.T.P was established	**NA**		
Notification all cases (rate)	**10.3**	**/100,000**	Year of Rifampicin introduction	**1969**		
Estimated incidence (all cases)	**10.3**	**/100,000**	Year of Isoniazid introduction			
Notification new sputum smear +	**139**		Use of Standardized Regimens	**Yes**		
Notification new sputum smear + (rate)	**2.6**	**/100,000**	% Use of Short Course Chemotherapy	**Yes**	**99**	**%**
Treatment Success	**88**	**%**	Use of Directly Observed Therapy	**Yes**	**10**	**%**
Retreatment cases	**34**		During continuation phase			
Retreatment as % of NTP	**6.2**	**%**	Use of Fixed Dose Combination	**No**		**%**
Estimated HIV positive TB cases	**5.46**	**%**	Treatment in private sector	**Cat 1**		

Category 1: virtually all TB patients public sector
Category 2: <15% in private sector
Category 3: 15% or more in private sector

TB drugs available on the private market	**Rx only**

CHARACTERISTICS OF THE SURVEY/SURVEILLANCE PROGRAMME

Study Duration	**12 Months**
Target Area	**Countrywide**
Sampling Method	**All cases**
Culture Media	**Löwenstein-Jensen and BACTEC**
DST Method	**BACTEC**
Supranational Reference Laboratory	**Reference Laboratory Mycobacteriology, Statens Serum Institut (SSI), Denmark under SIIDC, Sweden**

*Notations to accompany profile: Estimated HIV positive TB cases is a WHO estimate
Data from Denmark exclude Greenland and the Faroe Islands

*For survey settings where less than 100% of cases are sampled, combined estimates are based on the rates of new and previously treated cases obtained in the survey, but weighted by the absolute number of new and previously treated sputum positive TB cases, as published by the national authorities.

COUNTRY PROFILES

PREVALENCE OF DRUG RESISTANCE

Countrywide: 2000

	New		Previous		Combined	
	N	%	N	%	N	%
Total number of strains tested	392	100.0	33	100.0	425	100.0
SUSCEPTIBLE TO ALL 4 DRUGS	**345**	**88.0**	**24**	**72.7**	**369**	**86.8**
ANY RESISTANCE	**47**	**12.0**	**9**	**27.2**	**56**	**13.2**
- Isoniazid (INH)	29	7.4	8	24.2	37	8.7
- Rifampicin (RMP)	2	0.5	1	3.0	3	0.7
- Ethambutol (EMB)	3	0.8	1	3.0	4	0.0
- Streptomycin (SM)	34	8.7	8	24.2	42	9.9
MONORESISTANCE	**28**	**7.1**	**1**	**3.0**	**29**	**6.8**
- Isoniazid (INH)	11	2.8	0	0.0	11	2.6
- Rifampicin (RMP)	0	0.0	0	0.0	0	0.0
- Ethambutol (EMB)	0	0.0	0	0.0	0	0.0
- Streptomycin (SM)	17	4.3	1	3.0	18	4.2
MULTIDRUG RESISTANCE	**1**	**0.3**	**1**	**3.0**	**2**	**0.4**
- INH + RMP	0	0.0	0	0.0	0	0.0
- INH + RMP + EMB	0	0.0	1	3.0	1	0.2
- INH + RMP + SM	0	0.0	0	0.0	0	0.0
- INH + RMP + EMB + SM	1	0.3	0	0.0	1	0.2
OTHER PATTERNS	**18**	**4.6**	**7**	**21.2**	**25**	**5.9**
- INH + EMB	1	0.3	0	0.0	1	0.2
- INH + SM	16	4.1	7	21.2	23	5.4
- INH + EMB + SM	0	0.0	0	0.0	0	0.0
- RMP + EMB	1	0.3	0	0.0	1	0.2
- RMP + SM	0	0.0	0	0.0	0	0.0
- RMP + EMB + SM	0	0.0	0	0.0	0	0.0
- EMB + SM	0	0.0	0	0.0	0	0.0
NUMBER OF DRUGS RESISTANT TO:						
susceptible to 4 drugs	345	88.0	24	72.7	369	86.8
resistant to 1 drug	28	7.1	1	3.0	29	6.8
resistant to 2 drugs	18	4.6	7	21.2	25	5.9
resistant to 3 drugs	0	0.0	1	3.0	1	0.2
resistant to 4 drugs	1	0.3	0	0.0	1	0.2

ECUADOR

Countrywide: 2002

PROFILE OF THE COUNTRY AND ITS CONTROL PROGRAMME

Population in year of survey	**12,880,000**		Year N.T.P was established	**1973**		
Notification all cases (rate)	**47**	**/100,000**	Year of Rifampicin introduction	**1983**		
Estimated incidence (all cases)		**/100,000**	Year of Isoniazid introduction	**1973**		
Notification new sputum smear +	**4439**		Use of Standardized Regimens	**Yes**		
Notification new sputum smear + (rate)	**34.47**	**/100,000**	% Use of Short Course Chemotherapy	**Yes**	**100**	**%**
Treatment Success	**NA**	**%**	Use of Directly Observed Therapy	**Yes**	**26**	**%**
Retreatment cases	**590**		During continuation phase	**No**		
Retreatment as % of NTP		**%**	Use of Fixed Dose Combination	**Yes**	**100**	**%**
Estimated HIV positive TB cases	**1.12**	**%**	Treatment in private sector	**NA**		
			Category 1: virtually all TB patients public sector Category 2: <15% in private sector Category 3: 15% or more in private sector			
			TB drugs available on the private market	**All drugs**		

CHARACTERISTICS OF THE SURVEY/SURVEILLANCE PROGRAMME

Study Duration	**12 Months**
Target Area	**Countrywide**
Sampling Method	**All cases**
Culture Media	**Löwenstein-Jensen**
DST Method	**Proportion**
Supranational Reference Laboratory	**Instituto de Salud Pública de Chile, Santiago, Chile**

*Notations to accompany profile: Estimated HIV positive TB cases is a WHO estimate

*For survey settings where less than 100% of cases are sampled, combined estimates are based on the rates of new and previously treated cases obtained in the survey, but weighted by the absolute number of new and previously treated sputum positive TB cases, as published by the national authorities.

COUNTRY PROFILES

PREVALENCE OF DRUG RESISTANCE

Countrywide: 2002

	New		Previous		Combined	
	N	%	N	%	N	%
Total number of strains tested	812	100.0	185	100.0		100.0
SUSCEPTIBLE TO ALL 4 DRUGS	**649**	**80.0**	**104**	**56.2**		**77.1**
ANY RESISTANCE	**163**	**20.0**	**81**	**43.8**		**22.9**
- Isoniazid (INH)	89	11.0	56	30.3		13.2
- Rifampicin (RMP)	59	7.3	62	33.5		10.3
- Ethambutol (EMB)	10	1.2	10	5.4		1.7
- Streptomycin (SM)	92	11.3	38	20.5		12.4
MONORESISTANCE	**99**	**12.2**	**24**	**13.0**		**12.3**
- Isoniazid (INH)	29	3.6	5	2.7		3.5
- Rifampicin (RMP)	15	1.8	11	5.9		2.3
- Ethambutol (EMB)	2	0.2	0	0.0		0.2
- Streptomycin (SM)	53	6.5	8	4.3		6.3
MULTIDRUG RESISTANCE	**40**	**4.9**	**45**	**24.3**		**7.2**
- INH + RMP	20	2.5	23	12.4		3.6
- INH + RMP + EMB	4	0.5	3	1.6		0.6
- INH + RMP + SM	14	1.7	16	8.6		2.5
- INH + RMP + EMB + SM	2	0.2	3	1.6		0.4
OTHER PATTERNS	**24**	**3.0**	**12**	**6.5**		**3.4**
- INH + EMB	0	0.0	0	0.0		0.0
- INH + SM	20	2.5	3	1.6		2.4
- INH + EMB + SM	0	0.0	3	1.6		0.2
- RMP + EMB	1	0.1	1	0.5		0.2
- RMP + SM	2	0.2	5	2.7		0.5
- RMP + EMB + SM	1	0.1	0	0.0		0.1
- EMB + SM	0	0.0	0	0.0		0.0
NUMBER OF DRUGS RESISTANT TO:						
susceptible to 4 drugs	649	80.0	104	56.2		77.1
resistant to 1 drug	99	12.2	24	12.9		12.3
resistant to 2 drugs	43	5.3	32	17.3		6.7
resistant to 3 drugs	19	2.3	22	11.9		3.5
resistant to 4 drugs	2	0.2	3	1.6		0.4

COUNTRY PROFILES

EGYPT

Countrywide: 2002

PROFILE OF THE COUNTRY AND ITS CONTROL PROGRAMME

Population in year of survey	**68,355,826**		Year N.T.P was established	**1989**		
Notification all cases (rate)	**16**	**/100,000**	Year of Rifampicin introduction	**1980**		
Estimated incidence (all cases)	**29**	**/100,000**	Year of Isoniazid introduction	**1970s**		
Notification new sputum smear +	**4889**		Use of Standardized Regimens	**Yes**		
Notification new sputum smear + (rate)	**7.2**	**/100,000**	% Use of Short Course Chemotherapy	**Yes**	**100**	**%**
Treatment Success	**87**	**%**	Use of Directly Observed Therapy	**Yes**	**100**	**%**
Retreatment cases	**848**		During continuation phase	**Yes**		
Retreatment as % of NTP		**%**	Use of Fixed Dose Combination	**Yes**		**%**
Estimated HIV positive TB cases	**0.08**	**%**	Treatment in private sector	**Cat 3**		
			Category 1: virtually all TB patients public sector Category 2: <15% in private sector Category 3: 15% or more in private sector			
			TB drugs available on the private market	**All first line**		

CHARACTERISTICS OF THE SURVEY/SURVEILLANCE PROGRAMME

Study Duration	**12 Months**
Target Area	**Countrywide**
Sampling Method	**Proportionate cluster**
Culture Media	**Löwenstein-Jensen**
DST Method	**Proportion**
Supranational Reference Laboratory	**Laboratoire de la Tuberculose Institut Pasteur d'Algérie-Alger, Alger, Algeria**

*Notations to accompany profile: Estimated HIV positive TB cases is a WHO estimate
Retreatment indicates sputum smear positive pulmonary cases only

*For survey settings where less than 100% of cases are sampled, combined estimates are based on the rates of new and previously treated cases obtained in the survey, but weighted by the absolute number of new and previously treated sputum positive TB cases, as published by the national authorities.

COUNTRY PROFILES

PREVALENCE OF DRUG RESISTANCE

Countrywide: 2002

	New		Previous		Combined	
	N	%	N	%	N	%
Total number of strains tested	632	100.0	217	100.0		100.0
SUSCEPTIBLE TO ALL 4 DRUGS	**439**	**69.5**	**69**	**31.8**		**63.9**
ANY RESISTANCE	**193**	**30.5**	**148**	**68.2**		**36.1**
- Isoniazid (INH)	62	9.8	101	46.5		15.2
- Rifampicin (RMP)	44	7.0	110	50.7		13.4
- Ethambutol (EMB)	18	2.8	67	30.9		7.0
- Streptomycin (SM)	149	23.6	117	53.9		28.1
MONORESISTANCE	**137**	**21.7**	**40**	**18.4**		**21.2**
- Isoniazid (INH)	17	2.7	6	2.8		2.7
- Rifampicin (RMP)	22	3.5	15	6.9		4.0
- Ethambutol (EMB)	3	0.5	2	0.9		0.5
- Streptomycin (SM)	95	15.0	17	7.8		14.0
MULTIDRUG RESISTANCE	**14**	**2.2**	**83**	**38.4**		**7.5**
- INH + RMP	0	0.0	5	2.3		0.5
- INH + RMP + EMB	0	0.0	2	0.9		0.1
- INH + RMP + SM	5	0.8	21	9.7		2.1
- INH + RMP + EMB + SM	9	1.4	55	25.3		5.0
OTHER PATTERNS	**42**	**6.7**	**25**	**11.5**		**7.4**
- INH + EMB	2	0.3	1	0.5		0.3
- INH + SM	28	4.4	7	3.2		4.3
- INH + EMB + SM	1	0.2	4	1.8		0.4
- RMP + EMB	0	0.0	0	0.0		0.0
- RMP + SM	8	1.3	10	4.6		1.8
- RMP + EMB + SM	0	0.0	2	0.9		0.1
- EMB + SM	3	0.5	1	0.5		0.5
NUMBER OF DRUGS RESISTANT TO:						
susceptible to 4 drugs	439	69.5	69	31.8		63.9
resistant to 1 drug	137	21.7	40	18.4		21.2
resistant to 2 drugs	41	6.5	24	11.0		7.2
resistant to 3 drugs	6	0.9	29	13.4		2.8
resistant to 4 drugs	9	1.4	55	25.3		5.0

COUNTRY PROFILES

EL SALVADOR

Countrywide: 2001

PROFILE OF THE COUNTRY AND ITS CONTROL PROGRAMME

Population in year of survey	6,276,037		Year N.T.P was established	1942		
Notification all cases (rate)	23	/100,000	Year of Rifampicin introduction	1975		
Estimated incidence (all cases)	33	/100,000	Year of Isoniazid introduction	1952		
Notification new sputum smear +	1003		Use of Standardized Regimens	Yes		
Notification new sputum smear + (rate)	16	/100,000	% Use of Short Course Chemotherapy	Yes	100	%
Treatment Success	79	%	Use of Directly Observed Therapy	Yes	100	%
Retreatment cases	83		During continuation phase	Yes		
Retreatment as % of NTP		%	Use of Fixed Dose Combination	No		%
Estimated HIV positive TB cases	1.99	%	Treatment in private sector	NA		

Category 1: virtually all TB patients public sector
Category 2: <15% in private sector
Category 3: 15% or more in private sector

TB drugs available on the private market **No**

CHARACTERISTICS OF THE SURVEY/SURVEILLANCE PROGRAMME

Study Duration	**12 Months**
Target Area	**Countrywide**
Sampling Method	**All cases**
Culture Media	**Löwenstein-Jensen**
DST Method	**Proportion**
Supranational Reference Laboratory	**Instituto de Salud Pública de Chile, Santiago, Chile**

*Notations to accompany profile: Estimated HIV positive TB cases is a WHO estimate
Retreatment indicates sputum smear positive pulmonary cases only

*For survey settings where less than 100% of cases are sampled, combined estimates are based on the rates of new and previously treated cases obtained in the survey, but weighted by the absolute number of new and previously treated sputum positive TB cases, as published by the national authorities.

PREVALENCE OF DRUG RESISTANCE

Countrywide: 2001

	New		Previous		Combined	
	N	%	N	%	N	%
Total number of strains tested	611	100.0	100	100.0		100.0
SUSCEPTIBLE TO ALL 4 DRUGS	**576**	**94.3**	**78**	**78.0**		**93.0**
ANY RESISTANCE	**35**	**5.7**	**22**	**22.0**		**7.0**
- Isoniazid (INH)	8	1.3	12	12.0		2.1
- Rifampicin (RMP)	7	1.1	13	13.0		2.1
- Ethambutol (EMB)	2	0.3	3	3.0		0.5
- Streptomycin (SM)	23	3.8	9	9.0		4.2
MONORESISTANCE	**30**	**4.9**	**12**	**12.0**		**5.5**
- Isoniazid (INH)	3	0.5	3	3.0		0.7
- Rifampicin (RMP)	5	0.8	5	5..0		1.1
- Ethambutol (EMB)	2	0.3	1	1.0		0.4
- Streptomycin (SM)	20	3.3	3	3.0		3.3
MULTIDRUG RESISTANCE	**2**	**0.3**	**7**	**7.0**		**0.8**
- INH + RMP	2	0.3	3	3.0		6.3
- INH + RMP + EMB	0	0.0	1	1.0		0.1
- INH + RMP + SM	0	0.0	2	2.0		0.2
- INH + RMP + EMB + SM	0	0.0	1	1.0		0.1
OTHER PATTERNS	**3**	**0.5**	**3**	**3.0**		**0.7**
- INH + EMB	0	0.0	0	0.0		0.0
- INH + SM	3	0.5	2	2.0		0.6
- INH + EMB + SM	0	0.0	0	0.0		0.0
- RMP + EMB	0	0.0	0	0.0		0.0
- RMP + SM	0	0.0	1	1.0		0.1
- RMP + EMB + SM	0	0.0	0	0.0		0.0
- EMB + SM	0	0.0	0	0.0		0.0
NUMBER OF DRUGS RESISTANT TO:						
susceptible to 4 drugs	576	94.3	78	78.0		93.0
resistant to 1 drug	30	4.9	12	12.0		5.5
resistant to 2 drugs	5	0.8	6	6.0		1.2
resistant to 3 drugs	0	0.0	3	3.0		0.2
resistant to 4 drugs	0	0.0	1	1.0		0.1

COUNTRY PROFILES

ESTONIA

Countrywide: 2000

PROFILE OF THE COUNTRY AND ITS CONTROL PROGRAMME

Population in year of survey	**1,369,515**		Year N.T.P was established	**1997**		
Notification all cases (rate)	**55.5**	**/100,000**	Year of Rifampicin introduction	**1972**		
Estimated incidence (all cases)		**/100,000**	Year of Isoniazid introduction	**1956**		
Notification new sputum smear +	**255**		Use of Standardized Regimens	**Yes**		
Notification new sputum smear + (rate)	**18.6**	**/100,000**	% Use of Short Course Chemotherapy	**No**	**100**	**%**
Treatment Success	**66.2**	**%**	Use of Directly Observed Therapy	**Yes**	**98**	**%**
Retreatment cases	**39**		During continuation phase	**Yes**		
Retreatment as % of NTP		**%**	Use of Fixed Dose Combination	**Yes**	**75**	**%**
Estimated HIV positive TB cases	**0.15**	**%**	Treatment in private sector	**Cat 1**		

Category 1: virtually all TB patients public sector
Category 2: <15% in private sector
Category 3: 15% or more in private sector

TB drugs available on the private market	**No**

CHARACTERISTICS OF THE SURVEY/SURVEILLANCE PROGRAMME

Study Duration	**12 Months**
Target Area	**Countrywide**
Sampling Method	**All cases**
Culture Media	**Löwenstein-Jensen and BACTEC**
DST Method	**Proportion and BACTEC**
Supranational Reference Laboratory	**Swedish Institute for Infectious Disease Control (SIIDC), Karolinska, Stockholm, Sweden**

*Notations to accompany profile: Estimated HIV positive TB cases is a WHO estimate

*For survey settings where less than 100% of cases are sampled, combined estimates are based on the rates of new and previously treated cases obtained in the survey, but weighted by the absolute number of new and previously treated sputum positive TB cases, as published by the national authorities.

COUNTRY PROFILES

PREVALENCE OF DRUG RESISTANCE

Countrywide: 2000

	New		Previous		Combined	
	N	%	N	%	N	%
Total number of strains tested	410	100.0	117	100.0	527	100.0
SUSCEPTIBLE TO ALL 4 DRUGS	**293**	**71.5**	**49**	**41.9**	**342**	**64.9**
ANY RESISTANCE	**117**	**28.5**	**68**	**58.1**	**185**	**35.1**
- Isoniazid (INH)	94	22.9	64	54.7	158	30.0
- Rifampicin (RMP)	50	12.2	53	45.3	103	19.5
- Ethambutol (EMB)	54	13.2	49	41.9	103	19.5
- Streptomycin (SM)	92	22.4	57	48.7	149	28.3
MONORESISTANCE	**44**	**10.7**	**12**	**10.3**	**56**	**10.6**
- Isoniazid (INH)	21	5.1	8	6.8	29	5.5
- Rifampicin (RMP)	0	0.0	0	0.0	0	0.0
- Ethambutol (EMB)	0	0.0	0	0.0	0	0.0
- Streptomycin (SM)	23	5.6	4	3.4	27	5.1
MULTIDRUG RESISTANCE	**50**	**12.2**	**53**	**45.3**	**103**	**19.5**
- INH + RMP	0	0.0	2	1.7	2	0.4
- INH + RMP + EMB	3	0.7	1	0.9	4	0.8
- INH + RMP + SM	2	0.5	2	1.7	4	0.8
- INH + RMP + EMB + SM	45	11.0	48	41.0	93	17.6
OTHER PATTERNS	**23**	**5.6**	**3**	**2.6**	**26**	**4.9**
- INH + EMB	1	0.2	0	0.0	1	0.2
- INH + SM	17	4.1	3	2.6	20	3.8
- INH + EMB + SM	5	1.2	0	0.0	5	0.9
- RMP + EMB	0	0.0	0	0.0	0	0.0
- RMP + SM	0	0.0	0	0.0	0	0.0
- RMP + EMB + SM	0	0.0	0	0.0	0	0.0
- EMB + SM	0	0.0	0	0.0	0	0.0
NUMBER OF DRUGS RESISTANT TO:						
susceptible to 4 drugs	293	71.5	49	41.9	342	64.9
resistant to 1 drug	44	10.7	12	10.3	56	10.6
resistant to 2 drugs	18	4.4	5	4.3	23	4.4
resistant to 3 drugs	10	2.4	3	2.6	13	2.5
resistant to 4 drugs	45	11.0	48	41.0	93	17.6

COUNTRY PROFILES

FINLAND

Countrywide: 2000

PROFILE OF THE COUNTRY AND ITS CONTROL PROGRAMME

Population in year of survey	**5,172,000**		Year N.T.P was established	**1953**		
Notification all cases (rate)	**10.4**	**/100,000**	Year of Rifampicin introduction	**1972**		
Estimated incidence (all cases)		**/100,000**	Year of Isoniazid introduction	**NA**		
Notification new sputum smear +	**227**		Use of Standardized Regimens	**Yes**		
Notification new sputum smear + (rate)	**4.4**	**/100,000**	% Use of Short Course Chemotherapy	**Yes**	**100**	**%**
Treatment Success	**NA**	**%**	Use of Directly Observed Therapy	**No**		**%**
Retreatment cases	**NA**		During continuation phase	**No**		
Retreatment as % of NTP	**NA**	**%**	Use of Fixed Dose Combination	**No**		**%**
Estimated HIV positive TB cases	**1.54**	**%**	Treatment in private sector	**Cat 1**		
			Category 1: virtually all TB patients public sector Category 2: <15% in private sector Category 3: 15% or more in private sector			
			TB drugs available on the private market	**Rx only**		

CHARACTERISTICS OF THE SURVEY/SURVEILLANCE PROGRAMME

Study Duration	**12 Months**
Target Area	**Countrywide**
Sampling Method	**All cases**
Culture Media	**Löwenstein-Jensen**
DST Method	**Proportion**
Supranational Reference Laboratory	**Swedish Institute for Infectious Disease Control (SIIDC), Karolinska, Stockholm, Sweden**

*Notations to accompany profile: Estimated HIV positive TB cases is a WHO estimate
The combined column includes patients with unknown treatment history

*For survey settings where less than 100% of cases are sampled, combined estimates are based on the rates of new and previously treated cases obtained in the survey, but weighted by the absolute number of new and previously treated sputum positive TB cases, as published by the national authorities.

COUNTRY PROFILES

PREVALENCE OF DRUG RESISTANCE

Countrywide: 2000

	New		Previous		Combined	
	N	%	N	%	N	%
Total number of strains tested	374	100.0	29	100.0	437	100.0
SUSCEPTIBLE TO ALL 4 DRUGS	**357**	**95.5**	**25**	**86.2**	**415**	**95.0**
ANY RESISTANCE	**17**	**4.5**	**4**	**13.8**	**22**	**5.0**
- Isoniazid (INH)	10	2.7	4	13.8	15	3.4
- Rifampicin (RMP)	3	0.8	1	3.4	4	0.9
- Ethambutol (EMB)	1	0.3	0	0.0	1	0.2
- Streptomycin (SM)	9	2.4	0	0.0	9	2.1
MONORESISTANCE	**12**	**3.2**	**3**	**10.3**	**16**	**3.7**
- Isoniazid (INH)	5	1.3	3	10.3	9	2.1
- Rifampicin (RMP)	2	0.5	0	0.0	2	0.5
- Ethambutol (EMB)	0	0.0	0	0.0	0	0.0
- Streptomycin (SM)	5	1.3	0	0.0	5	1.1
MULTIDRUG RESISTANCE	**1**	**0.3**	**1**	**3.4**	**2**	**0.4**
- INH + RMP	0	0.0	1	3.4	1	0.2
- INH + RMP + EMB	0	0.0	0	0.0	0	0.0
- INH + RMP + SM	1	0.3	0	0.0	1	0.2
- INH + RMP + EMB + SM	0	0.0	0	0.0	0	0.0
OTHER PATTERNS	**4**	**1.1**	**0**	**0.0**	**4**	**0.9**
- INH + EMB	1	0.3	0	0.0	1	0.2
- INH + SM	3	0.8	0	0.0	3	0.7
- INH + EMB + SM	0	0.0	0	0.0	0	0.0
- RMP + EMB	0	0.0	0	0.0	0	0.0
- RMP + SM	0	0.0	0	0.0	0	0.0
- RMP + EMB + SM	0	0.0	0	0.0	0	0.0
- EMB + SM	0	0.0	0	0.0	0	0.0
NUMBER OF DRUGS RESISTANT TO:						
susceptible to 4 drugs	357	95.5	25	86.2	415	95.0
resistant to 1 drug	12	3.2	3	10.3	16	3.7
resistant to 2 drugs	4	1.1	1	3.4	5	1.1
resistant to 3 drugs	1	0.3	0	0.0	1	0.2
resistant to 4 drugs	0	0.0	0	0.0	0	0.0

COUNTRY PROFILES

FRANCE

15 Regions: 2000

PROFILE OF THE COUNTRY AND ITS CONTROL PROGRAMME

Population in year of survey	**59,296,000**		Year N.T.P was established	**NA**	
Notification all cases (rate)	**/100,000**		Year of Rifampicin introduction	**1967**	
Estimated incidence (all cases)	**/100,000**		Year of Isoniazid introduction	**NA**	
Notification new sputum smear +	**1815**		Use of Standardized Regimens	**Yes**	
Notification new sputum smear + (rate)	**/100,000**		% Use of Short Course Chemotherapy	**Yes**	**100** **%**
Treatment Success	**%**		Use of Directly Observed Therapy	**No**	**%**
Retreatment cases			During continuation phase	**No**	
Retreatment as % of NTP	**%**		Use of Fixed Dose Combination	**Yes**	**50** **%**
Estimated HIV positive TB cases	**12.14** **%**		Treatment in private sector	**Cat 2**	

Category 1: virtually all TB patients public sector
Category 2: <15% in private sector
Category 3: 15% or more in private sector

TB drugs available on the private market

CHARACTERISTICS OF THE SURVEY/SURVEILLANCE PROGRAMME

Study Duration	**12 Months**
Target Area	**Sentinel sites**
Sampling Method	**All cases**
Culture Media	**Löwenstein-Jensen and BACTEC**
DST Method	**Proportion**
Supranational Reference Laboratory	**Institut Pasteur, Centre National de Référence des Mycobacteries, Paris, France**

*Notations to accompany profile: Estimated HIV positive TB cases is a WHO estimate
The combined column includes patients with unknown treatment history

*For survey settings where less than 100% of cases are sampled, combined estimates are based on the rates of new and previously treated cases obtained in the survey, but weighted by the absolute number of new and previously treated sputum positive TB cases, as published by the national authorities.

COUNTRY PROFILES

PREVALENCE OF DRUG RESISTANCE

15 Regions: 2000

	New		Previous		Combined	
	N	%	N	%	N	%
Total number of strains tested	947	100.0	82	100.0	1,191	100.0
SUSCEPTIBLE TO ALL 4 DRUGS	**859**	**90.7**	**59**	**72.0**	**1,061**	**89.1**
ANY RESISTANCE	**88**	**9.3**	**23**	**28.0**	**130**	**10.9**
- Isoniazid (INH)	24	2.5	15	18.3	45	3.8
- Rifampicin (RMP)	8	0.8	9	11.0	18	1.5
- Ethambutol (EMB)	20	2.1	2	2.4	23	1.9
- Streptomycin (SM)	61	6.4	13	15.9	88	7.4
MONORESISTANCE	**69**	**7.3**	**11**	**13.4**	**96**	**8.1**
- Isoniazid (INH)	5	0.5	4	4.9	12	1.0
- Rifampicin (RMP)	0	0.0	1	1.2	2	0.2
- Ethambutol (EMB)	8	0.8	1	1.2	10	0.8
- Streptomycin (SM)	56	5.9	5	6.1	72	6.0
MULTIDRUG RESISTANCE	**8**	**0.8**	**7**	**8.5**	**15**	**1.3**
- INH + RMP	4	0.4	3	3.7	7	0.6
- INH + RMP + EMB	2	0.2	1	1.2	3	0.3
- INH + RMP + SM	1	0.1	3	3.7	4	0.3
- INH + RMP + EMB + SM	1	0.1	0	0.0	1	0.1
OTHER PATTERNS	**11**	**1.2**	**5**	**6.1**	**19**	**1.6**
- INH + EMB	8	0.8	0	0.0	8	0.7
- INH + SM	2	0.2	4	4.9	9	0.8
- INH + EMB + SM	1	0.1	0	0.0	1	0.1
- RMP + EMB	0	0.0	0	0.0	0	0.0
- RMP + SM	0	0.0	1	1.2	1	0.1
- RMP + EMB + SM	0	0.0	0	0.0	0	0.0
- EMB + SM	0	0.0	0	0.0	0	0.0
NUMBER OF DRUGS RESISTANT TO:						
susceptible to 4 drugs	859	90.7	59	72.0	1,061	89.1
resistant to 1 drug	69	7.3	11	13.4	96	8.1
resistant to 2 drugs	14	1.5	8	9.8	25	2.1
resistant to 3 drugs	4	0.4	4	4.9	8	0.7
resistant to 4 drugs	1	0.1	0	0.0	1	0.1

COUNTRY PROFILES

THE GAMBIA

Countrywide: 1999-2000

PROFILE OF THE COUNTRY AND ITS CONTROL PROGRAMME

Population in year of survey	**1,280,000**		Year N.T.P was established	**1986**		
Notification all cases (rate)	**119**	**/100,000**	Year of Rifampicin introduction	**1986**		
Estimated incidence (all cases)		**/100,000**	Year of Isoniazid introduction	**1950**		
Notification new sputum smear +	**850**		Use of Standardized Regimens	**Yes**		
Notification new sputum smear + (rate)	**66**	**/100,000**	% Use of Short Course Chemotherapy	**Yes**	**100**	**%**
Treatment Success	**65**	**%**	Use of Directly Observed Therapy	**Yes**	**100**	**%**
Retreatment cases	**26**		During continuation phase	**Yes**		
Retreatment as % of NTP		**%**	Use of Fixed Dose Combination	**Yes**	**100**	**%**
Estimated HIV positive TB cases	**7.64**	**%**	Treatment in private sector	**Cat 1**		

Category 1: virtually all TB patients public sector
Category 2: <15% in private sector
Category 3: 15% or more in private sector

TB drugs available on the private market	**No**

CHARACTERISTICS OF THE SURVEY/SURVEILLANCE PROGRAMME

Study Duration	**7 Months**
Target Area	**Countrywide**
Sampling Method	**All diagnostic centers**
Culture Media	**Löwenstein-Jensen and BACTEC**
DST Method	**Resistance Ratio**
Supranational Reference Laboratory	**Health Protection Agency Mycobacterium Reference Unit (HPA MRU), London, UK**

*Notations to accompany profile: Estimated HIV positive TB cases is a WHO estimate
Retreatment indicates sputum smear positive pulmonary cases only

*For survey settings where less than 100% of cases are sampled, combined estimates are based on the rates of new and previously treated cases obtained in the survey, but weighted by the absolute number of new and previously treated sputum positive TB cases, as published by the national authorities.

PREVALENCE OF DRUG RESISTANCE

Countrywide: 1999-2000

	New		Previous		Combined	
	N	%	N	%	N	%
Total number of strains tested	210	100.0	15	100.0		100.0
SUSCEPTIBLE TO ALL 4 DRUGS	**201**	**95.7**	**15**	**100.0**		**95.9**
ANY RESISTANCE	**9**	**4.3**	**0**	**0.0**		**4.1**
- Isoniazid (INH)	5	2.4	0	0.0		2.3
- Rifampicin (RMP)	2	0.9	0	0.0		0.9
- Ethambutol (EMB)	0	0.0	0	0.0		0.0
- Streptomycin (SM)	3	1.4	0	0.0		1.4
MONORESISTANCE	**8**	**3.8**	**0**	**0.0**		**3.7**
- Isoniazid (INH)	4	1.9	0	0.0		1.8
- Rifampicin (RMP)	1	0.5	0	0.0		0.5
- Ethambutol (EMB)	0	0.0	0	0.0		0.0
- Streptomycin (SM)	3	1.4	0	0.0		1.4
MULTIDRUG RESISTANCE	**1**	**0.5**	**0**	**0.0**		**0.5**
- INH + RMP	1	0.5	0	0.0		0.0
- INH + RMP + EMB	0	0.0	0	0.0		0.0
- INH + RMP + SM	0	0.0	0	0.0		0.0
- INH + RMP + EMB + SM	0	0.0	0	0.0		0.0
OTHER PATTERNS	**0**	**0.0**	**0**	**0.0**		**0.0**
- INH + EMB	0	0.0	0	0.0		0.0
- INH + SM	0	0.0	0	0.0		0.0
- INH + EMB + SM	0	0.0	0	0.0		0.0
- RMP + EMB	0	0.0	0	0.0		0.0
- RMP + SM	0	0.0	0	0.0		0.0
- RMP + EMB + SM	0	0.0	0	0.0		0.0
- EMB + SM	0	0.0	0	0.0		0.0
NUMBER OF DRUGS RESISTANT TO:						
susceptible to 4 drugs	201	95.7	15	100.0		95.9
resistant to 1 drug	8	3.8	0	0.0		3.7
resistant to 2 drugs	1	0.5	0	0.0		0.5
resistant to 3 drugs	0	0.0	0	0.0		0.0
resistant to 4 drugs	0	0.0	0	0.0		0.0

GERMANY

Countrywide: 2000

PROFILE OF THE COUNTRY AND ITS CONTROL PROGRAMME

Population in year of survey	**82,282,000**	Year N.T.P was established	**NA**	
Notification all cases (rate)	**/100,000**	Year of Rifampicin introduction	**1969**	
Estimated incidence (all cases)	**/100,000**	Year of Isoniazid introduction		
Notification new sputum smear +	**3963**	Use of Standardized Regimens	**Yes**	
Notification new sputum smear + (rate)	**/100,000**	% Use of Short Course Chemotherapy	**Yes** **100** **%**	
Treatment Success	**%**	Use of Directly Observed Therapy	**No** **%**	
Retreatment cases		During continuation phase		
Retreatment as % of NTP	**%**	Use of Fixed Dose Combination	**Yes** **20** **%**	
Estimated HIV positive TB cases	**3.16** **%**	Treatment in private sector	**Cat 3**	
		Category 1: virtually all TB patients public sector Category 2: <15% in private sector Category 3: 15% or more in private sector		
		TB drugs available on the private market	**Rx required**	

CHARACTERISTICS OF THE SURVEY/SURVEILLANCE PROGRAMME

Study Duration	**12 Months**
Target Area	**Countrywide**
Sampling Method	**All cases**
Culture Media	**Löwenstein-Jensen and BACTEC**
DST Method	**Proportion and BACTEC**
Supranational Reference Laboratory	**National Reference Center for Mycobacteria, Borstel, Germany**

*Notations to accompany profile: Estimated HIV positive TB cases is a WHO estimate
The combined column includes patients with unknown treatment history
The study area covered 55% of all health departments.

*For survey settings where less than 100% of cases are sampled, combined estimates are based on the rates of new and previously treated cases obtained in the survey, but weighted by the absolute number of new and previously treated sputum positive TB cases, as published by the national authorities.

COUNTRY PROFILES

PREVALENCE OF DRUG RESISTANCE

Countrywide: 2000

	New		Previous		Combined	
	N	%	N	%	N	%
Total number of strains tested	1,743	100.0	257	100.0	2,780	100.0
SUSCEPTIBLE TO ALL 4 DRUGS	**1,628**	**93.4**	**206**	**80.2**	**2,540**	**91.4**
ANY RESISTANCE	**115**	**6.6**	**51**	**19.8**	**240**	**8.6**
- Isoniazid (INH)	67	3.8	44	17.1	166	6.0
- Rifampicin (RMP)	17	1.0	21	8.2	54	1.9
- Ethambutol (EMB)	17	1.0	14	5.4	43	1.5
- Streptomycin (SM)	72	4.1	35	13.6	151	5.4
MONORESISTANCE	**76**	**4.4**	**17**	**6.6**	**134**	**4.8**
- Isoniazid (INH)	29	1.7	11	4.3	62	2.2
- Rifampicin (RMP)	3	0.2	1	0.4	6	0.2
- Ethambutol (EMB)	5	0.3	0	0.0	6	0.2
- Streptomycin (SM)	39	2.2	5	1.9	60	2.2
MULTIDRUG RESISTANCE	**14**	**0.8**	**19**	**7.4**	**47**	**1.7**
- INH + RMP	4	0.2	3	1.2	11	0.4
- INH + RMP + EMB	2	0.1	1	0.4	4	0.1
- INH + RMP + SM	4	0.2	5	1.9	14	0.5
- INH + RMP + EMB + SM	4	0.2	10	3.9	18	0.6
OTHER PATTERNS	**25**	**1.4**	**15**	**5.8**	**59**	**2.1**
- INH + EMB	0	0.0	0	0.0	0	0.0
- INH + SM	19	1.1	11	4.3	43	1.5
- INH + EMB + SM	5	0.3	3	1.2	14	0.5
- RMP + EMB	0	0.0	0	0.0	0	0.0
- RMP + SM	0	0.0	1	0.4	1	0.0
- RMP + EMB + SM	0	0.0	0	0.0	0	0.0
- EMB + SM	1	0.1	0	0.0	1	0.0
NUMBER OF DRUGS RESISTANT TO:						
susceptible to 4 drugs	1,628	93.4	206	80.2	2,540	91.4
resistant to 1 drug	76	4.4	17	6.6	134	4.8
resistant to 2 drugs	24	1.4	15	5.8	56	2.0
resistant to 3 drugs	11	0.6	9	3.1	32	1.2
resistant to 4 drugs	4	0.2	10	3.9	18	0.6

COUNTRY PROFILES

HONDURAS

Countrywide: 2002

PROFILE OF THE COUNTRY AND ITS CONTROL PROGRAMME

Population in year of survey	**6,216,939**		Year N.T.P was established	**1950**		
Notification all cases (rate)	**72**	**/100,000**	Year of Rifampicin introduction	**1985**		
Estimated incidence (all cases)	**>80**	**/100,000**	Year of Isoniazid introduction	**1970**		
Notification new sputum smear +	**2802**		Use of Standardized Regimens	**Yes**		
Notification new sputum smear + (rate)	**45.1**	**/100,000**	% Use of Short Course Chemotherapy	**Yes**	**100**	**%**
Treatment Success	**89**	**%**	Use of Directly Observed Therapy	**Yes**	**100**	**%**
Retreatment cases	**103**		During continuation phase	**Yes**		
Retreatment as % of NTP		**%**	Use of Fixed Dose Combination	**Yes**	**100**	**%**
Estimated HIV positive TB cases	**9.0**	**%**	Treatment in private sector	**Cat 2**		

Category 1: virtually all TB patients public sector
Category 2: <15% in private sector
Category 3: 15% or more in private sector

TB drugs available on the private market	**No**

CHARACTERISTICS OF THE SURVEY/SURVEILLANCE PROGRAMME

Study Duration	**14 Months**
Target Area	**Countrywide**
Sampling Method	**Cluster**
Culture Media	**Löwenstein-Jensen**
DST Method	**Proportion**
Supranational Reference Laboratory	**Instituto de Salud Pública de Chile, Santiago, Chile**

*Notations to accompany profile: Retreatment indicates sputum smear positive pulmonary cases only
Preliminary data

*For survey settings where less than 100% of cases are sampled, combined estimates are based on the rates of new and previously treated cases obtained in the survey, but weighted by the absolute number of new and previously treated sputum positive TB cases, as published by the national authorities.

COUNTRY PROFILES

PREVALENCE OF DRUG RESISTANCE

Countrywide: 2002

	New		Previous		Combined	
	N	%	N	%	N	%
Total number of strains tested	169	100.0	29	100.0		100.0
SUSCEPTIBLE TO ALL 4 DRUGS	**140**	**82.8**	**17**	**58.6**		**82.0**
ANY RESISTANCE	**29**	**17.2**	**12**	**41.4**		**18.0**
- Isoniazid (INH)	11	6.5	5	17.2		6.9
- Rifampicin (RMP)	4	2.4	5	17.2		2.9
- Ethambutol (EMB)	2	1.2	1	3.4		1.3
- Streptomycin (SM)	25	14.8	8	27.6		15.2
MONORESISTANCE	**19**	**11.2**	**8**	**27.6**		**11.8**
- Isoniazid (INH)	2	1.2	2	6.9		1.4
- Rifampicin (RMP)	0	0.0	2	6.9		0.2
- Ethambutol (EMB)	0	0.0	0	0.0		0.0
- Streptomycin (SM)	17	10.1	4	13.8		10.2
MULTIDRUG RESISTANCE	**3**	**1.8**	**2**	**6.9**		**2.0**
- INH + RMP	1	0.6	0	0.0		3.3
- INH + RMP + EMB	0	0.0	0	0.0		0.0
- INH + RMP + SM	1	0.6	1	3.4		0.7
- INH + RMP + EMB + SM	1	0.6	1	3.4		0.7
OTHER PATTERNS	**7**	**4.1**	**2**	**6.9**		**4.2**
- INH + EMB	1	0.6	0	0.0		0.6
- INH + SM	5	3.0	1	3.4		3.0
- INH + EMB + SM	0	0.0	0	0.0		0.0
- RMP + EMB	0	0.0	0	0.0		0.0
- RMP + SM	1	0.6	1	3.4		0.7
- RMP + EMB + SM	0	0.0	0	0.0		0.0
- EMB + SM	0	0.0	0	0.0		0.0
NUMBER OF DRUGS RESISTANT TO:						
susceptible to 4 drugs	140	82.8	17	58.6		82.0
resistant to 1 drug	19	11.2	8	27.6		11.8
resistant to 2 drugs	8	4.7	2	6.9		4.8
resistant to 3 drugs	1	0.6	1	3.4		0.7
resistant to 4 drugs	1	0.6	1	3.4		0.7

ICELAND

Countrywide: 2000

PROFILE OF THE COUNTRY AND ITS CONTROL PROGRAMME

Population in year of survey	**282,000**	Year N.T.P was established	
Notification all cases (rate)	**/100,000**	Year of Rifampicin introduction	
Estimated incidence (all cases)	**/100,000**	Year of Isoniazid introduction	
Notification new sputum smear +	**1**	Use of Standardized Regimens	
Notification new sputum smear + (rate)	**/100,000**	% Use of Short Course Chemotherapy	**%**
Treatment Success	**%**	Use of Directly Observed Therapy	**%**
Retreatment cases		During continuation phase	
Retreatment as % of NTP	**%**	Use of Fixed Dose Combination	**%**
Estimated HIV positive TB cases	**4.5 %**	Treatment in private sector	

Category 1: virtually all TB patients public sector
Category 2: <15% in private sector
Category 3: 15% or more in private sector

TB drugs available on the private market

CHARACTERISTICS OF THE SURVEY/SURVEILLANCE PROGRAMME

Study Duration	**12 Months**
Target Area	**Countrywide**
Sampling Method	**All cases**
Culture Media	
DST Method	
Supranational Reference Laboratory	**Reference Laboratory Mycobacteriology, Statens Serum Institut (SSI), Denmark under SIIDC, Sweden**

*Notations to accompany profile: Estimated HIV positive TB cases is a WHO estimate

*For survey settings where less than 100% of cases are sampled, combined estimates are based on the rates of new and previously treated cases obtained in the survey, but weighted by the absolute number of new and previously treated sputum positive TB cases, as published by the national authorities.

COUNTRY PROFILES

PREVALENCE OF DRUG RESISTANCE

Countrywide: 2000

	New		Previous		Combined	
	N	%	N	%	N	%
Total number of strains tested	8	100.0	1	100.0	9	100.0
SUSCEPTIBLE TO ALL 4 DRUGS	**8**	**100.0**	**1**	**100.0**	**9**	**100.0**
ANY RESISTANCE	**0**	**0.0**	**0**	**0.0**	**0**	**0.0**
- Isoniazid (INH)	0	0.0	0	0.0	0	0.0
- Rifampicin (RMP)	0	0.0	0	0.0	0	0.0
- Ethambutol (EMB)	0	0.0	0	0.0	0	0.0
- Streptomycin (SM)	0	0.0	0	0.0	0	0.0
MONORESISTANCE	**0**	**0.0**	**0**	**0.0**	**0**	**0.0**
- Isoniazid (INH)	0	0.0	0	0.0	0	0.0
- Rifampicin (RMP)	0	0.0	0	0.0	0	0.0
- Ethambutol (EMB)	0	0.0	0	0.0	0	0.0
- Streptomycin (SM)	0	0.0	0	0.0	0	0.0
MULTIDRUG RESISTANCE	**0**	**0.0**	**0**	**0.0**	**0**	**0.0**
- INH + RMP	0	0.0	0	0.0	0	0.0
- INH + RMP + EMB	0	0.0	0	0.0	0	0.0
- INH + RMP + SM	0	0.0	0	0.0	0	0.0
- INH + RMP + EMB + SM	0	0.0	0	0.0	0	0.0
OTHER PATTERNS	**0**	**0.0**	**0**	**0.0**	**0**	**0.0**
- INH + EMB	0	0.0	0	0.0	0	0.0
- INH + SM	0	0.0	0	0.0	0	0.0
- INH + EMB + SM	0	0.0	0	0.0	0	0.0
- RMP + EMB	0	0.0	0	0.0	0	0.0
- RMP + SM	0	0.0	0	0.0	0	0.0
- RMP + EMB + SM	0	0.0	0	0.0	0	0.0
- EMB + SM	0	0.0	0	0.0	0	0.0
NUMBER OF DRUGS RESISTANT TO:						
susceptible to 4 drugs	8	100.0	1	100.0	9	100.0
resistant to 1 drug	0	0.0	0	0.0	0	0.0
resistant to 2 drugs	0	0.0	0	0.0	0	0.0
resistant to 3 drugs	0	0.0	0	0.0	0	0.0
resistant to 4 drugs	0	0.0	0	0.0	0	0.0

COUNTRY PROFILES

INDIA

Wardha District, Maharashtra State: 2000-2001

PROFILE OF THE COUNTRY AND ITS CONTROL PROGRAMME

Population in year of survey	**1,230,640**		Year N.T.P was established	**1962**		
Notification all cases (rate)	**120**	**/100,000**	Year of Rifampicin introduction	**1969**		
Estimated incidence (all cases)	**190.9**	**/100,000**	Year of Isoniazid introduction	**1961**		
Notification new sputum smear +	**954**		Use of Standardized Regimens	**Yes**		
Notification new sputum smear + (rate)	**75.5**	**/100,000**	% Use of Short Course Chemotherapy	**Yes**	**41**	**%**
Treatment Success		**%**	Use of Directly Observed Therapy	**No**		**%**
Retreatment cases	**97**		During continuation phase	**No**		
Retreatment as % of NTP		**%**	Use of Fixed Dose Combination	**No**		**%**
Estimated HIV positive TB cases	**NA**	**%**	Treatment in private sector Category 1: virtually all TB patients public sector Category 2: <15% in private sector Category 3: 15% or more in private sector	**Cat 3**		
			TB drugs available on the private market	**All 1st line, some 2nd line**		

CHARACTERISTICS OF THE SURVEY/SURVEILLANCE PROGRAMME

Study Duration	**10 Months**
Target Area	**Districtwide**
Sampling Method	**All diagnostic centers**
Culture Media	**Löwenstein-Jensen**
DST Method	**Proportion**
Supranational Reference Laboratory	**Tuberculosis Research Centre, Chennai, India**

*Notations to accompany profile: Retreatment indicates sputum smear positive pulmonary cases only

*For survey settings where less than 100% of cases are sampled, combined estimates are based on the rates of new and previously treated cases obtained in the survey, but weighted by the absolute number of new and previously treated sputum positive TB cases, as published by the national authorities.

COUNTRY PROFILES

PREVALENCE OF DRUG RESISTANCE

Wardha District, Maharashtra State: 2000-2001

	New		Previous		Combined	
	N	%	N	%	N	%
Total number of strains tested	197	100.0				
SUSCEPTIBLE TO ALL 4 DRUGS	**158**	**80.2**				
ANY RESISTANCE	**39**	**19.8**				
- Isoniazid (INH)	30	15.2				
- Rifampicin (RMP)	1	0.5				
- Ethambutol (EMB)	2	1.0				
- Streptomycin (SM)	15	7.6				
MONORESISTANCE	**30**	**15.3**				
- Isoniazid (INH)	21	10.7				
- Rifampicin (RMP)	0	0.0				
- Ethambutol (EMB)	0	0.0				
- Streptomycin (SM)	9	4.6				
MULTIDRUG RESISTANCE	**1**	**0.5**				
- INH + RMP	1	0.5				
- INH + RMP + EMB	0	0.0				
- INH + RMP + SM	0	0.0				
- INH + RMP + EMB + SM	0	0.0				
OTHER PATTERNS	**8**	**4.0**				
- INH + EMB	2	1.0				
- INH + SM	6	3.0				
- INH + EMB + SM	0	0.0				
- RMP + EMB	0	0.0				
- RMP + SM	0	0.0				
- RMP + EMB + SM	0	0.0				
- EMB + SM	0	0.0				
NUMBER OF DRUGS RESISTANT TO:						
susceptible to 4 drugs	158	80.2				
resistant to 1 drug	30	15.3				
resistant to 2 drugs	9	4.5				
resistant to 3 drugs	0	0.0				
resistant to 4 drugs	0	0.0				

INDIA

Raichur District, Karnataka State: 1999

PROFILE OF THE COUNTRY AND ITS CONTROL PROGRAMME

Population in year of survey	**1,783,822**		Year N.T.P was established	**1962**		
Notification all cases (rate)	**162**	**/100,000**	Year of Rifampicin introduction	**1983**		
Estimated incidence (all cases)	**127**	**/100,000**	Year of Isoniazid introduction	**1962**		
Notification new sputum smear +	**1209**		Use of Standardized Regimens	**Yes**		
Notification new sputum smear + (rate)	**73**	**/100,000**	% Use of Short Course Chemotherapy	**Yes**	**90**	**%**
Treatment Success		**%**	Use of Directly Observed Therapy	**Yes**	**30**	**%**
Retreatment cases	**NA**		During continuation phase	**Yes**		
Retreatment as % of NTP		**%**	Use of Fixed Dose Combination	**No**		**%**
Estimated HIV positive TB cases	**NA**	**%**	Treatment in private sector	**Cat 3**		

Category 1: virtually all TB patients public sector
Category 2: <15% in private sector
Category 3: 15% or more in private sector

TB drugs available on the private market — **All 1st line, some 2nd line**

CHARACTERISTICS OF THE SURVEY/SURVEILLANCE PROGRAMME

Study Duration	**6 Months**
Target Area	**Districtwide**
Sampling Method	**All diagnostic centers**
Culture Media	**Löwenstein-Jensen**
DST Method	**Proportion**
Supranational Reference Laboratory	**Tuberculosis Research Centre, Chennai, India**

*Notations to accompany profile: Patient numbers refers to treated not notified

*For survey settings where less than 100% of cases are sampled, combined estimates are based on the rates of new and previously treated cases obtained in the survey, but weighted by the absolute number of new and previously treated sputum positive TB cases, as published by the national authorities.

COUNTRY PROFILES

PREVALENCE OF DRUG RESISTANCE

Raichur District, Karnataka State: 1999

	New		Previous		Combined	
	N	%	N	%	N	%
Total number of strains tested	278	100.0				
SUSCEPTIBLE TO ALL 4 DRUGS	**217**	**78.1**				
ANY RESISTANCE	**61**	**21.9**				
- Isoniazid (INH)	52	18.7				
- Rifampicin (RMP)	7	2.5				
- Ethambutol (EMB)	9	3.2				
- Streptomycin (SM)	20	7.2				
MONORESISTANCE	**43**	**15.5**				
- Isoniazid (INH)	34	12.3				
- Rifampicin (RMP)	0	0.0				
- Ethambutol (EMB)	0	0.0				
- Streptomycin (SM)	9	3.2				
MULTIDRUG RESISTANCE	**7**	**2.5**				
- INH + RMP	2	0.7				
- INH + RMP + EMB	2	0.7				
- INH + RMP + SM	1	0.4				
- INH + RMP + EMB + SM	2	0.7				
OTHER PATTERNS	**11**	**4.0**				
- INH + EMB	3	1.1				
- INH + SM	6	2.2				
- INH + EMB + SM	2	0.7				
- RMP + EMB	0	0.0				
- RMP + SM	0	0.0				
- RMP + EMB + SM	0	0.0				
- EMB + SM	0	0.0				
NUMBER OF DRUGS RESISTANT TO:						
susceptible to 4 drugs	217	78.1				
resistant to 1 drug	43	15.5				
resistant to 2 drugs	11	4.0				
resistant to 3 drugs	5	1.8				
resistant to 4 drugs	2	0.7				

COUNTRY PROFILES

INDIA

North Arcot District, Tamil Nadu State: 1999

PROFILE OF THE COUNTRY AND ITS CONTROL PROGRAMME

Population in year of survey	**5,664,823**		Year N.T.P was established	**1962**		
Notification all cases (rate)	**NA**	**/100,000**	Year of Rifampicin introduction	**1983**		
Estimated incidence (all cases)	**400**	**/100,000**	Year of Isoniazid introduction	**1962**		
Notification new sputum smear +	**26532**		Use of Standardized Regimens	**Yes**		
Notification new sputum smear + (rate)	**43**	**/100,000**	% Use of Short Course Chemotherapy	**Yes**	**90**	**%**
Treatment Success		**%**	Use of Directly Observed Therapy	**Yes**		**%**
Retreatment cases	**NA**		During continuation phase	**Yes**		
Retreatment as % of NTP		**%**	Use of Fixed Dose Combination	**No**		**%**
Estimated HIV positive TB cases	**NA**	**%**	Treatment in private sector	**Cat 3**		

Category 1: virtually all TB patients public sector
Category 2: <15% in private sector
Category 3: 15% or more in private sector

TB drugs available on the private market	**All 1st line, some 2nd line**

CHARACTERISTICS OF THE SURVEY/SURVEILLANCE PROGRAMME

Study Duration	**3 Months**
Target Area	**Districtwide**
Sampling Method	**All diagnostic centers**
Culture Media	**Löwenstein-Jensen**
DST Method	**Proportion**
Supranational Reference Laboratory	**Tuberculosis Research Centre, Chennai, India**

*Notations to accompany profile:

*For survey settings where less than 100% of cases are sampled, combined estimates are based on the rates of new and previously treated cases obtained in the survey, but weighted by the absolute number of new and previously treated sputum positive TB cases, as published by the national authorities.

PREVALENCE OF DRUG RESISTANCE

North Arcot District, Tamil Nadu State: 1999

	New		Previous		Combined	
	N	%	N	%	N	%
Total number of strains tested	282	100.0				
SUSCEPTIBLE TO ALL 4 DRUGS	**204**	**72.3**				
ANY RESISTANCE	**78**	**27.7**				
- Isoniazid (INH)	66	23.4				
- Rifampicin (RMP)	8	2.8				
- Ethambutol (EMB)	13	4.6				
- Streptomycin (SM)	35	12.4				
MONORESISTANCE	**47**	**16.7**				
- Isoniazid (INH)	36	12.8				
- Rifampicin (RMP)	0	0.0				
- Ethambutol (EMB)	1	0.4				
- Streptomycin (SM)	10	3.5				
MULTIDRUG RESISTANCE	**8**	**2.8**				
- INH + RMP	0	0.0				
- INH + RMP + EMB	2	0.7				
- INH + RMP + SM	4	1.4				
- INH + RMP + EMB + SM	2	0.7				
OTHER PATTERNS	**23**	**7.8**				
- INH + EMB	4	1.4				
- INH + SM	15	5.3				
- INH + EMB + SM	3	1.1				
- RMP + EMB	0	0.0				
- RMP + SM	0	0.0				
- RMP + EMB + SM	0	0.0				
- EMB + SM	1	0.4				
NUMBER OF DRUGS RESISTANT TO:						
susceptible to 4 drugs	204	72.3				
resistant to 1 drug	47	16.7				
resistant to 2 drugs	20	6.7				
resistant to 3 drugs	9	2.1				
resistant to 4 drugs	2	0.7				

IRELAND

Countrywide: 2000

PROFILE OF THE COUNTRY AND ITS CONTROL PROGRAMME

Population in year of survey	**3,596,543**		Year N.T.P was established	**1947**		
Notification all cases (rate)	**10.9**	**/100,000**	Year of Rifampicin introduction	**1969**		
Estimated incidence (all cases)	**10.8**	**/100,000**	Year of Isoniazid introduction	**1940s**		
Notification new sputum smear +	**127**		Use of Standardized Regimens	**Yes**		
Notification new sputum smear + (rate)	**3.5**	**/100,000**	% Use of Short Course Chemotherapy	**Yes**	**100**	**%**
Treatment Success	**49.6**	**%**	Use of Directly Observed Therapy	**No**		**%**
Retreatment cases	**17**		During continuation phase	**No**		
Retreatment as % of NTP	**4.3**	**%**	Use of Fixed Dose Combination	**NA**		**%**
Estimated HIV positive TB cases	**3.39**	**%**	Treatment in private sector	**Cat 1**		

Category 1: virtually all TB patients public sector
Category 2: <15% in private sector
Category 3: 15% or more in private sector

TB drugs available on the private market

CHARACTERISTICS OF THE SURVEY/SURVEILLANCE PROGRAMME

Study Duration	**12 Months**
Target Area	**Ireland**
Sampling Method	**All cases**
Culture Media	**Löwenstein-Jensen and BACTEC**
DST Method	**Resistance Ratio**
Supranational Reference Laboratory	**Health Protection Agency Mycobacterium Reference Unit (HPA MRU), London, United Kingdom**

*Notations to accompany profile: Estimated HIV positive TB cases is a WHO estimate
The combined column includes patients with unknown treatment history

*For survey settings where less than 100% of cases are sampled, combined estimates are based on the rates of new and previously treated cases obtained in the survey, but weighted by the absolute number of new and previously treated sputum positive TB cases, as published by the national authorities.

COUNTRY PROFILES

PREVALENCE OF DRUG RESISTANCE

Countrywide: 2000

	New		Previous		Combined	
	N	%	N	%	N	%
Total number of strains tested	138	100.0	26	100.0	225	100.0
SUSCEPTIBLE TO ALL 4 DRUGS	**134**	**97.1**	**24**	**92.3**	**218**	**96.8**
ANY RESISTANCE	**4**	**2.9**	**2**	**7.7**	**7**	**3.1**
- Isoniazid (INH)	4	2.9	1	3.8	6	2.7
- Rifampicin (RMP)	1	0.7	1	3.8	3	1.3
- Ethambutol (EMB)	0	0.0	0	0.0	0	0.0
- Streptomycin (SM)	0	0.0	1	3.8	1	0.4
MONORESISTANCE	**3**	**2.2**	**1**	**3.8**	**4**	**1.7**
- Isoniazid (INH)	3	2.2	0	0.0	3	1.3
- Rifampicin (RMP)	0	0.0	0	0.0	0	0.0
- Ethambutol (EMB)	0	0.0	0	0.0	0	0.0
- Streptomycin (SM)	0	0.0	1	3.8	1	0.4
MULTIDRUG RESISTANCE	**1**	**0.7**	**1**	**3.8**	**3**	**1.3**
- INH + RMP	1	0.7	1	3.8	3	1.3
- INH + RMP + EMB	0	0.0	0	0.0	0	0.0
- INH + RMP + SM	0	0.0	0	0.0	0	0.0
- INH + RMP + EMB + SM	0	0.0	0	0.0	0	0.0
OTHER PATTERNS	**0**	**0.0**	**0**	**0.0**	**0**	**0.0**
- INH + EMB	0	0.0	0	0.0	0	0.0
- INH + SM	0	0.0	0	0.0	0	0.0
- INH + EMB + SM	0	0.0	0	0.0	0	0.0
- RMP + EMB	0	0.0	0	0.0	0	0.0
- RMP + SM	0	0.0	0	0.0	0	0.0
- RMP + EMB + SM	0	0.0	0	0.0	0	0.0
- EMB + SM	0	0.0	0	0.0	0	0.0
NUMBER OF DRUGS RESISTANT TO:						
susceptible to 4 drugs	134	97.1	24	92.3	218	96.8
resistant to 1 drug	3	2.2	1	3.8	4	1.7
resistant to 2 drugs	1	0.7	1	3.8	3	1.3
resistant to 3 drugs	0	0.0	0	0.0	0	0.0
resistant to 4 drugs	0	0.0	0	0.0	0	0.0

ISRAEL

Countrywide: 2000

PROFILE OF THE COUNTRY AND ITS CONTROL PROGRAMME

Population in year of survey	**6,369,300**		Year N.T.P was established	**1997**		
Notification all cases (rate)	**9.3**	**/100,000**	Year of Rifampicin introduction	**NA**		
Estimated incidence (all cases)	**9.3**	**/100,000**	Year of Isoniazid introduction	**NA**		
Notification new sputum smear +	**253**		Use of Standardized Regimens	**Yes**		
Notification new sputum smear + (rate)	**0.42**	**/100,000**	% Use of Short Course Chemotherapy	**Yes**	**100**	**%**
Treatment Success	**78.5**	**%**	Use of Directly Observed Therapy	**Yes**	**100**	**%**
Retreatment cases	**24**		During continuation phase	**Yes**		
Retreatment as % of NTP		**%**	Use of Fixed Dose Combination	**No**		**%**
Estimated HIV positive TB cases	**2.52**	**%**	Treatment in private sector	**Cat 1**		

Category 1: virtually all TB patients public sector
Category 2: <15% in private sector
Category 3: 15% or more in private sector

TB drugs available on the private market

CHARACTERISTICS OF THE SURVEY/SURVEILLANCE PROGRAMME

Study Duration	**12 Months**
Target Area	**Countrywide**
Sampling Method	**All cases**
Culture Media	**Löwenstein-Jensen**
DST Method	**Resistance Ratio**
Supranational Reference Laboratory	**Health Protection Agency Mycobacterium Reference Unit (HPA MRU), London, United Kingdom**

*Notations to accompany profile:
Estimated HIV positive TB cases is a WHO estimate
Indicators refer to culture positivity rather than smear positivity.
The combined column includes patients with unknown treatment history.
Data from Israel contain DST results on isolates taken during treatment (i.e. those transferred from abroad). This may lead to an overestimate of resistance. The precise number is not available.

*For survey settings where less than 100% of cases are sampled, combined estimates are based on the rates of new and previously treated cases obtained in the survey, but weighted by the absolute number of new and previously treated sputum positive TB cases, as published by the national authorities.

COUNTRY PROFILES

PREVALENCE OF DRUG RESISTANCE

Countrywide: 2000

	New		Previous		Combined	
	N	%	N	%	N	%
Total number of strains tested	253	100.0	24	100.0	281	100.0
SUSCEPTIBLE TO ALL 4 DRUGS	**174**	**68.8**	**14**	**58.3**	**191**	**68.0**
ANY RESISTANCE	**79**	**31.2**	**10**	**41.7**	**90**	**32.0**
- Isoniazid (INH)	65	25.7	9	37.5	74	26.3
- Rifampicin (RMP)	37	14.6	5	20.8	42	14.9
- Ethambutol (EMB)	25	9.9	2	8.3	28	10.0
- Streptomycin (SM)	56	22.1	7	8.3	63	22.4
MONORESISTANCE	**30**	**11.9**	**4**	**16.7**	**35**	**12.5**
- Isoniazid (INH)	16	6.3	3	12.5	19	6.8
- Rifampicin (RMP)	1	0.4	0	0.0	1	0.4
- Ethambutol (EMB)	3	1.2	0	0.0	4	1.4
- Streptomycin (SM)	10	4.0	1	4.2	11	3.9
MULTIDRUG RESISTANCE	**36**	**14.2**	**5**	**20.8**	**41**	**14.6**
- INH + RMP	3	1.2	0	0.0	3	1.1
- INH + RMP + EMB	0	0.0	0	0.0	0	0.0
- INH + RMP + SM	15	5.9	3	12.5	18	6.4
- INH + RMP + EMB + SM	18	7.1	2	8.3	20	7.1
OTHER PATTERNS	**13**	**5.1**	**1**	**4.2**	**14**	**5.0**
- INH + EMB	0	0.0	0	0.0	0	0.0
- INH + SM	9	3.6	1	4.2	10	3.6
- INH + EMB + SM	4	1.6	0	0.0	4	1.4
- RMP + EMB	0	0.0	0	0.0	0	0.0
- RMP + SM	0	0.0	0	0.0	0	0.0
- RMP + EMB + SM	0	0.0	0	0.0	0	0.0
- EMB + SM	0	0.0	0	0.0	0	0.0
NUMBER OF DRUGS RESISTANT TO:						
susceptible to 4 drugs	174	68.8	14	58.3	191	68.0
resistant to 1 drug	30	11.9	4	16.7	35	12.5
resistant to 2 drugs	12	4.7	1	4.2	13	4.6
resistant to 3 drugs	19	7.5	3	12.5	22	7.8
resistant to 4 drugs	18	7.1	2	8.3	20	7.1

COUNTRY PROFILES

ITALY

10 Regions: 2000

PROFILE OF THE COUNTRY AND ITS CONTROL PROGRAMME

Population in year of survey	**57,536,000**		Year N.T.P was established	**1995**		
Notification all cases (rate)	**6**	**/100,000**	Year of Rifampicin introduction	**1966**		
Estimated incidence (all cases)	**10**	**/100,000**	Year of Isoniazid introduction	**1952**		
Notification new sputum smear +	**687**		Use of Standardized Regimens	**Yes**		
Notification new sputum smear + (rate)	**1**	**/100,000**	% Use of Short Course Chemotherapy	**Yes**	**80**	**%**
Treatment Success	**74**	**%**	Use of Directly Observed Therapy	**Yes**	**Yes**	**%**
Retreatment cases	**72**		During continuation phase	**No**		
Retreatment as % of NTP		**%**	Use of Fixed Dose Combination	**Yes**	**>10**	**%**
Estimated HIV positive TB cases	**10.05**	**%**	Treatment in private sector Category 1: virtually all TB patients public sector Category 2: <15% in private sector Category 3: 15% or more in private sector	**Cat 2**		
			TB drugs available on the private market	**Rx required**		

CHARACTERISTICS OF THE SURVEY/SURVEILLANCE PROGRAMME

Study Duration	**12 Months**
Target Area	**Half of country**
Sampling Method	**Cluster**
Culture Media	**Löwenstein-Jensen and BACTEC**
DST Method	**Proportion and BACTEC**
Supranational Reference Laboratory	**Instituto Superiore di Sanità, Rome, Italy**

*Notations to accompany profile: Estimated HIV positive TB cases is a WHO estimate

*For survey settings where less than 100% of cases are sampled, combined estimates are based on the rates of new and previously treated cases obtained in the survey, but weighted by the absolute number of new and previously treated sputum positive TB cases, as published by the national authorities.

COUNTRY PROFILES

PREVALENCE OF DRUG RESISTANCE

10 Regions: 2000

	New		Previous		Combined	
	N	%	N	%	N	%
Total number of strains tested	688	100.0	108	100.0		100.0
SUSCEPTIBLE TO ALL 4 DRUGS	**610**	**88.7**	**57**	**52.8**		**85.3**
ANY RESISTANCE	**78**	**11.3**	**51**	**47.2**		**14.7**
- Isoniazid (INH)	44	6.4	39	36.1		9.2
- Rifampicin (RMP)	11	1.6	32	29.6		4.3
- Ethambutol (EMB)	10	1.5	12	11.1		2.4
- Streptomycin (SM)	54	7.8	25	23.1		9.3
MONORESISTANCE	**48**	**7.0**	**18**	**16.7**		**7.9**
- Isoniazid (INH)	14	2.0	6	5.6		2.4
- Rifampicin (RMP)	3	0.4	6	5.6		0.9
- Ethambutol (EMB)	4	0.6	1	0.9		0.6
- Streptomycin (SM)	27	3.9	5	4.6		4.0
MULTIDRUG RESISTANCE	**8**	**1.2**	**26**	**24.1**		**3.3**
- INH + RMP	2	0.3	9	8.3		4.0
- INH + RMP + EMB	0	0.0	3	2.8		0.3
- INH + RMP + SM	2	0.3	7	6.5		0.9
- INH + RMP + EMB + SM	4	0.6	7	6.5		1.1
OTHER PATTERNS	**22**	**3.2**	**7**	**6.5**		**3.5**
- INH + EMB	1	0.1	1	0.9		0.2
- INH + SM	20	2.9	6	5.6		3.2
- INH + EMB + SM	1	0.1	0	0.0		0.1
- RMP + EMB	0	0.0	0	0.0		0.0
- RMP + SM	0	0.0	0	0.0		0.0
- RMP + EMB + SM	0	0.0	0	0.0		0.0
- EMB + SM	0	0.0	0	0.0		0.0
NUMBER OF DRUGS RESISTANT TO:						
susceptible to 4 drugs	610	88.7	57	52.8		85.3
resistant to 1 drug	48	7.0	18	16.7		7.9
resistant to 2 drugs	23	3.3	16	14.8		4.4
resistant to 3 drugs	3	0.4	10	9.3		1.3
resistant to 4 drugs	4	0.6	7	6.5		1.1

COUNTRY PROFILES

JAPAN

Countrywide: 1997

PROFILE OF THE COUNTRY AND ITS CONTROL PROGRAMME

Population in year of survey	**126,166,000**		Year N.T.P was established	**1951**		
Notification all cases (rate)	**33.4**	**/100,000**	Year of Rifampicin introduction	**1971**		
Estimated incidence (all cases)	**NA**	**/100,000**	Year of Isoniazid introduction	**1952**		
Notification new sputum smear +	**13571**		Use of Standardized Regimens	**Yes**	**1st line**	
Notification new sputum smear + (rate)	**10.8**	**/100,000**	% Use of Short Course Chemotherapy	**Yes**	**91**	**%**
Treatment Success	**NA**	**%**	Use of Directly Observed Therapy	**No**		**%**
Retreatment cases	**827**		During continuation phase	**No**		
Retreatment as % of NTP	**5.7**	**%**	Use of Fixed Dose Combination	**No**		**%**
Estimated HIV positive TB cases	**0.32**	**%**	Treatment in private sector	**100% regulated**		

Category 1: virtually all TB patients public sector
Category 2: <15% in private sector
Category 3: 15% or more in private sector

TB drugs available on the private market	**No**	

CHARACTERISTICS OF THE SURVEY/SURVEILLANCE PROGRAMME

Study Duration	**6 Months**
Target Area	**Countrywide**
Sampling Method	**Sentinel surveillance**
Culture Media	**Ogawa**
DST Method	**Proportion**
Supranational Reference Laboratory	**Research Institute of Tuberculosis (RIT), Tokyo, Japan**

*Notations to accompany profile: Estimated HIV positive TB cases is a WHO estimate
Retreatment indicates sputum smear positive pulmonary cases only

*For survey settings where less than 100% of cases are sampled, combined estimates are based on the rates of new and previously treated cases obtained in the survey, but weighted by the absolute number of new and previously treated sputum positive TB cases, as published by the national authorities.

COUNTRY PROFILES

PREVALENCE OF DRUG RESISTANCE

Countrywide: 1997

	New		Previous		Combined	
	N	%	N	%	N	%
Total number of strains tested	1,374	100.0	264	100.0	1,638	100.0
SUSCEPTIBLE TO ALL 4 DRUGS	**1,233**	**89.7**	**152**	**57.6**	**1,385**	**84.6**
ANY RESISTANCE	**141**	**10.3**	**112**	**42.4**	**253**	**15.4**
- Isoniazid (INH)	61	4.4	87	33.0	148	9.0
- Rifampicin (RMP)	19	1.4	57	21.6	76	4.6
- Ethambutol (EMB)	6	0.4	40	15.2	46	2.8
- Streptomycin (SM)	103	7.5	64	24.2	167	10.2
MONORESISTANCE	**104**	**7.6**	**40**	**15.2**	**144**	**8.8**
- Isoniazid (INH)	28	2.0	18	6.8	46	2.8
- Rifampicin (RMP)	3	0.2	2	0.8	5	0.3
- Ethambutol (EMB)	1	0.1	0	0.0	1	0.1
- Streptomycin (SM)	72	5.2	20	7.6	92	5.6
MULTIDRUG RESISTANCE	**12**	**0.9**	**52**	**19.7**	**64**	**3.9**
- INH + RMP	5	0.4	13	4.9	18	1.1
- INH + RMP + EMB	0	0.0	13	4.9	13	0.8
- INH + RMP + SM	4	0.3	7	2.7	11	0.7
- INH + RMP + EMB + SM	3	0.2	19	7.2	22	1.3
OTHER PATTERNS	**25**	**1.8**	**20**	**7.6**	**45**	**2.7**
- INH + EMB	1	0.1	1	0.4	2	0.1
- INH + SM	20	1.5	11	4.2	31	1.9
- INH + EMB + SM	0	0.0	5	1.9	5	0.3
- RMP + EMB	0	0.0	1	0.4	1	0.1
- RMP + SM	3	0.2	1	0.4	4	0.2
- RMP + EMB + SM	1	0.1	1	0.4	2	0.1
- EMB + SM	0	0.1	0	0.0	0	0.0
NUMBER OF DRUGS RESISTANT TO:						
susceptible to 4 drugs	1,233	89.7	152	57.6	1,385	84.6
resistant to 1 drug	104	7.6	40	15.2	144	8.8
resistant to 2 drugs	29	2.1	27	10.2	56	3.4
resistant to 3 drugs	5	0.4	26	9.8	31	1.9
resistant to 4 drugs	3	0.2	19	7.2	22	1.3

COUNTRY PROFILES

KAZAKHSTAN

Countrywide: 2001

PROFILE OF THE COUNTRY AND ITS CONTROL PROGRAMME

Population in year of survey	**14,831,400**		Year N.T.P was established	**Revised 1998**		
Notification all cases (rate)	**193.6**	**/100,000**	Year of Rifampicin introduction	**1973**		
Estimated incidence (all cases)	**155.7**	**/100,000**	Year of Isoniazid introduction	**1960s**		
Notification new sputum smear +	**9079**		Use of Standardized Regimens	**Yes**		
Notification new sputum smear + (rate)	**61.2**	**/100,000**	% Use of Short Course Chemotherapy	**Yes**	**76.5**	**%**
Treatment Success	**82.5**	**%**	Use of Directly Observed Therapy	**Yes**		**%**
Retreatment cases	**2996**		During continuation phase	**Yes**		
Retreatment as % of NTP		**%**	Use of Fixed Dose Combination	**Yes**		**%**
Estimated HIV positive TB cases	**0.17**	**%**	Treatment in private sector	**NA**		
			Category 1: virtually all TB patients public sector Category 2: <15% in private sector Category 3: 15% or more in private sector			
			TB drugs available on the private market	**No**		

CHARACTERISTICS OF THE SURVEY/SURVEILLANCE PROGRAMME

Study Duration	**2 Months**
Target Area	**Countrywide**
Sampling Method	**All diagnostic units**
Culture Media	**Löwenstein-Jensen**
DST Method	**Absolute Concentration**
Supranational Reference Laboratory	**National Reference Center for Mycobacteria, Borstel, Germany**

*Notations to accompany profile: Estimated HIV positive TB cases is a WHO estimate
Retreatment indicates sputum smear positive pulmonary cases only

*For survey settings where less than 100% of cases are sampled, combined estimates are based on the rates of new and previously treated cases obtained in the survey, but weighted by the absolute number of new and previously treated sputum positive TB cases, as published by the national authorities.

PREVALENCE OF DRUG RESISTANCE

Countrywide: 2001

	New		Previous		Combined	
	N	%	N	%	N	%
Total number of strains tested	359	100.0	319	100.0		100.0
SUSCEPTIBLE TO ALL 4 DRUGS	**154**	**42.9**	**57**	**17.9**		**36.7**
ANY RESISTANCE	**205**	**57.1**	**262**	**82.1**		**63.3**
- Isoniazid (INH)	153	42.6	216	67.7		48.8
- Rifampicin (RMP)	56	15.6	196	61.4		27.0
- Ethambutol (EMB)	89	24.8	173	54.2		32.1
- Streptomycin (SM)	185	51.5	246	77.1		57.9
MONORESISTANCE	**50**	**13.9**	**26**	**8.2**		**12.5**
- Isoniazid (INH)	11	3.1	3	0.9		2.5
- Rifampicin (RMP)	1	0.3	1	0.3		0.3
- Ethambutol (EMB)	3	0.8	4	1.3		0.9
- Streptomycin (SM)	35	9.7	18	5.6		8.7
MULTIDRUG RESISTANCE	**51**	**14.2**	**180**	**56.4**		**24.7**
- INH + RMP	2	0.6	6	1.9		1.3
- INH + RMP + EMB	0	0.0	1	0.3		0.1
- INH + RMP + SM	17	4.7	39	12.2		6.6
- INH + RMP + EMB + SM	32	8.9	134	42.0		17.1
OTHER PATTERNS	**104**	**29.0**	**56**	**17.6**		**26.1**
- INH + EMB	2	0.6	0	0.0		0.4
- INH + SM	50	13.9	18	5.6		11.9
- INH + EMB + SM	39	10.9	15	4.7		9.3
- RMP + EMB	1	0.3	1	0.3		0.3
- RMP + SM	0	0.0	4	1.3		0.3
- RMP + EMB + SM	3	0.8	10	3.1		1.4
- EMB + SM	9	2.5	8	2.5		2.5
NUMBER OF DRUGS RESISTANT TO:						
susceptible to 4 drugs	154	42.9	57	17.9		36.7
resistant to 1 drug	50	13.9	26	8.2		12.5
resistant to 2 drugs	64	17.8	37	11.6		16.3
resistant to 3 drugs	59	16.4	65	20.4		17.4
resistant to 4 drugs	32	8.9	134	42.0		17.1

LATVIA

Countrywide: 2000

PROFILE OF THE COUNTRY AND ITS CONTROL PROGRAMME

Population in year of survey	**2,373,000**		Year N.T.P was established	**1995**		
Notification all cases (rate)	**82**	**/100,000**	Year of Rifampicin introduction	**1975**		
Estimated incidence (all cases)		**/100,000**	Year of Isoniazid introduction			
Notification new sputum smear +	**637**		Use of Standardized Regimens	**Yes**		
Notification new sputum smear + (rate)	**26**	**/100,000**	% Use of Short Course Chemotherapy	**Yes**	**92**	**%**
Treatment Success		**%**	Use of Directly Observed Therapy	**Yes**	**100**	**%**
Retreatment cases	**192**		During continuation phase	**Yes**		
Retreatment as % of NTP		**%**	Use of Fixed Dose Combination	**Yes**		**%**
Estimated HIV positive TB cases	**0.47**	**%**	Treatment in private sector	**Cat 1**		

Category 1: virtually all TB patients public sector
Category 2: <15% in private sector
Category 3: 15% or more in private sector

TB drugs available on the private market

CHARACTERISTICS OF THE SURVEY/SURVEILLANCE PROGRAMME

Study Duration	**12 Months**
Target Area	**Countrywide**
Sampling Method	**All cases**
Culture Media	**Löwenstein-Jensen**
DST Method	**Absolute concentration**
Supranational Reference Laboratory	**Swedish Institute for Infectious Disease Control (SIIDC), Karolinska, Stockholm, Sweden**

*Notations to accompany profile: Estimated HIV positive TB cases is a WHO estimate

COUNTRY PROFILES

PREVALENCE OF DRUG RESISTANCE

Countrywide: 2000

	New		Previous		Combined	
	N	%	N	%	N	%
Total number of strains tested	897	100.0	247	100.0	1,144	100.0
SUSCEPTIBLE TO ALL 4 DRUGS	**613**	**68.3**	**153**	**61.9**	**766**	**67.0**
ANY RESISTANCE	**284**	**31.7**	**94**	**38.1**	**378**	**33.0**
- Isoniazid (INH)	260	29.0	87	35.2	347	30.3
- Rifampicin (RMP)	83	9.3	67	27.1	150	13.1
- Ethambutol (EMB)	56	6.2	37	15.0	93	8.1
- Streptomycin (SM)	219	24.4	81	32.8	300	26.2
MONORESISTANCE	**83**	**9.3**	**16**	**6.5**	**99**	**8.7**
- Isoniazid (INH)	59	6.6	9	3.6	68	5.9
- Rifampicin (RMP)	0	0.0	0	0.0	0	0.0
- Ethambutol (EMB)	2	0.2	0	0.0	2	0.2
- Streptomycin (SM)	22	2.5	7	2.8	29	2.5
MULTIDRUG RESISTANCE	**83**	**9.3**	**67**	**27.1**	**150**	**13.1**
- INH + RMP	3	0.3	3	1.2	6	0.5
- INH + RMP + EMB	1	0.1	0	0.0	1	0.1
- INH + RMP + SM	38	4.2	28	11.3	66	5.8
- INH + RMP + EMB + SM	41	4.6	36	14.6	77	6.7
OTHER PATTERNS	**118**	**13.2**	**11**	**4.5**	**129**	**11.3**
- INH + EMB	0	0.0	1	0.4	1	0.1
- INH + SM	106	11.8	10	4.0	116	10.1
- INH + EMB + SM	12	1.3	0	0.0	12	1.0
- RMP + EMB	0	0.0	0	0.0	0	0.0
- RMP + SM	0	0.0	0	0.0	0	0.0
- RMP + EMB + SM	0	0.0	0	0.0	0	0.0
- EMB + SM	0	0.0	0	0.0	0	0.0
NUMBER OF DRUGS RESISTANT TO:						
susceptible to 4 drugs	613	68.3	153	61.9	766	67.0
resistant to 1 drug	83	9.3	16	6.5	99	8.7
resistant to 2 drugs	109	12.2	14	5.7	123	10.8
resistant to 3 drugs	51	5.7	28	11.3	79	7.8
resistant to 4 drugs	41	4.6	36	14.6	77	6.7

COUNTRY PROFILES

LITHUANIA

Countrywide: 2002

PROFILE OF THE COUNTRY AND ITS CONTROL PROGRAMME

Population in year of survey	**3,487,00**		Year N.T.P was established	**1998**		
Notification all cases (rate)		**/100,000**	Year of Rifampicin introduction	**1972**		
Estimated incidence (all cases)	**74.7**	**/100,000**	Year of Isoniazid introduction	**1960**		
Notification new sputum smear +	**822**		Use of Standardized Regimens	**Yes**		
Notification new sputum smear + (rate)	**23.6**	**/100,000**	% Use of Short Course Chemotherapy	**Yes**	**95**	**%**
Treatment Success		**%**	Use of Directly Observed Therapy	**Yes**	**79**	**%**
Retreatment cases	**380**		During continuation phase	**Yes**		
Retreatment as % of NTP		**%**	Use of Fixed Dose Combination	**Yes**	**100**	**%**
Estimated HIV positive TB cases	**0.07**	**%**	Treatment in private sector	**Cat 1**		

Category 1: virtually all TB patients public sector
Category 2: <15% in private sector
Category 3: 15% or more in private sector

TB drugs available on the private market	**All drugs**

CHARACTERISTICS OF THE SURVEY/SURVEILLANCE PROGRAMME

Study Duration	**12 Months**
Target Area	**Countrywide**
Sampling Method	**All cases**
Culture Media	**Löwenstein-Jensen**
DST Method	**BACTEC 460**
Supranational Reference Laboratory	**Reference Laboratory Mycobacteriology, Statens Serum Institut (SSI), Denmark under SIIDC, Sweden**

*Notations to accompany profile: Estimated HIV positive TB cases is a WHO estimate
Retreatment indicates sputum smear positive pulmonary cases only

*For survey settings where less than 100% of cases are sampled, combined estimates are based on the rates of new and previously treated cases obtained in the survey, but weighted by the absolute number of new and previously treated sputum positive TB cases, as published by the national authorities.

PREVALENCE OF DRUG RESISTANCE

Countrywide: 2002

	New		Previous		Combined	
	N	%	N	%	N	%
Total number of strains tested	819	100.0	321	100.0	1,140	100.0
SUSCEPTIBLE TO ALL 4 DRUGS	**580**	**70.8**	**103**	**32.1**	**683**	**59.9**
ANY RESISTANCE	**239**	**29.2**	**218**	**67.9**	**457**	**40.1**
- Isoniazid (INH)	208	25.4	210	65.4	418	36.7
- Rifampicin (RMP)	80	9.8	171	53.3	251	22.0
- Ethambutol (EMB)	60	7.3	122	38.0	182	16.0
- Streptomycin (SM)	178	21.7	188	58.6	366	32.1
MONORESISTANCE	**85**	**10.4**	**28**	**8.7**	**113**	**9.9**
- Isoniazid (INH)	54	6.6	20	6.2	74	6.5
- Rifampicin (RMP)	3	0.4	0	0.0	3	0.3
- Ethambutol (EMB)	0	0.0	0	0.0	0	0.0
- Streptomycin (SM)	28	3.4	8	2.5	36	3.1
MULTIDRUG RESISTANCE	**77**	**9.4**	**171**	**53.3**	**248**	**21.8**
- INH + RMP	2	0.2	7	2.2	9	0.8
- INH + RMP + EMB	1	0.1	2	0.6	3	0.3
- INH + RMP + SM	28	3.4	47	14.6	75	6.6
- INH + RMP + EMB + SM	46	5.6	115	35.8	161	14.1
OTHER PATTERNS	**77**	**9.4**	**19**	**2.3**	**96**	**8.4**
- INH + EMB	1	0.1	1	0.3	2	0.2
- INH + SM	64	7.8	14	4.4	78	6.8
- INH + EMB + SM	12	1.5	4	1.2	16	1.4
- RMP + EMB	0	0.0	0	0.0	0	0.0
- RMP + SM	0	0.0	0	0.0	0	0.0
- RMP + EMB + SM	0	0.0	0	0.0	0	0.0
- EMB + SM	0	0.0	0	0.0	0	0.0
NUMBER OF DRUGS RESISTANT TO:						
susceptible to 4 drugs	580	70.8	103	32.1	683	59.9
resistant to 1 drug	85	10.4	28	8.7	113	9.9
resistant to 2 drugs	67	8.2	22	6.9	89	7.8
resistant to 3 drugs	41	5.0	53	16.5	94	8.2
resistant to 4 drugs	46	5.6	115	35.8	161	14.1

COUNTRY PROFILES

LUXEMBOURG

Countrywide: 2000

PROFILE OF THE COUNTRY AND ITS CONTROL PROGRAMME

Population in year of survey	**435,000**	Year N.T.P was established		
Notification all cases (rate)	**/100,000**	Year of Rifampicin introduction	**NA**	
Estimated incidence (all cases)	**/100,000**	Year of Isoniazid introduction	**NA**	
Notification new sputum smear +	**21**	Use of Standardized Regimens	**No**	
Notification new sputum smear + (rate)	**/100,000**	% Use of Short Course Chemotherapy	**No**	**.5-1** **%**
Treatment Success	**%**	Use of Directly Observed Therapy	**Yes**	**%**
Retreatment cases		During continuation phase		
Retreatment as % of NTP	**%**	Use of Fixed Dose Combination	**Yes**	**%**
Estimated HIV positive TB cases	**4.99 %**	Treatment in private sector		

Treatment in private sector
Category 1: virtually all TB patients public sector
Category 2: <15% in private sector
Category 3: 15% or more in private sector

TB drugs available on the private market **No**

CHARACTERISTICS OF THE SURVEY/SURVEILLANCE PROGRAMME

Study Duration	**Months**
Target Area	
Sampling Method	**All cases**
Culture Media	
DST Method	
Supranational Reference Laboratory	

*Notations to accompany profile: Estimated HIV positive TB cases is a WHO estimate

*For survey settings where less than 100% of cases are sampled, combined estimates are based on the rates of new and previously treated cases obtained in the survey, but weighted by the absolute number of new and previously treated sputum positive TB cases, as published by the national authorities.

COUNTRY PROFILES

PREVALENCE OF DRUG RESISTANCE

Countrywide: 2000

	New		Previous		Combined	
	N	%	N	%	N	%
Total number of strains tested	39	100.0	5	100.0	44	100.0
SUSCEPTIBLE TO ALL 4 DRUGS	**36**	**92.3**	**5**	**100.0**	**41**	**93.2**
ANY RESISTANCE	**3**	**7.7**	**0**	**0.0**	**3**	**6.8**
- Isoniazid (INH)	2	5.1	0	0.0	2	4.5
- Rifampicin (RMP)	0	0.0	0	0.0	0	0.0
- Ethambutol (EMB)	0	0.0	0	0.0	0	0.0
- Streptomycin (SM)	1	2.6	0	0.0	1	2.3
MONORESISTANCE	**3**	**7.7**	**0**	**0.0**	**3**	**6.8**
- Isoniazid (INH)	2	5.1	0	0.0	2	4.5
- Rifampicin (RMP)	0	0.0	0	0.0	0	0.0
- Ethambutol (EMB)	0	0.0	0	0.0	0	0.0
- Streptomycin (SM)	1	2.6	0	0.0	1	2.3
MULTIDRUG RESISTANCE	**0**	**0.0**	**0**	**0.0**	**0**	**0.0**
- INH + RMP	0	0.0	0	0.0	0	0.0
- INH + RMP + EMB	0	0.0	0	0.0	0	0.0
- INH + RMP + SM	0	0.0	0	0.0	0	0..0
- INH + RMP + EMB + SM	0	0.0	0	0.0	0	0.0
OTHER PATTERNS	**0**	**0.0**	**0**	**0.0**	**0**	**0.0**
- INH + EMB	0	0.0	0	0.0	0	0.0
- INH + SM	0	0.0	0	0.0	0	0.0
- INH + EMB + SM	0	0.0	0	0.0	0	0.0
- RMP + EMB	0	0.0	0	0.0	0	0.0
- RMP + SM	0	0.0	0	0.0	0	0.0
- RMP + EMB + SM	0	0.0	0	0.0	0	0.0
- EMB + SM	0	0.0	0	0.0	0	0.0
NUMBER OF DRUGS RESISTANT TO:						
susceptible to 4 drugs	36	92.3	5	100.0	41	93.2
resistant to 1 drug	3	7.7	0	0.0	3	6.8
resistant to 2 drugs	0	0.0	0	0.0	0	0.0
resistant to 3 drugs	0	0.0	0	0.0	0	0.0
resistant to 4 drugs	0	0.0	0	0.0	0	0.0

COUNTRY PROFILES

MALTA

Countrywide: 2000

PROFILE OF THE COUNTRY AND ITS CONTROL PROGRAMME

Population in year of survey	**389,000**	Year N.T.P was established		
Notification all cases (rate)	**/100,000**	Year of Rifampicin introduction		
Estimated incidence (all cases)	**/100,000**	Year of Isoniazid introduction		
Notification new sputum smear +	**5**	Use of Standardized Regimens	**Yes**	
Notification new sputum smear + (rate)	**/100,000**	% Use of Short Course Chemotherapy	**Yes**	**100** **%**
Treatment Success	**%**	Use of Directly Observed Therapy	**Yes**	**100** **%**
Retreatment cases		During continuation phase	**NA**	
Retreatment as % of NTP	**%**	Use of Fixed Dose Combination	**Yes**	**100** **%**
Estimated HIV positive TB cases	**3.73** **%**	Treatment in private sector		

Treatment in private sector
Category 1: virtually all TB patients public sector
Category 2: <15% in private sector
Category 3: 15% or more in private sector

TB drugs available on the private market   **No**

CHARACTERISTICS OF THE SURVEY/SURVEILLANCE PROGRAMME

Study Duration	**Months**
Target Area	
Sampling Method	**All cases**
Culture Media	
DST Method	
Supranational Reference Laboratory	**Health Protection Agency Mycobacterium Reference Unit (HPA MRU), London, United Kingdom**

*Notations to accompany profile: Estimated HIV positive TB cases is a WHO estimate

*For survey settings where less than 100% of cases are sampled, combined estimates are based on the rates of new and previously treated cases obtained in the survey, but weighted by the absolute number of new and previously treated sputum positive TB cases, as published by the national authorities.

PREVALENCE OF DRUG RESISTANCE

Countrywide: 2000

	New		Previous		Combined	
	N	%	N	%	N	%
Total number of strains tested	9	100.0	1	100.0	10	100.0
SUSCEPTIBLE TO ALL 4 DRUGS	**9**	**100.0**	**1**	**100.0**	**10**	**100.0**
ANY RESISTANCE	**0**	**0.0**	**0**	**0.0**	**0**	**0.0**
- Isoniazid (INH)	0	0.0	0	0.0	0	0.0
- Rifampicin (RMP)	0	0.0	0	0.0	0	0.0
- Ethambutol (EMB)	0	0.0	0	0.0	0	0.0
- Streptomycin (SM)	0	0.0	0	0.0	0	0.0
MONORESISTANCE	**0**	**0.0**	**0**	**0.0**	**0**	**0.0**
- Isoniazid (INH)	0	0.0	0	0.0	0	0.0
- Rifampicin (RMP)	0	0.0	0	0.0	0	0.0
- Ethambutol (EMB)	0	0.0	0	0.0	0	0.0
- Streptomycin (SM)	0	0.0	0	0.0	0	0.0
MULTIDRUG RESISTANCE	**0**	**0.0**	**0**	**0.0**	**0**	**0.0**
- INH + RMP	0	0.0	0	0.0	0	0.0
- INH + RMP + EMB	0	0.0	0	0.0	0	0.0
- INH + RMP + SM	0	0.0	0	0.0	0	0.0
- INH + RMP + EMB + SM	0	0.0	0	0.0	0	0.0
OTHER PATTERNS	**0**	**0.0**	**0**	**0.0**	**0**	**0.0**
- INH + EMB	0	0.0	0	0.0	0	0.0
- INH + SM	0	0.0	0	0.0	0	0.0
- INH + EMB + SM	0	0.0	0	0.0	0	0.0
- RMP + EMB	0	0.0	0	0.0	0	0.0
- RMP + SM	0	0.0	0	0.0	0	0.0
- RMP + EMB + SM	0	0.0	0	0.0	0	0.0
- EMB + SM	0	0.0	0	0.0	0	0.0
NUMBER OF DRUGS RESISTANT TO:						
susceptible to 4 drugs	9	100.0	1	100.0	10	100.0
resistant to 1 drug	0	0.0	0	0.0	0	0.0
resistant to 2 drugs	0	0.0	0	0.0	0	0.0
resistant to 3 drugs	0	0.0	0	0.0	0	0.0
resistant to 4 drugs	0	0.0	0	0.0	0	0.0

COUNTRY PROFILES

MONGOLIA

Countrywide: 1999

PROFILE OF THE COUNTRY AND ITS CONTROL PROGRAMME

Population in year of survey	2,448,220		Year N.T.P was established	Revised 1994		
Notification all cases (rate)	136.8	/100,000	Year of Rifampicin introduction	1988		
Estimated incidence (all cases)	244	/100,000	Year of Isoniazid introduction	1959		
Notification new sputum smear +	1513		Use of Standardized Regimens	Yes		
Notification new sputum smear + (rate)	61.8	/100,000	% Use of Short Course Chemotherapy	Yes	100	%
Treatment Success	86	%	Use of Directly Observed Therapy	Yes	100	%
Retreatment cases	127		During continuation phase	Yes		
Retreatment as % of NTP	3.8	%	Use of Fixed Dose Combination	Yes	100	%
Estimated HIV positive TB cases	0.01	%	Treatment in private sector	Cat 1		

Category 1: virtually all TB patients public sector
Category 2: <15% in private sector
Category 3: 15% or more in private sector

TB drugs available on the private market — **Yes (INH, RMP)**

CHARACTERISTICS OF THE SURVEY/SURVEILLANCE PROGRAMME

Study Duration	**7 Months**
Target Area	**Countrywide**
Sampling Method	**All diagnostic units**
Culture Media	**Ogawa and subcultured on LJ for DST**
DST Method	**Proportion**
Supranational Reference Laboratory	**Research Institute of Tuberculosis (RIT), Tokyo, Japan**

*Notations to accompany profile: Estimated HIV positive TB cases is a WHO estimate
Retreatment indicates sputum smear positive pulmonary cases only

*For survey settings where less than 100% of cases are sampled, combined estimates are based on the rates of new and previously treated cases obtained in the survey, but weighted by the absolute number of new and previously treated sputum positive TB cases, as published by the national authorities.

COUNTRY PROFILES

PREVALENCE OF DRUG RESISTANCE

Countrywide: 1999

	New		Previous		Combined	
	N	%	N	%	N	%
Total number of strains tested	405	100.0				
SUSCEPTIBLE TO ALL 4 DRUGS	**286**	**70.6**				
ANY RESISTANCE	**119**	**29.4**				
- Isoniazid (INH)	62	15.3				
- Rifampicin (RMP)	5	1.2				
- Ethambutol (EMB)	7	1.7				
- Streptomycin (SM)	98	24.2				
MONORESISTANCE	**74**	**18.3**				
- Isoniazid (INH)	18	4.4				
- Rifampicin (RMP)	1	0.2				
- Ethambutol (EMB)	0	0.0				
- Streptomycin (SM)	55	13.6				
MULTIDRUG RESISTANCE	**4**	**1.0**				
- INH + RMP	1	0.2				
- INH + RMP + EMB	0	0.0				
- INH + RMP + SM	1	0.2				
- INH + RMP + EMB + SM	2	0.5				
OTHER PATTERNS	**41**	**10.1**				
- INH + EMB	1	0.2				
- INH + SM	36	8.9				
- INH + EMB + SM	3	0.7				
- RMP + EMB	0	0.0				
- RMP + SM	0	0.0				
- RMP + EMB + SM	0	0.0				
- EMB + SM	1	0.2				
NUMBER OF DRUGS RESISTANT TO:						
susceptible to 4 drugs	286	70.6				
resistant to 1 drug	74	18.3				
resistant to 2 drugs	39	9.6				
resistant to 3 drugs	4	1.0				
resistant to 4 drugs	2	0.5				

NEPAL

Countrywide: 2001

PROFILE OF THE COUNTRY AND ITS CONTROL PROGRAM

Population in year of survey	23,593,000		Year N.T.P was established	1989	
Notification all cases (rate)	125	/100,000	Year of Rifampicin introduction	1990	
Estimated incidence (all cases)	201	/100,000	Year of Isoniazid introduction	1965	
Notification new sputum smear +	13683		Use of Standardized Regimens	Yes	
Notification new sputum smear + (rate)	58	/100,000	% Use of Short Course Chemotherapy	Yes	%
Treatment Success	86	%	Use of Directly Observed Therapy	Yes	70.5 %
Retreatment cases	2044		During continuation phase	No	
Retreatment as % of NTP		%	Use of Fixed Dose Combination	No	%
Estimated HIV positive TB cases	1.15	%	Treatment in private sector	Cat 3	

Category 1: virtually all TB patients public sector
Category 2: <15% in private sector
Category 3: 15% or more in private sector

TB drugs available on the private market	All drugs

CHARACTERISTICS OF THE SURVEY/SURVEILLANCE PROGRAMME

Study Duration	10 Months
Target Area	Countrywide
Sampling Method	Cluster
Culture Media	Löwenstein-Jensen
DST Method	Proportion
Supranational Reference Laboratory	Kuratorium Tuberkulose in der Welt E.V., Gauting, Germany

*Notations to accompany profile: Estimated HIV positive TB cases is a WHO estimate
Retreatment indicates sputum smear positive pulmonary cases only

*For survey settings where less than 100% of cases are sampled, combined estimates are based on the rates of new and previously treated cases obtained in the survey, but weighted by the absolute number of new and previously treated sputum positive TB cases, as published by the national authorities.

COUNTRY PROFILES

PREVALENCE OF DRUG RESISTANCE

Countrywide: 2001

	New		Previous		Combined	
	N	%	N	%	N	%
Total number of strains tested	755	100.0	171	100.0		100.0
SUSCEPTIBLE TO ALL 4 DRUGS	**672**	**89.0**	**101**	**59.1**		**84.3**
ANY RESISTANCE	**83**	**11.0**	**70**	**40.9**		**15.7**
- Isoniazid (INH)	41	5.4	57	33.3		9.8
- Rifampicin (RMP)	13	1.7	35	20.5		4.7
- Ethambutol (EMB)	7	0.9	17	9.9		2.3
- Streptomycin (SM)	67	8.9	53	31.0		12.4
MONORESISTANCE	**53**	**7.0**	**22**	**13.0**		**7.9**
- Isoniazid (INH)	12	1.6	9	5.0		2.2
- Rifampicin (RMP)	2	0.3	0	0.0		0.2
- Ethambutol (EMB)	0	0.0	0	0.0		0.0
- Streptomycin (SM)	39	5.2	13	8.0		5.5
MULTIDRUG RESISTANCE	**10**	**1.3**	**35**	**20.5**		**4.3**
- INH + RMP	1	0.1	7	4.1		2.6
- INH + RMP + EMB	0	0.0	1	0.6		0.1
- INH + RMP + SM	3	0.4	11	6.4		1.3
- INH + RMP + EMB + SM	6	0.8	16	9.4		2.1
OTHER PATTERNS	**20**	**2.6**	**13**	**7.6**		**3.4**
- INH + EMB	1	0.1	0	0.0		0.1
- INH + SM	18	2.4	13	7.6		3.2
- INH + EMB + SM	0	0..0	0	0.0		0.0
- RMP + EMB	0	0..0	0	0.0		0.0
- RMP + SM	1	0.1	0	0.0		0.1
- RMP + EMB + SM	0	0.0	0	0.0		0.0
- EMB + SM	0	0.0	0	0.0		0.0
NUMBER OF DRUGS RESISTANT TO:						
susceptible to 4 drugs	672	89.0	101	59.1		84.3
resistant to 1 drug	53	7.0	22	12.9		7.9
resistant to 2 drugs	21	2.8	20	11.7		4.2
resistant to 3 drugs	3	0.4	12	7.0		1.4
resistant to 4 drugs	6	0.8	16	9.4		2.1

COUNTRY PROFILES

NETHERLANDS

Countrywide: 2000

PROFILE OF THE COUNTRY AND ITS CONTROL PROGRAMME

Population in year of survey	**15,864,000**		Year N.T.P was established	**1953**		
Notification all cases (rate)	**8.85**	**/100,000**	Year of Rifampicin introduction	**1966**		
Estimated incidence (all cases)	**8.85**	**/100,000**	Year of Isoniazid introduction	**1955**		
Notification new sputum smear +	**312**		Use of Standardized Regimens	**Yes**		
Notification new sputum smear + (rate)	**1.97**	**/100,000**	% Use of Short Course Chemotherapy	**Yes**	**88**	**%**
Treatment Success		**%**	Use of Directly Observed Therapy	**Yes**	**7.4**	**%**
Retreatment cases	**12**		During continuation phase	**Yes**		
Retreatment as % of NTP		**%**	Use of Fixed Dose Combination	**Yes**	**NA**	**%**
Estimated HIV positive TB cases	**5.94**	**%**	Treatment in private sector	**Cat 3**		

Category 1: virtually all TB patients public sector
Category 2: <15% in private sector
Category 3: 15% or more in private sector

TB drugs available on the private market	**Rx required**

CHARACTERISTICS OF THE SURVEY/SURVEILLANCE PROGRAMME

Study Duration	**12 Months**
Target Area	**Countrywide**
Sampling Method	**All cases**
Culture Media	**Various**
DST Method	**Absolute concentration**
Supranational Reference Laboratory	**National Institute of Public Health and the Environment (RIVM), Bilthoven, The Netherlands**

*Notations to accompany profile: Estimated HIV positive TB cases is a WHO estimate

*For survey settings where less than 100% of cases are sampled, combined estimates are based on the rates of new and previously treated cases obtained in the survey, but weighted by the absolute number of new and previously treated sputum positive TB cases, as published by the national authorities.

COUNTRY PROFILES

PREVALENCE OF DRUG RESISTANCE

Countrywide: 2000

	New		Previous		Combined	
	N	%	N	%	N	%
Total number of strains tested	768	100.0	95	100.0	863	100.0
SUSCEPTIBLE TO ALL 4 DRUGS	**686**	**89.3**	**87**	**91.6**	**773**	**89.6**
ANY RESISTANCE	**82**	**10.7**	**8**	**8.4**	**90**	**10.4**
- Isoniazid (INH)	43	5.6	8	8.4	51	5.9
- Rifampicin (RMP)	7	0.9	1	1.1	8	0.9
- Ethambutol (EMB)	5	0.7	2	2.1	7	0.8
- Streptomycin (SM)	53	6.9	4	4.2	57	6.6
MONORESISTANCE	**60**	**7.8**	**4**	**4.2**	**64**	**7.4**
- Isoniazid (INH)	21	2.7	4	4.2	25	2.9
- Rifampicin (RMP)	0	0.0	0	0.0	0	0.0
- Ethambutol (EMB)	1	0.1	0	0.0	1	0.1
- Streptomycin (SM)	38	4.9	0	0.0	38	4.4
MULTIDRUG RESISTANCE	**7**	**0.9**	**1**	**1.1**	**8**	**0.9**
- INH + RMP	5	0.7	0	0.0	5	0.6
- INH + RMP + EMB	1	0.1	0	0.0	1	0.1
- INH + RMP + SM	0	0.0	0	0.0	0	0.0
- INH + RMP + EMB + SM	1	0.1	1	1.1	2	0.2
OTHER PATTERNS	**15**	**2.0**	**3**	**3.2**	**18**	**2.1**
- INH + EMB	1	0.1	0	0.0	1	0.1
- INH + SM	13	1.7	2	2.1	15	1.7
- INH + EMB + SM	1	0.1	1	1.1	2	0.2
- RMP + EMB	0	0.0	0	0.0	0	0.0
- RMP + SM	0	0.0	0	0.0	0	0.0
- RMP + EMB + SM	0	0.0	0	0.0	0	0.0
- EMB + SM	0	0.0	0	0.0	0	0.0
NUMBER OF DRUGS RESISTANT TO:						
susceptible to 4 drugs	686	89.3	87	91.6	773	89.6
resistant to 1 drug	60	7.8	4	4.2	64	7.4
resistant to 2 drugs	19	2.5	2	2.1	21	2.4
resistant to 3 drugs	2	0.2	1	1.0	3	0.3
resistant to 4 drugs	1	0.1	1	1.0	2	0.2

NEW ZEALAND

Countrywide: 2001

PROFILE OF THE COUNTRY AND ITS CONTROL PROGRAMME

Population in year of survey	**3,737,490**		Year N.T.P was established	**NA**		
Notification all cases (rate)	**10.1**	**/100,000**	Year of Rifampicin introduction	**NA**		
Estimated incidence (all cases)	**11-15**	**/100,000**	Year of Isoniazid introduction	**NA**		
Notification new sputum smear +	**157**		Use of Standardized Regimens	**Yes, recommended**		
Notification new sputum smear + (rate)	**4.2**	**/100,000**	% Use of Short Course Chemotherapy	**Yes**	**95**	**%**
Treatment Success	**>90**	**%**	Use of Directly Observed Therapy	**Yes**	**35**	**%**
Retreatment cases	**19**		During continuation phase	**Yes**		
Retreatment as % of NTP	**7.2**	**%**	Use of Fixed Dose Combination	**Yes**	**95**	**%**
Estimated HIV positive TB cases	**1.13**	**%**	Treatment in private sector	**Cat 1**		
			Category 1: virtually all TB patients public sector Category 2: <15% in private sector Category 3: 15% or more in private sector			
			TB drugs available on the private market	**Rx required**		

CHARACTERISTICS OF THE SURVEY/SURVEILLANCE PROGRAMME

Study Duration	**12 Months**
Target Area	**Countrywide**
Sampling Method	**All cases**
Culture Media	**BACTEC**
DST Method	**BACTEC**
Supranational Reference Laboratory	**Queensland Mycobacterium Reference Laboratory, Australia**

*Notations to accompany profile: Estimated HIV positive TB cases is a WHO estimate
Retreatment indicates sputum smear positive pulmonary cases only

*For survey settings where less than 100% of cases are sampled, combined estimates are based on the rates of new and previously treated cases obtained in the survey, but weighted by the absolute number of new and previously treated sputum positive TB cases, as published by the national authorities.

COUNTRY PROFILES

PREVALENCE OF DRUG RESISTANCE

Countrywide: 2001

	New		Previous		Combined	
	N	%	N	%	N	%
Total number of strains tested	272	100.0	22	100.0	294	100.0
SUSCEPTIBLE TO ALL 4 DRUGS	**241**	**88.6**	**20**	**90.9**	**261**	**88.8**
ANY RESISTANCE	**31**	**11.4**	**2**	**9.1**	**33**	**11.2**
- Isoniazid (INH)	17	6.3	1	4.6	18	6.1
- Rifampicin (RMP)	1	0.4	0	0.0	1	0.3
- Ethambutol (EMB)	2	0.7	0	0.0	2	0.7
- Streptomycin (SM)	17	6.3	2	9.1	19	6.5
MONORESISTANCE	**25**	**9.2**	**1**	**4.6**	**26**	**8.8**
- Isoniazid (INH)	12	4.4	0	0.0	12	4.1
- Rifampicin (RMP)	0	0.0	0	0.0	0	0.0
- Ethambutol (EMB)	1	0.4	0	0.0	1	0.3
- Streptomycin (SM)	12	4.4	1	4.6	13	4.4
MULTIDRUG RESISTANCE	**0**	**0.0**	**0**	**0.0**	**0**	**0.0**
- INH + RMP	0	0.0	0	0.0	0	0.0
- INH + RMP + EMB	0	0.0	0	0.0	0	0.0
- INH + RMP + SM	0	0.0	0	0.0	0	0.0
- INH + RMP + EMB + SM	0	0.0	0	0.0	0	0.0
OTHER PATTERNS	**6**	**2.2**	**1**	**4.6**	**7**	**2.4**
- INH + EMB	0	0.0	0	0.0	0	0.0
- INH + SM	5	1.8	1	4.6	6	2.0
- INH + EMB + SM	0	0.0	0	0.0	0	0.0
- RMP + EMB	1	0.4	0	0.0	1	0.3
- RMP + SM	0	0.0	0	0.0	0	0.0
- RMP + EMB + SM	0	0.0	0	0.0	0	0.0
- EMB + SM	0	0.0	0	0.0	0	0.0
NUMBER OF DRUGS RESISTANT TO:						
susceptible to 4 drugs	241	88.6	20	90.9	261	88.8
resistant to 1 drug	25	9.2	1	4.6	26	8.8
resistant to 2 drugs	6	2.2	1	4.6	7	2.4
resistant to 3 drugs	0	0.0	0	0.0	0	0.0
resistant to 4 drugs	0	0.0	0	0.0	0	0.0

NORWAY

Countrywide: 2000

PROFILE OF THE COUNTRY AND ITS CONTROL PROGRAMME

Population in year of survey	**4,473,000**		Year N.T.P was established	**1900**		
Notification all cases (rate)	**5**	**/100,000**	Year of Rifampicin introduction	**1968**		
Estimated incidence (all cases)	**6**	**/100,000**	Year of Isoniazid introduction	**1952**		
Notification new sputum smear +	**37**		Use of Standardized Regimens	**Yes**		
Notification new sputum smear + (rate)	**1**	**/100,000**	% Use of Short Course Chemotherapy	**Yes**	**100**	**%**
Treatment Success	**70**	**%**	Use of Directly Observed Therapy	**Yes**		**%**
Retreatment cases	**3**		During continuation phase	**Yes**		
Retreatment as % of NTP		**%**	Use of Fixed Dose Combination	**Yes**	**50**	**%**
Estimated HIV positive TB cases	**2.46**	**%**	Treatment in private sector	**Cat 1**		

Category 1: virtually all TB patients public sector
Category 2: <15% in private sector
Category 3: 15% or more in private sector

TB drugs available on the private market **No**

CHARACTERISTICS OF THE SURVEY/SURVEILLANCE PROGRAMME

Study Duration	**12 Months**
Target Area	**Countrywide**
Sampling Method	**All cases**
Culture Media	**Löwenstein-Jensen**
DST Method	**BACTEC**
Supranational Reference Laboratory	**Swedish Institute for Infectious Disease Control (SIIDC), Stockholm, Sweden**

*Notations to accompany profile: Estimated HIV positive TB cases is a WHO estimate

*For survey settings where less than 100% of cases are sampled, combined estimates are based on the rates of new and previously treated cases obtained in the survey, but weighted by the absolute number of new and previously treated sputum positive TB cases, as published by the national authorities.

COUNTRY PROFILES

PREVALENCE OF DRUG RESISTANCE

Countrywide: 2000

	New		Previous		Combined	
	N	%	N	%	N	%
Total number of strains tested	160	100.0	10	100.0	170	100.0
SUSCEPTIBLE TO ALL 4 DRUGS	**122**	**76.2**	**9**	**90.0**	**131**	**77.0**
ANY RESISTANCE	**38**	**23.8**	**1**	**10.0**	**39**	**23.0**
- Isoniazid (INH)	21	13.1	0	0.0	21	12.4
- Rifampicin (RMP)	4	2.5	0	0.0	4	2.4
- Ethambutol (EMB)	11	6.9	0	0.0	11	6.5
- Streptomycin (SM)	18	11.3	1	10.0	19	11.2
MONORESISTANCE	**24**	**15.0**	**1**	**10.0**	**25**	**14.7**
- Isoniazid (INH)	7	4.4	0	0.0	7	4.1
- Rifampicin (RMP)	0	0.0	0	0.0	0	0.0
- Ethambutol (EMB)	8	5.0	0	0.0	8	4.7
- Streptomycin (SM)	9	5.6	1	10.0	10	5.9
MULTIDRUG RESISTANCE	**3**	**1.9**	**0**	**0.0**	**3**	**1.8**
- INH + RMP	3	1.9	0	0.0	3	1.8
- INH + RMP + EMB	0	0.0	0	0.0	0	0.0
- INH + RMP + SM	0	0.0	0	0.0	0	0.0
- INH + RMP + EMB + SM	0	0.0	0	0.0	0	0.0
OTHER PATTERNS	**11**	**6.8**	**0**	**0.0**	**11**	**6.5**
- INH + EMB	3	1.9	0	0.0	3	1.8
- INH + SM	8	5.0	0	0.0	8	4.7
- INH + EMB + SM	0	0.0	0	0.0	0	0.0
- RMP + EMB	0	0.0	0	0.0	0	0.0
- RMP + SM	0	0.0	0	0.0	0	0.0
- RMP + EMB + SM	0	0.0	0	0.0	0	0.0
- EMB + SM	0	0.0	0	0.0	0	0.0
NUMBER OF DRUGS RESISTANT TO:						
susceptible to 4 drugs	122	76.2	9	90.0	131	77.0
resistant to 1 drug	24	15.0	1	10.0	25	14.7
resistant to 2 drugs	14	9.3	0	0.0	14	8.8
resistant to 3 drugs	0	0.0	0	0.0	0	0.0
resistant to 4 drugs	0	0.0	0	0.0	0	0.0

COUNTRY PROFILES

OMAN

Countrywide: 2001

PROFILE OF THE COUNTRY AND ITS CONTROL PROGRAMME

Population in year of survey	**2,401,256**		Year N.T.P was established	**1981**		
Notification all cases (rate)	**11.13**	**/100,000**	Year of Rifampicin introduction	**1982**		
Estimated incidence (all cases)	**12.36**	**/100,000**	Year of Isoniazid introduction	**1981**		
Notification new sputum smear +	**109**		Use of Standardized Regimens	**Yes**		
Notification new sputum smear + (rate)	**5.96**	**/100,000**	% Use of Short Course Chemotherapy	**Yes**		**%**
Treatment Success	**93**	**%**	Use of Directly Observed Therapy	**Yes**	**100**	**%**
Retreatment cases	**5**		During continuation phase	**Not entirely**		
Retreatment as % of NTP		**%**	Use of Fixed Dose Combination	**Yes**	**100**	**%**
Estimated HIV positive TB cases	**0.39**	**%**	Treatment in private sector	**Cat 1**		

Category 1: virtually all TB patients public sector
Category 2: <15% in private sector
Category 3: 15% or more in private sector

TB drugs available on the private market	**No**

CHARACTERISTICS OF THE SURVEY/SURVEILLANCE PROGRAMME

Study Duration	**12 Months**
Target Area	**Countrywide**
Sampling Method	**All cases**
Culture Media	**Löwenstein-Jensen**
DST Method	**Critical proportion**
Supranational Reference Laboratory	**Instituto Superiore di Sanità, Rome, Italy**

*Notations to accompany profile: Estimated HIV positive TB cases is a WHO estimate
Retreatment indicates sputum smear positive pulmonary cases only

*For survey settings where less than 100% of cases are sampled, combined estimates are based on the rates of new and previously treated cases obtained in the survey, but weighted by the absolute number of new and previously treated sputum positive TB cases, as published by the national authorities.

COUNTRY PROFILES

PREVALENCE OF DRUG RESISTANCE

Countrywide: 2001

	New		Previous		Combined	
	N	%	N	%	N	%
Total number of strains tested	171	100.0	12	100.0	183	100.0
SUSCEPTIBLE TO ALL 4 DRUGS	**162**	**94.7**	**5**	**41.7**	**167**	**91.3**
ANY RESISTANCE	**9**	**5.3**	**7**	**58.3**	**16**	**8.7**
- Isoniazid (INH)	7	4.1	7	58.3	14	8.0
- Rifampicin (RMP)	1	0.6	7	58.3	8	4.4
- Ethambutol (EMB)	0	0.0	3	25.0	3	1.6
- Streptomycin (SM)	2	1.2	7	58.3	9	4.9
MONORESISTANCE	**8**	**4.7**	**0**	**0.0**	**8**	**4.4**
- Isoniazid (INH)	6	3.5	0	0.0	6	3.3
- Rifampicin (RMP)	1	0.6	0	0.0	1	0.5
- Ethambutol (EMB)	0	0.0	0	0.0	0	0.0
- Streptomycin (SM)	1	0.6	0	0.0	1	0.5
MULTIDRUG RESISTANCE	**0**	**0.0**	**7**	**58.3**	**7**	**4.0**
- INH + RMP	0	0.0	0	0.0	0	0.0
- INH + RMP + EMB	0	0.0	0	0.0	0	0.0
- INH + RMP + SM	0	0.0	4	33.0	4	2.2
- INH + RMP + EMB + SM	0	0.0	3	25.0	3	2.0
OTHER PATTERNS	**1**	**0.6**	**0**	**0.0**	**1**	**0.5**
- INH + EMB	0	0.0	0	0.0	0	0.0
- INH + SM	1	0.6	0	0.0	1	0.5
- INH + EMB + SM	0	0.0	0	0.0	0	0.0
- RMP + EMB	0	0.0	0	0.0	0	0.0
- RMP + SM	0	0.0	0	0.0	0	0.0
- RMP + EMB + SM	0	0.0	0	0.0	0	0.0
- EMB + SM	0	0.0	0	0.0	0	0.0
NUMBER OF DRUGS RESISTANT TO:						
susceptible to 4 drugs	162	94.7	5	41.7	167	91.3
resistant to 1 drug	8	4.7	0	0..0	8	4.4
resistant to 2 drugs	1	0.6	0	0.0	1	0.5
resistant to 3 drugs	0	0.0	4	33.3	4	2.2
resistant to 4 drugs	0	0.0	3	25.0	3	1.6

COUNTRY PROFILES

POLAND

Countrywide: 2001

PROFILE OF THE COUNTRY AND ITS CONTROL PROGRAMME

Population in year of survey	**38,671,000**		Year N.T.P was established	**1963**		
Notification all cases (rate)	**28**	**/100,000**	Year of Rifampicin introduction	**1970**		
Estimated incidence (all cases)	**28.5**	**/100,000**	Year of Isoniazid introduction	**1952**		
Notification new sputum smear +	**3180**		Use of Standardized Regimens	**Yes**		
Notification new sputum smear + (rate)	**8**	**/100,000**	% Use of Short Course Chemotherapy	**Yes**	**80**	**%**
Treatment Success	**86.7**	**%**	Use of Directly Observed Therapy	**Yes**	**>90**	**%**
Retreatment cases	**632**		During continuation phase	**40%**		
Retreatment as % of NTP	**13**	**%**	Use of Fixed Dose Combination	**Yes**	**90**	**%**
Estimated HIV positive TB cases	**0.27**	**%**	Treatment in private sector Category 1: virtually all TB patients public sector Category 2: <15% in private sector Category 3: 15% or more in private sector	**Cat 1**		
			TB drugs available on the private market	**No**		

CHARACTERISTICS OF THE SURVEY/SURVEILLANCE PROGRAMME

Study Duration	**12 Months**
Target Area	**Countrywide**
Sampling Method	**All cases/ selected laboratories**
Culture Media	**Löwenstein-Jensen and BACTEC**
DST Method	**Proportion**
Supranational Reference Laboratory	**National Institute of Public Health and the Environment (RIVM), Bilthoven, The Netherlands**

*Notations to accompany profile: Estimated HIV positive TB cases is a WHO estimate

*For survey settings where less than 100% of cases are sampled, combined estimates are based on the rates of new and previously treated cases obtained in the survey, but weighted by the absolute number of new and previously treated sputum positive TB cases, as published by the national authorities.

COUNTRY PROFILES

PREVALENCE OF DRUG RESISTANCE

Countrywide: 2001

	New		Previous		Combined	
	N	%	N	%	N	%
Total number of strains tested	3,037	100.0	668	100.0	3,705	100.0
SUSCEPTIBLE TO ALL 4 DRUGS	**2,851**	**93.9**	**557**	**83.4**	**3,408**	**92.0**
ANY RESISTANCE	**186**	**6.1**	**111**	**16.6**	**297**	**8.0**
- Isoniazid (INH)	125	4.1	96	14.4	221	6.0
- Rifampicin (RMP)	44	1.4	60	9.0	104	2.8
- Ethambutol (EMB)	19	0.6	22	3.3	41	1.1
- Streptomycin (SM)	103	3.4	67	10.0	170	4.6
MONORESISTANCE	**121**	**4.0**	**38**	**5.7**	**159**	**4.3**
- Isoniazid (INH)	62	2.0	23	3.4	85	2.3
- Rifampicin (RMP)	8	0.3	3	0.4	11	0.3
- Ethambutol (EMB)	0	0.0	0	0.0	0	0.0
- Streptomycin (SM)	51	1.7	12	1.8	63	1.7
MULTIDRUG RESISTANCE	**35**	**1.2**	**57**	**8.5**	**92**	**2.5**
- INH + RMP	11	0.4	11	1.6	22	0.6
- INH + RMP + EMB	2	0.1	7	1.0	9	0.2
- INH + RMP + SM	7	0.2	25	3.7	32	0.9
- INH + RMP + EMB + SM	15	0.5	14	2.1	29	0.8
OTHER PATTERNS	**30**	**1.0**	**16**	**2.4**	**46**	**1.2**
- INH + EMB	0	0.0	0	0.0	0	0.0
- INH + SM	27	0.9	15	2.2	42	1.1
- INH + EMB + SM	1	0.1	1	0.1	2	0.1
- RMP + EMB	0	0.0	0	0.0	0	0.0
- RMP + SM	1	0.1	0	0.0	1	0.1
- RMP + EMB + SM	0	0.0	0	0.0	0	0.0
- EMB + SM	1	0.1	0	0.0	1	0.1
NUMBER OF DRUGS RESISTANT TO:						
susceptible to 4 drugs	2,851	93.9	557	83.4	3,408	92.0
resistant to 1 drug	121	4.0	38	5.7	159	4.3
resistant to 2 drugs	40	0.1	26	0.4	66	1.8
resistant to 3 drugs	10	0.1	33	0.5	43	1.7
resistant to 4 drugs	15	0.1	14	0.2	29	0.7

COUNTRY PROFILES

PUERTO RICO

Countrywide: 2001

PROFILE OF THE COUNTRY AND ITS CONTROL PROGRAMME

Population in year of survey	**3,839,810**		Year N.T.P was established	**1931**		
Notification all cases (rate)	**3**	**/100,000**	Year of Rifampicin introduction	**1971**		
Estimated incidence (all cases)	**3.2**	**/100,000**	Year of Isoniazid introduction	**1952**		
Notification new sputum smear +	**71**		Use of Standardized Regimens	**Yes**		
Notification new sputum smear + (rate)	**1.8**	**/100,000**	% Use of Short Course Chemotherapy	**Yes**	**95**	**%**
Treatment Success	**72**	**%**	Use of Directly Observed Therapy	**Yes**	**64**	**%**
Retreatment cases	**NA**		During continuation phase	**Yes**		
Retreatment as % of NTP		**%**	Use of Fixed Dose Combination	**No**		**%**
Estimated HIV positive TB cases	**28.0**	**%**	Treatment in private sector	**Cat 3**		

Category 1: virtually all TB patients public sector
Category 2: <15% in private sector
Category 3: 15% or more in private sector

TB drugs available on the private market	**All drugs**

CHARACTERISTICS OF THE SURVEY/SURVEILLANCE PROGRAMME

Study Duration	**12 Months**
Target Area	**Countrywide**
Sampling Method	**All cases**
Culture Media	**BACTEC**
DST Method	**Proportion and BACTEC**
Supranational Reference Laboratory	**Centers for Disease Control and Prevention (CDC), Atlanta, United States of America**

*Notations to accompany profile:

*For survey settings where less than 100% of cases are sampled, combined estimates are based on the rates of new and previously treated cases obtained in the survey, but weighted by the absolute number of new and previously treated sputum positive TB cases, as published by the national authorities.

PREVALENCE OF DRUG RESISTANCE

Countrywide: 2001

	New		Previous		Combined	
	N	%	N	%	N	%
Total number of strains tested	100	100.0				
SUSCEPTIBLE TO ALL 4 DRUGS	**88**	**88.0**				
ANY RESISTANCE	**12**	**12.0**				
- Isoniazid (INH)	8	8.0				
- Rifampicin (RMP)	3	3.0				
- Ethambutol (EMB)	1	1.0				
- Streptomycin (SM)	8	8.0				
MONORESISTANCE	**6**	**6.0**				
- Isoniazid (INH)	3	3.0				
- Rifampicin (RMP)	0	0.0				
- Ethambutol (EMB)	0	0.0				
- Streptomycin (SM)	3	3.0				
MULTIDRUG RESISTANCE	**2**	**2.0**				
- INH + RMP	1	1.0				
- INH + RMP + EMB	0	0.0				
- INH + RMP + SM	0	0.0				
- INH + RMP + EMB + SM	1	1.0				
OTHER PATTERNS	**4**	**4.0**				
- INH + EMB	0	0.0				
- INH + SM	3	3.0				
- INH + EMB + SM	0	0.0				
- RMP + EMB	0	0.0				
- RMP + SM	1	1.0				
- RMP + EMB + SM	0	0.0				
- EMB + SM	0	0.0				
NUMBER OF DRUGS RESISTANT TO:						
susceptible to 4 drugs	88	88.0				
resistant to 1 drug	6	6.0				
resistant to 2 drugs	5	5.0				
resistant to 3 drugs	0	0.0				
resistant to 4 drugs	1	1.0				

COUNTRY PROFILES

QATAR

Countrywide: 2001

PROFILE OF THE COUNTRY AND ITS CONTROL PROGRAMME

Population in year of survey	**610,000**		Year N.T.P was established	**1997**		
Notification all cases (rate)	**46.55**	**/100,000**	Year of Rifampicin introduction	**Early 1970s**		
Estimated incidence (all cases)	**25**	**/100,000**	Year of Isoniazid introduction	**Early 1970s**		
Notification new sputum smear +	**77**		Use of Standardized Regimens	**Yes**		
Notification new sputum smear + (rate)	**12.6**	**/100,000**	% Use of Short Course Chemotherapy	**Yes**	**90**	**%**
Treatment Success	**66**	**%**	Use of Directly Observed Therapy	**Yes**	**100**	**%**
Retreatment cases	**1**		During continuation phase	**Yes**		
Retreatment as % of NTP		**%**	Use of Fixed Dose Combination	**Yes**	**>90**	**%**
Estimated HIV positive TB cases	**0.32**	**%**	Treatment in private sector	**Cat 1**		

Category 1: virtually all TB patients public sector
Category 2: <15% in private sector
Category 3: 15% or more in private sector

TB drugs available on the private market	**No**	

CHARACTERISTICS OF THE SURVEY/SURVEILLANCE PROGRAMME

Study Duration	**12 Months**
Target Area	**Countrywide**
Sampling Method	**All cases**
Culture Media	**Bact/Alert 3D and Löwenstein-Jensen**
DST Method	**Bact/Alert 3D**
Supranational Reference Laboratory	**Instituto Superiore di Sanità, Rome, Italy**

*Notations to accompany profile: Estimated HIV positive TB cases is a WHO estimate

*For survey settings where less than 100% of cases are sampled, combined estimates are based on the rates of new and previously treated cases obtained in the survey, but weighted by the absolute number of new and previously treated sputum positive TB cases, as published by the national authorities.

PREVALENCE OF DRUG RESISTANCE

Countrywide: 2001

	New		Previous		Combined	
	N	%	N	%	N	%
Total number of strains tested	284	100.0				
SUSCEPTIBLE TO ALL 4 DRUGS	**256**	**90.0**				
ANY RESISTANCE	**28**	**9.9**				
- Isoniazid (INH)	19	6.7				
- Rifampicin (RMP)	3	1.1				
- Ethambutol (EMB)	5	1.8				
- Streptomycin (SM)	9	3.2				
MONORESISTANCE	**20**	**7.0**				
- Isoniazid (INH)	12	4.2				
- Rifampicin (RMP)	1	0.4				
- Ethambutol (EMB)	2	0.7				
- Streptomycin (SM)	5	1.8				
MULTIDRUG RESISTANCE	**1**	**0.4**				
- INH + RMP	1	0.4				
- INH + RMP + EMB	0	0.0				
- INH + RMP + SM	0	0.0				
- INH + RMP + EMB + SM	0	0.0				
OTHER PATTERNS	**7**	**2.5**				
- INH + EMB	2	0.7				
- INH + SM	4	1.4				
- INH + EMB + SM	0	0.0				
- RMP + EMB	1	0.4				
- RMP + SM	0	0.0				
- RMP + EMB + SM	0	0.0				
- EMB + SM	0	0.0				
NUMBER OF DRUGS RESISTANT TO:						
susceptible to 4 drugs	256	90.0				
resistant to 1 drug	20	7.0				
resistant to 2 drugs	8	2.8				
resistant to 3 drugs	0	0.0				
resistant to 4 drugs	0	0.0				

COUNTRY PROFILES

RUSSIAN FEDERATION

Tomsk Oblast: 2002

PROFILE OF THE COUNTRY AND ITS CONTROL PROGRAMME

Population in year of survey	**941,278**		Year N.T.P was established	**1920**		
Notification all cases (rate)	**93**	**/100,000**	Year of Rifampicin introduction	**1972**		
Estimated incidence (all cases)		**/100,000**	Year of Isoniazid introduction	**1950s**		
Notification new sputum smear +	**380**		Use of Standardized Regimens	**Yes**		
Notification new sputum smear + (rate)	**40.4**	**/100,000**	% Use of Short Course Chemotherapy	**Yes**	**100**	**%**
Treatment Success		**%**	Use of Directly Observed Therapy	**Yes**	**60-70**	**%**
Retreatment cases	**97**		During continuation phase	**Yes**		
Retreatment as % of NTP	**17.3**	**%**	Use of Fixed Dose Combination	**Yes**		**%**
Estimated HIV positive TB cases	**NA**	**%**	Treatment in private sector	**Cat 1**		

Category 1: virtually all TB patients public sector
Category 2: <15% in private sector
Category 3: 15% or more in private sector

TB drugs available on the private market	**All drugs**

CHARACTERISTICS OF THE SURVEY/SURVEILLANCE PROGRAMME

Study Duration	**12 Months**
Target Area	**Countrywide**
Sampling Method	**All cases**
Culture Media	**Löwenstein-Jensen**
DST Method	**Absolute concentration**
Supranational Reference Laboratory	**Massachusetts State Laboratory, Boston, United States of America**

*Notations to accompany profile: Retreatment indicates sputum smear positive pulmonary cases only

*For survey settings where less than 100% of cases are sampled, combined estimates are based on the rates of new and previously treated cases obtained in the survey, but weighted by the absolute number of new and previously treated sputum positive TB cases, as published by the national authorities.

COUNTRY PROFILES

PREVALENCE OF DRUG RESISTANCE

Tomsk Oblast: 2002

	New		Previous		Combined	
	N	%	N	%	N	%
Total number of strains tested	533	100.0	117	100.0	650	100.0
SUSCEPTIBLE TO ALL 4 DRUGS	**334**	**62.7**	**46**	**39.3**	**380**	**58.5**
ANY RESISTANCE	**199**	**37.3**	**71**	**60.7**	**270**	**41.5**
- Isoniazid (INH)	155	29.1	60	51.3	215	33.0
- Rifampicin (RMP)	76	14.3	56	47.9	132	20.3
- Ethambutol (EMB)	23	4.3	16	13.7	39	6.0
- Streptomycin (SM)	182	34.1	67	57.3	249	38.3
MONORESISTANCE	**56**	**10.5**	**8**	**6.8**	**64**	**98.4**
- Isoniazid (INH)	13	2.4	0	0.0	13	2.0
- Rifampicin (RMP)	2	0.4	2	1.7	4	0.6
- Ethambutol (EMB)	0	0.0	0	0.0	0	0.0
- Streptomycin (SM)	41	7.7	6	5.1	47	7.2
MULTIDRUG RESISTANCE	**73**	**13.7**	**51**	**43.6**	**124**	**19.0**
- INH + RMP	2	0.4	2	1.7	4	0.6
- INH + RMP + EMB	0	0.0	0	0.0	0	0.0
- INH + RMP + SM	49	9.2	33	28.2	82	12.6
- INH + RMP + EMB + SM	22	4.1	16	13.7	38	5.8
OTHER PATTERNS	**70**	**13.1**	**12**	**10.3**	**82**	**12.6**
- INH + EMB	0	0.0	0	0.0	0	0.0
- INH + SM	68	12.8	9	7.7	77	11.8
- INH + EMB + SM	1	0.2	0	0.0	1	0.1
- RMP + EMB	0	0.0	0	0.0	0	0.0
- RMP + SM	1	0.2	3	2.6	4	0.6
- RMP + EMB + SM	0	0.0	0	0.0	0	0.0
- EMB + SM	0	0.0	0	0.0	0	0.0
NUMBER OF DRUGS RESISTANT TO:						
susceptible to 4 drugs	334	62.7	46	39.3	380	58.5
resistant to 1 drug	56	10.5	8	6.8	64	9.8
resistant to 2 drugs	71	13.3	14	12.0	85	13.0
resistant to 3 drugs	50	9.3	33	28.2	83	12.8
resistant to 4 drugs	22	4.1	16	13.7	38	5.8

RUSSIAN FEDERATION

Orel Oblast: 2002

PROFILE OF THE COUNTRY AND ITS CONTROL PROGRAMME

Population in year of survey	**890,700**		Year N.T.P was established	**1997**		
Notification all cases (rate)		**/100,000**	Year of Rifampicin introduction	**NA**		
Estimated incidence (all cases)	**67**	**/100,000**	Year of Isoniazid introduction	**NA**		
Notification new sputum smear +	**286**		Use of Standardized Regimens	**Yes**		
Notification new sputum smear + (rate)		**/100,000**	% Use of Short Course Chemotherapy	**Yes**	**100**	**%**
Treatment Success		**%**	Use of Directly Observed Therapy	**Yes**	**100**	**%**
Retreatment cases	**43**		During continuation phase	**Yes**		
Retreatment as % of NTP		**%**	Use of Fixed Dose Combination	**Yes**	**<1**	**%**
Estimated HIV positive TB cases	**NA**	**%**	Treatment in private sector	**Cat 1**		

Category 1: virtually all TB patients public sector
Category 2: <15% in private sector
Category 3: 15% or more in private sector

TB drugs available on the private market	**No**

CHARACTERISTICS OF THE SURVEY/SURVEILLANCE PROGRAMME

Study Duration	**12 Months**
Target Area	**Oblast**
Sampling Method	**All cases**
Culture Media	**Löwenstein-Jensen**
DST Method	**Absolute concentration**
Supranational Reference Laboratory	**Centers for Disease Control and Prevention (CDC), Atlanta, United States of America**

*Notations to accompany profile: Retreatment indicates sputum smear positive pulmonary cases only

*For survey settings where less than 100% of cases are sampled, combined estimates are based on the rates of new and previously treated cases obtained in the survey, but weighted by the absolute number of new and previously treated sputum positive TB cases, as published by the national authorities.

PREVALENCE OF DRUG RESISTANCE

Orel Oblast: 2002

	New		Previous		Combined	
	N	%	N	%	N	%
Total number of strains tested	379	100.0	210	100.0	589	100.0
SUSCEPTIBLE TO ALL 4 DRUGS	**299**	**78.9**	**56**	**26.7**	**355**	**60.3**
ANY RESISTANCE	**80**	**21.1**	**154**	**73.3**	**234**	**39.7**
- Isoniazid (INH)	68	17.9	149	71.0	217	36.8
- Rifampicin (RMP)	10	2.6	89	42.4	99	16.8
- Ethambutol (EMB)	18	4.7	92	43.8	110	18.7
- Streptomycin (SM)	72	19.0	139	66.2	211	35.8
MONORESISTANCE	**20**	**5.3**	**15**	**7.1**	**35**	**5.9**
- Isoniazid (INH)	8	2.1	10	4.8	18	3.1
- Rifampicin (RMP)	0	0.0	0	0.0	0	0.0
- Ethambutol (EMB)	0	0.0	1	0.5	1	0.2
- Streptomycin (SM)	12	3.2	4	1.9	16	2.7
MULTIDRUG RESISTANCE	**10**	**2.6**	**89**	**42.4**	**99**	**16.8**
- INH + RMP	0	0.0	1	0.5	1	0.2
- INH + RMP + EMB	0	0.0	2	1.0	2	0.3
- INH + RMP + SM	5	1.3	21	10.0	26	4.4
- INH + RMP + EMB + SM	5	1.3	65	31.0	70	11.9
OTHER PATTERNS	**50**	**13.2**	**50**	**23.8**	**100**	**17.0**
- INH + EMB	0	0.0	1	0.5	1	0.2
- INH + SM	37	9.8	26	12.4	63	10.7
- INH + EMB + SM	13	3.4	23	11.0	36	6.1
- RMP + EMB	0	0.0	0	0.0	0	0.0
- RMP + SM	0	0.0	0	0.0	0	0.0
- RMP + EMB + SM	0	0.0	0	0.0	0	0.0
- EMB + SM	0	0.0	0	0.0	0	0.0
NUMBER OF DRUGS RESISTANT TO:						
susceptible to 4 drugs	299	78.9	56	26.7	355	60.3
resistant to 1 drug	20	5.3	15	7.1	35	5.9
resistant to 2 drugs	37	9.8	28	13.3	65	11.0
resistant to 3 drugs	18	4.7	46	21.9	64	10.9
resistant to 4 drugs	5	1.3	65	31.0	70	11.9

COUNTRY PROFILES

SERBIA AND MONTENEGRO

Belgrade: 2000

PROFILE OF THE COUNTRY AND ITS CONTROL PROGRAMME

Population in year of survey		Year N.T.P was established		
Notification all cases (rate)	/100,000	Year of Rifampicin introduction		
Estimated incidence (all cases)	/100,000	Year of Isoniazid introduction		
Notification new sputum smear +		Use of Standardized Regimens		
Notification new sputum smear + (rate)	/100,000	% Use of Short Course Chemotherapy		%
Treatment Success	%	Use of Directly Observed Therapy		%
Retreatment cases		During continuation phase		
Retreatment as % of NTP	%	Use of Fixed Dose Combination		%
Estimated HIV positive TB cases	NA %	Treatment in private sector		

Category 1: virtually all TB patients public sector
Category 2: <15% in private sector
Category 3: 15% or more in private sector

TB drugs available on the private market

CHARACTERISTICS OF THE SURVEY/SURVEILLANCE PROGRAMME

Study Duration	**12 Months**
Target Area	**Regionwide**
Sampling Method	**All cases**
Culture Media	
DST Method	
Supranational Reference Laboratory	**National Reference Center for Mycobacteria, Borstel, Germany**

*Notations to accompany profile:

*For survey settings where less than 100% of cases are sampled, combined estimates are based on the rates of new and previously treated cases obtained in the survey, but weighted by the absolute number of new and previously treated sputum positive TB cases, as published by the national authorities.

PREVALENCE OF DRUG RESISTANCE

Belgrade: 2000

	New		Previous		Combined	
	N	%	N	%	N	%
Total number of strains tested	249	100.0	30	100.0	279	100.0
SUSCEPTIBLE TO ALL 4 DRUGS	**235**	**94.4**	**25**	**83.4**	**260**	**93.2**
ANY RESISTANCE	**14**	**5.6**	**5**	**16.7**	**19**	**6.8**
- Isoniazid (INH)	4	1.6	3	10.0	7	2.5
- Rifampicin (RMP)	5	2.0	0	0.0	5	1.8
- Ethambutol (EMB)	2	0.8	2	6.7	4	1.4
- Streptomycin (SM)	6	2.4	1	3.3	7	2.5
MONORESISTANCE	**12**	**4.8**	**4**	**13.3**	**16**	**5.7**
- Isoniazid (INH)	3	1.2	2	6.7	5	1.8
- Rifampicin (RMP)	4	1.6	0	0.0	4	1.4
- Ethambutol (EMB)	1	0.4	2	6.7	3	1.1
- Streptomycin (SM)	4	1.6	0	0.0	4	1.4
MULTIDRUG RESISTANCE	**1**	**0.4**	**0**	**0.0**	**1**	**0.4**
- INH + RMP	0	0.0	0	0.0	0	0.0
- INH + RMP + EMB	0	0.0	0	0.0	0	0.0
- INH + RMP + SM	1	0.4	0	0.0	1	0.4
- INH + RMP + EMB + SM	0	0.0	0	0.0	0	0.0
OTHER PATTERNS	**1**	**0.4**	**1**	**3.3**	**2**	**0.7**
- INH + EMB	0	0.0	0	0.0	0	0.0
- INH + SM	0	0.0	1	3.3	1	0.4
- INH + EMB + SM	0	0.0	0	0.0	0	0.0
- RMP + EMB	0	0.0	0	0.0	0	0.0
- RMP + SM	0	0.0	0	0.0	0	0.0
- RMP + EMB + SM	0	0.0	0	0.0	0	0.0
- EMB + SM	1	0.4	0	0.0	1	0.4
NUMBER OF DRUGS RESISTANT TO:						
susceptible to 4 drugs	235	94.4	25	83.4	260	93.2
resistant to 1 drug	12	4.8	4	13.3	16	5.7
resistant to 2 drugs	1	0.4	1	3.3	2	0.7
resistant to 3 drugs	1	0.4	0	0	1	0.4
resistant to 4 drugs	0	0.0	0	0	0	0.0

COUNTRY PROFILES

SINGAPORE

Countrywide: 2001

PROFILE OF THE COUNTRY AND ITS CONTROL PROGRAMME

Population in year of survey	**3,319,000**		Year N.T.P was established	**1957**		
Notification all cases (rate)		**/100,000**	Year of Rifampicin introduction	**1970s**		
Estimated incidence (all cases)	**44.4**	**/100,000**	Year of Isoniazid introduction	**1950s**		
Notification new sputum smear +	**357**		Use of Standardized Regimens	**Yes**		
Notification new sputum smear + (rate)	**10.8**	**/100,000**	% Use of Short Course Chemotherapy	**Yes**	**76**	**%**
Treatment Success		**%**	Use of Directly Observed Therapy	**Yes**	**41**	**%**
Retreatment cases	**62**		During continuation phase	**Yes**		
Retreatment as % of NTP		**%**	Use of Fixed Dose Combination	**No**		**%**
Estimated HIV positive TB cases	**3.29**	**%**	Treatment in private sector	**Cat 2**		

Category 1: virtually all TB patients public sector
Category 2: <15% in private sector
Category 3: 15% or more in private sector

TB drugs available on the private market	**Yes**

CHARACTERISTICS OF THE SURVEY/SURVEILLANCE PROGRAMME

Study Duration	**12 Months**
Target Area	**Countrywide**
Sampling Method	**All cases**
Culture Media	**Löwenstein-Jensen and BACTEC**
DST Method	**BACTEC**
Supranational Reference Laboratory	**Research Institute of Tuberculosis (RIT), Tokyo, Japan**

*Notations to accompany profile: Estimated HIV positive TB cases is a WHO estimate
Retreatment indicates sputum smear positive pulmonary cases only

*For survey settings where less than 100% of cases are sampled, combined estimates are based on the rates of new and previously treated cases obtained in the survey, but weighted by the absolute number of new and previously treated sputum positive TB cases, as published by the national authorities.

COUNTRY PROFILES

PREVALENCE OF DRUG RESISTANCE

Countrywide: 2001

	New		Previous		Combined	
	N	%	N	%	N	%
Total number of strains tested	823	100.0	126	100.0	949	100.0
SUSCEPTIBLE TO ALL 4 DRUGS	**782**	**95.0**	**111**	**88.1**	**893**	**94.1**
ANY RESISTANCE	**41**	**5.0**	**15**	**11.9**	**56**	**5.9**
- Isoniazid (INH)	27	3.5	8	6.3	35	3.9
- Rifampicin (RMP)	5	0.5	3	2.4	8	0.7
- Ethambutol (EMB)	6	0.7	1	0.8	7	0.7
- Streptomycin (SM)	25	3.0	7	5.6	32	3.4
MONORESISTANCE	**26**	**3.1**	**12**	**9.5**	**38**	**4.0**
- Isoniazid (INH)	13	1.6	5	4.0	18	1.9
- Rifampicin (RMP)	0	0.0	2	1.6	2	0.2
- Ethambutol (EMB)	1	0.1	0	0.0	1	0.1
- Streptomycin (SM)	12	1.5	5	4.0	17	1.8
MULTIDRUG RESISTANCE	**4**	**0.9**	**1**	**0.8**	**5**	**0.5**
- INH + RMP	1	0.1	0	0.0	1	0.1
- INH + RMP + EMB	0	0.0	0	0.0	0	0.0
- INH + RMP + SM	1	0.1	1	0.8	2	0.2
- INH + RMP + EMB + SM	2	0.2	0	0.0	2	0.2
OTHER PATTERNS	**11**	**1.3**	**2**	**1.6**	**13**	**1.4**
- INH + EMB	1	0.1	1	0.8	2	0.2
- INH + SM	7	0.9	1	0.8	8	0.8
- INH + EMB + SM	2	0.2	0	0.0	2	0.2
- RMP + EMB	0	0.0	0	0.0	0	0.0
- RMP + SM	1	0.1	0	0.0	1	0.1
- RMP + EMB + SM	0	0.0	0	0.0	0	0.0
- EMB + SM	0	0.0	0	0.0	0	0.0
NUMBER OF DRUGS RESISTANT TO:						
susceptible to 4 drugs	782	95.0	111	88.1	893	94.1
resistant to 1 drug	26	3.1	12	9.5	38	4.0
resistant to 2 drugs	10	1.2	2	1.6	12	1.3
resistant to 3 drugs	3	0.4	1	0.8	4	0.4
resistant to 4 drugs	2	0.2	0	0.0	2	0.2

COUNTRY PROFILES

SLOVAKIA

Countrywide: 2000

PROFILE OF THE COUNTRY AND ITS CONTROL PROGRAMME

Population in year of survey	**5,391,000**		Year N.T.P was established	**1982**		
Notification all cases (rate)	**19**	**/100,000**	Year of Rifampicin introduction	**1970**		
Estimated incidence (all cases)		**/100,000**	Year of Isoniazid introduction	**1952**		
Notification new sputum smear +	**236**		Use of Standardized Regimens	**No**		
Notification new sputum smear + (rate)	**4**	**/100,000**	% Use of Short Course Chemotherapy	**Yes**	**100**	**%**
Treatment Success	**82**	**%**	Use of Directly Observed Therapy	**Yes**	**100**	**%**
Retreatment cases	**62**		During continuation phase	**Yes**		
Retreatment as % of NTP		**%**	Use of Fixed Dose Combination	**No**		**%**
Estimated HIV positive TB cases	**0.04**	**%**	Treatment in private sector	**Cat 1**		

Category 1: virtually all TB patients public sector
Category 2: <15% in private sector
Category 3: 15% or more in private sector

TB drugs available on the private market	**No**

CHARACTERISTICS OF THE SURVEY/SURVEILLANCE PROGRAMME

Study Duration	**12 Months**
Target Area	**Countrywide**
Sampling Method	**All cases**
Culture Media	**Löwenstein-Jensen**
DST Method	**Proportion**
Supranational Reference Laboratory	

*Notations to accompany profile: Estimated HIV positive TB cases is a WHO estimate

*For survey settings where less than 100% of cases are sampled, combined estimates are based on the rates of new and previously treated cases obtained in the survey, but weighted by the absolute number of new and previously treated sputum positive TB cases, as published by the national authorities.

COUNTRY PROFILES

PREVALENCE OF DRUG RESISTANCE

Countrywide: 2000

	New		Previous		Combined	
	N	%	N	%	N	%
Total number of strains tested	465	100.0	110	100.0	575	100.0
SUSCEPTIBLE TO ALL 4 DRUGS	**446**	**95.9**	**95**	**86.4**	**541**	**94.1**
ANY RESISTANCE	**19**	**4.1**	**15**	**13.6**	**34**	**5.9**
- Isoniazid (INH)	15	3.2	12	10.9	27	4.7
- Rifampicin (RMP)	7	1.5	2	1.8	9	1.6
- Ethambutol (EMB)	1	0.2	1	0.9	2	0.3
- Streptomycin (SM)	6	1.3	6	5.5	12	2.1
MONORESISTANCE	**11**	**2.4**	**11**	**10.0**	**22**	**3.8**
- Isoniazid (INH)	8	1.7	8	7.3	16	2.8
- Rifampicin (RMP)	1	0.2	0	0.0	1	0.2
- Ethambutol (EMB)	0	0.0	0	0.0	0	0.0
- Streptomycin (SM)	2	0.4	3	2.7	5	0.9
MULTIDRUG RESISTANCE	**5**	**1.1**	**2**	**1.8**	**7**	**1.2**
- INH + RMP	3	0.6	1	0.9	4	0.7
- INH + RMP + EMB	1	0.2	0	0.0	1	0.2
- INH + RMP + SM	1	0.2	0	0.0	1	0.2
- INH + RMP + EMB + SM	0	0.0	1	0.9	1	0.2
OTHER PATTERNS	**3**	**0.6**	**2**	**1.8**	**5**	**0.9**
- INH + EMB	0	0.0	0	0.0	0	0.0
- INH + SM	2	0.4	2	1.8	4	0.7
- INH + EMB + SM	0	0.0	0	0.0	0	0.0
- RMP + EMB	0	0.0	0	0.0	0	0.0
- RMP + SM	1	0.2	0	0.0	1	0.2
- RMP + EMB + SM	0	0.0	0	0.0	0	0.0
- EMB + SM	0	0.0	0	0.0	0	0.0
NUMBER OF DRUGS RESISTANT TO:						
susceptible to 4 drugs	446	95.9	95	86.4	541	94.1
resistant to 1 drug	11	2.4	11	10.0	22	3.8
resistant to 2 drugs	6	1.3	3	2.7	9	1.6
resistant to 3 drugs	2	0.4	0	0.0	2	0.3
resistant to 4 drugs	0	0.0	1	0.9	1	0.2

COUNTRY PROFILES

SLOVENIA

Countrywide: 2000

PROFILE OF THE COUNTRY AND ITS CONTROL PROGRAMME

Population in year of survey	**1,990,000**		Year N.T.P was established	**1952**		
Notification all cases (rate)	**19**	**/100,000**	Year of Rifampicin introduction	**1973**		
Estimated incidence (all cases)	**23**	**/100,000**	Year of Isoniazid introduction	**1956**		
Notification new sputum smear +	**145**		Use of Standardized Regimens	**Yes**		
Notification new sputum smear + (rate)	**7**	**/100,000**	% Use of Short Course Chemotherapy	**Yes**	**93**	**%**
Treatment Success	**84**	**%**	Use of Directly Observed Therapy	**Yes**	**60**	**%**
Retreatment cases	**24**		During continuation phase	**No**		
Retreatment as % of NTP		**%**	Use of Fixed Dose Combination	**Yes**	**75**	**%**
Estimated HIV positive TB cases	**0.07**	**%**	Treatment in private sector	**Cat 1**		

Category 1: virtually all TB patients public sector
Category 2: <15% in private sector
Category 3: 15% or more in private sector

TB drugs available on the private market	**No**

CHARACTERISTICS OF THE SURVEY/SURVEILLANCE PROGRAMME

Study Duration	**12 Months**
Target Area	**Countrywide**
Sampling Method	**All cases**
Culture Media	**Löwenstein-Jensen**
DST Method	**Proportion**
Supranational Reference Laboratory	**National Reference Center for Mycobacteria, Borstel, Germany**

*Notations to accompany profile: Estimated HIV positive TB cases is a WHO estimate

*For survey settings where less than 100% of cases are sampled, combined estimates are based on the rates of new and previously treated cases obtained in the survey, but weighted by the absolute number of new and previously treated sputum positive TB cases, as published by the national authorities.

COUNTRY PROFILES

PREVALENCE OF DRUG RESISTANCE

Countrywide: 2000

	New		Previous		Combined	
	N	%	N	%	N	%
Total number of strains tested	282	100.0	38	100.0	320	100.0
SUSCEPTIBLE TO ALL 4 DRUGS	**275**	**97.5**	**34**	**89.5**	**309**	**96.6**
ANY RESISTANCE	**7**	**2.5**	**4**	**10.5**	**11**	**3.4**
- Isoniazid (INH)	6	2.1	3	7.9	9	2.8
- Rifampicin (RMP)	0	0.0	0	0.0	0	0..0
- Ethambutol (EMB)	0	0.0	1	2.6	1	0.3
- Streptomycin (SM)	3	1.1	2	5.3	5	1.6
MONORESISTANCE	**5**	**1.8**	**3**	**7.9**	**8**	**2.5**
- Isoniazid (INH)	4	1.4	2	5.3	6	1.9
- Rifampicin (RMP)	0	0.0	0	0.0	0	0.0
- Ethambutol (EMB)	0	0.0	0	0.0	0	0.0
- Streptomycin (SM)	1	0.4	1	2.6	2	0.6
MULTIDRUG RESISTANCE	**0**	**0.0**	**0**	**0.0**	**0**	**0.0**
- INH + RMP	0	0.0	0	0.0	0	0.0
- INH + RMP + EMB	0	0.0	0	0.0	0	0.0
- INH + RMP + SM	0	0.0	0	0.0	0	0.0
- INH + RMP + EMB + SM	0	0.0	0	0.0	0	0.0
OTHER PATTERNS	**2**	**0.7**	**1**	**2.6**	**3**	**0.9**
- INH + EMB	0	0.0	0	0.0	0	0.0
- INH + SM	2	0.7	0	0.0	2	0.6
- INH + EMB + SM	0	0.0	1	2.6	1	0.3
- RMP + EMB	0	0.0	0	0.0	0	0.0
- RMP + SM	0	0.0	0	0.0	0	0.0
- RMP + EMB + SM	0	0.0	0	0.0	0	0.0
- EMB + SM	0	0.0	0	0.0	0	0.0
NUMBER OF DRUGS RESISTANT TO:						
susceptible to 4 drugs	275	97.5	34	89.5	309	96.6
resistant to 1 drug	5	1.8	3	7.9	8	2.5
resistant to 2 drugs	2	0.7	0	0.0	2	0.6
resistant to 3 drugs	0	0.0	1	2.6	1	0.3
resistant to 4 drugs	0	0.0	0	0.0	0	0.0

COUNTRY PROFILES

SOUTH AFRICA

Kwazulu-Natal Province: 2001-2002

PROFILE OF THE COUNTRY AND ITS CONTROL PROGRAMME

Population in year of survey	9,146,297		Year N.T.P was established	**1999** **(revised programme)**
Notification all cases (rate)	**251**	**/100,000**	Year of Rifampicin introduction	**1979**
Estimated incidence (all cases)	**827**	**/100,000**	Year of Isoniazid introduction	**1968**
Notification new sputum smear +	**12393**		Use of Standardized Regimens	**Yes**
Notification new sputum smear + (rate)	**135**	**/100,000**	% Use of Short Course Chemotherapy	**Yes** **100** **%**
Treatment Success	**58.8**	**%**	Use of Directly Observed Therapy	**Yes** **60** **%**
Retreatment cases	**2727**		During continuation phase	**Variable**
Retreatment as % of NTP	**7**	**%**	Use of Fixed Dose Combination	**Yes** **100** **%**
Estimated HIV positive TB cases	**64.4**	**%**	Treatment in private sector	**Cat 1**

Category 1: virtually all TB patients public sector
Category 2: <15% in private sector
Category 3: 15% or more in private sector

TB drugs available on the private market — **No**

CHARACTERISTICS OF THE SURVEY/SURVEILLANCE PROGRAMME

Study Duration	**12 Months**
Target Area	**Kwazulu-Natal Province**
Sampling Method	**Multistage stratified cluster sampling**
Culture Media	**Löwenstein-Jensen**
DST Method	**Indirect proportion**
Supranational Reference Laboratory	**Medical Research Council (MRC) National TB Research Programme, South Africa**

*Notations to accompany profile: Retreatment indicates sputum smear positive pulmonary cases only

*For survey settings where less than 100% of cases are sampled, combined estimates are based on the rates of new and previously treated cases obtained in the survey, but weighted by the absolute number of new and previously treated sputum positive TB cases, as published by the national authorities.

PREVALENCE OF DRUG RESISTANCE

Kwazulu-Natal Province: 2001-2002

	New		Previous		Combined	
	N	%	N	%	N	%
Total number of strains tested	595	100.0	207	100.0		100.0
SUSCEPTIBLE TO ALL 4 DRUGS	**556**	**93.4**	**169**	**81.6**		**91.3**
ANY RESISTANCE	**39**	**6.6**	**38**	**18.4**		**8.7**
- Isoniazid (INH)	32	5.4	30	14.5		7.0
- Rifampicin (RMP)	11	1.8	18	8.7		3.1
- Ethambutol (EMB)	5	5.0	5	2.4		1.1
- Streptomycin (SM)	23	3.9	22	10.6		5.1
MONORESISTANCE	**22**	**3.7**	**17**	**8.2**		**4.5**
- Isoniazid (INH)	15	2.5	9	4.3		2.9
- Rifampicin (RMP)	1	0.2	2	1.0		0.3
- Ethambutol (EMB)	0	0.0	1	0.5		0.1
- Streptomycin (SM)	6	1.0	5	2.4		1.3
MULTIDRUG RESISTANCE	**10**	**1.7**	**16**	**7.7**		**2.8**
- INH + RMP	0	0.0	4	1.9		0.3
- INH + RMP + EMB	0	0.0	0	0.0		0.0
- INH + RMP + SM	6	1.0	8	3.9		1.5
- INH + RMP + EMB + SM	4	0.7	4	1.9		0.9
OTHER PATTERNS	**7**	**1.2**	**5**	**2.4**		**1.4**
- INH + EMB	0	0.0	0	0.0		0.0
- INH + SM	6	1.0	5	2.4		1.3
- INH + EMB + SM	1	0.2	0	0.0		0.1
- RMP + EMB	0	0.0	0	0.0		0.0
- RMP + SM	0	0.0	0	0.0		0.0
- RMP + EMB + SM	0	0.0	0	0.0		0.0
- EMB + SM	0	0.0	0	0.0		0.0
NUMBER OF DRUGS RESISTANT TO:						
susceptible to 4 drugs	556	93.4	169	81.6		91.3
resistant to 1 drug	22	3.7	17	8.2		4.5
resistant to 2 drugs	6	1.0	9	4.3		1.6
resistant to 3 drugs	7	1.2	8	3.9		1.7
resistant to 4 drugs	4	0.7	4	1.9		0.9

COUNTRY PROFILES

SOUTH AFRICA

Eastern Cape Province: 2001-2002

PROFILE OF THE COUNTRY AND ITS CONTROL PROGRAMME

Population in year of survey	**7,001,260**		Year N.T.P was established	**1996** **(revised programme)**		
Notification all cases (rate)	**400**	**/100,000**	Year of Rifampicin introduction	**1979**		
Estimated incidence (all cases)	**875**	**/100,000**	Year of Isoniazid introduction	**1968**		
Notification new sputum smear +	**15346**		Use of Standardized Regimens	**Yes**		
Notification new sputum smear + (rate)	**219**	**/100,000**	% Use of Short Course Chemotherapy	**Yes**	**100**	**%**
Treatment Success	**60.3**	**%**	Use of Directly Observed Therapy	**Yes**	**60**	**%**
Retreatment cases	**7540**		During continuation phase	**Variable**		
Retreatment as % of NTP	**12**	**%**	Use of Fixed Dose Combination	**Yes**	**100**	**%**
Estimated HIV positive TB cases	**30.5**	**%**	Treatment in private sector Category 1: virtually all TB patients public sector Category 2: <15% in private sector Category 3: 15% or more in private sector	**Cat 1**		
			TB drugs available on the private market	**No**		

CHARACTERISTICS OF THE SURVEY/SURVEILLANCE PROGRAMME

Study Duration	**12 Months**
Target Area	**Eastern Cape Province**
Sampling Method	**Multistage stratified cluster sampling**
Culture Media	**Löwenstein-Jensen**
DST Method	**Indirect proportion**
Supranational Reference Laboratory	**Medical Research Council (MRC) National TB Research Programme, South Africa**

*Notations to accompany profile: Retreatment indicates sputum smear positive pulmonary cases only

*For survey settings where less than 100% of cases are sampled, combined estimates are based on the rates of new and previously treated cases obtained in the survey, but weighted by the absolute number of new and previously treated sputum positive TB cases, as published by the national authorities.

COUNTRY PROFILES

PREVALENCE OF DRUG RESISTANCE

Eastern Cape Province: 2001-2002

	New		Previous		Combined	
	N	%	N	%	N	%
Total number of strains tested	506	100.0	283	100.0		100.0
SUSCEPTIBLE TO ALL 4 DRUGS	449	88.7	233	82.3		86.6
ANY RESISTANCE	57	11.3	50	17.7		13.4
- Isoniazid (INH)	36	7.1	38	13.4		9.2
- Rifampicin (RMP)	6	1.2	22	7.8		3.4
- Ethambutol (EMB)	3	0.6	4	1.4		0.9
- Streptomycin (SM)	34	6.7	25	8.8		7.4
MONORESISTANCE	40	7.9	21	7.4		7.7
- Isoniazid (INH)	19	3.8	9	3.2		3.6
- Rifampicin (RMP)	1	0.2	1	0.3		0.2
- Ethambutol (EMB)	0	0.0	0	0.0		0.0
- Streptomycin (SM)	20	4.0	11	3.9		3.9
MULTIDRUG RESISTANCE	5	1.0	21	7.8		3.1
- INH + RMP	3	0.6	13	4.6		1.9
- INH + RMP + EMB	0	0.0	1	0.4		0.1
- INH + RMP + SM	0	0.0	5	0.0		0.6
- INH + RMP + EMB + SM	2	0.4	2	0.7		0.5
OTHER PATTERNS	12	2.3	8	2.8		2.5
- INH + EMB	0	0.0	1	0.4		0.1
- INH + SM	11	2.1	7	2.5		2.3
- INH + EMB + SM	1	0.2	0	0.0		0.1
- RMP + EMB	0	0.0	0	0.0		0.0
- RMP + SM	0	0.0	0	0.0		0.0
- RMP + EMB + SM	0	0.0	0	0.0		0.0
- EMB + SM	0	0.0	0	0.0		0.0
NUMBER OF DRUGS RESISTANT TO:						
susceptible to 4 drugs	449	88.7	233	82.3		86.6
resistant to 1 drug	40	7.9	21	7.4		7.7
resistant to 2 drugs	14	2.8	21	7.4		4.3
resistant to 3 drugs	1	0.2	6	2.1		0.8
resistant to 4 drugs	2	0.4	2	0.7		0.5

COUNTRY PROFILES

SOUTH AFRICA

Mpumalanga: 2001-2002

PROFILE OF THE COUNTRY AND ITS CONTROL PROGRAMME

Population in year of survey	**3,111,069**		Year N.T.P was established	**1996** **(revised programme)**		
Notification all cases (rate)	**188**	**/100,000**	Year of Rifampicin introduction	**1979**		
Estimated incidence (all cases)	**578**	**/100,000**	Year of Isoniazid introduction	**1968**		
Notification new sputum smear +	**4296**		Use of Standardized Regimens	**Yes**		
Notification new sputum smear + (rate)	**138**	**/100,000**	% Use of Short Course Chemotherapy	**Yes**	**100**	**%**
Treatment Success	**67.2**	**%**	Use of Directly Observed Therapy	**Yes**	**60**	**%**
Retreatment cases	**618**		During continuation phase	**Variable**		
Retreatment as % of NTP	**8**	**%**	Use of Fixed Dose Combination	**Yes**	**100**	**%**
Estimated HIV positive TB cases	**67.2**	**%**	Treatment in private sector	**Cat 1**		
			Category 1: virtually all TB patients public sector Category 2: <15% in private sector Category 3: 15% or more in private sector			
			TB drugs available on the private market	**No**		

CHARACTERISTICS OF THE SURVEY/SURVEILLANCE PROGRAMME

Study Duration	**12 Months**
Target Area	**Mpumalanga**
Sampling Method	**Multistage stratified cluster sampling**
Culture Media	**Löwenstein-Jensen**
DST Method	**Indirect proportion**
Supranational Reference Laboratory	**Medical Research Council (MRC), Unit for TB Operational Research and Policy, Pretoria, South Africa**

*Notations to accompany profile:

*For survey settings where less than 100% of cases are sampled, combined estimates are based on the rates of new and previously treated cases obtained in the survey, but weighted by the absolute number of new and previously treated sputum positive TB cases, as published by the national authorities.

COUNTRY PROFILES

PREVALENCE OF DRUG RESISTANCE

Mpumalanga: 2001-2002

	New		Previous		Combined	
	N	%	N	%	N	%
Total number of strains tested	702	100.0	175	100.0		100.0
SUSCEPTIBLE TO ALL 4 DRUGS	**636**	**90.9**	**134**	**76.6**		**88.8**
ANY RESISTANCE	**66**	**9.1**	**41**	**23.4**		**11.2**
- Isoniazid (INH)	49	7.0	33	18.9		8.5
- Rifampicin (RMP)	22	3.1	28	16.0		4.8
- Ethambutol (EMB)	7	1.0	16	9.1		2.0
- Streptomycin (SM)	29	4.1	25	14.3		5.4
MONORESISTANCE	**39**	**5.5**	**12**	**6.9**		**5.7**
- Isoniazid (INH)	22	3.1	4	2.3		3.0
- Rifampicin (RMP)	4	0.6	4	2.3		0.8
- Ethambutol (EMB)	0	0.0	0	0.0		0.0
- Streptomycin (SM)	13	1.9	4	2.3		1.9
MULTIDRUG RESISTANCE	**18**	**2.6**	**24**	**13.7**		**4.0**
- INH + RMP	6	0.9	6	3.4		1.2
- INH + RMP + EMB	4	0.6	2	1.1		0.6
- INH + RMP + SM	6	0.9	4	2.3		1.0
- INH + RMP + EMB + SM	2	0.3	12	6.9		1.1
OTHER PATTERNS	**9**	**1.2**	**5**	**2.9**		**1.5**
- INH + EMB	1	0.1	0	0.0		0.1
- INH + SM	8	1.1	3	1.7		1.2
- INH + EMB + SM	0	0.0	2	1.1		0.1
- RMP + EMB	0	0.0	0	0.0		0.0
- RMP + SM	0	0.0	0	0.0		0.0
- RMP + EMB + SM	0	0.0	0	0.0		0.0
- EMB + SM	0	0.0	0	0.0		0.0
NUMBER OF DRUGS RESISTANT TO:						
susceptible to 4 drugs	636	90.9	134	76.6		88.8
resistant to 1 drug	39	5.5	12	6.9		5.7
resistant to 2 drugs	15	2.1	9	5.2		2.5
resistant to 3 drugs	10	1.4	8	4.6		1.8
resistant to 4 drugs	2	0.3	12	6.9		1.1

COUNTRY PROFILES

SOUTH AFRICA

Gauteng Province: 2001-2002

PROFILE OF THE COUNTRY AND ITS CONTROL PROGRAMME

Population in year of survey	**8,020,408**		Year N.T.P was established	**1996 (revised programme)**		
Notification all cases (rate)	**299**	**/100,000**	Year of Rifampicin introduction	**1979**		
Estimated incidence (all cases)	**670**	**/100,000**	Year of Isoniazid introduction	**1968**		
Notification new sputum smear +	**14742**		Use of Standardized Regimens	**Yes**		
Notification new sputum smear + (rate)	**184**	**/100,000**	% Use of Short Course Chemotherapy	**Yes**	**100**	**%**
Treatment Success	**68**	**%**	Use of Directly Observed Therapy	**Yes**	**60**	**%**
Retreatment cases	**2909**		During continuation phase	**Variable**		
Retreatment as % of NTP	**9**	**%**	Use of Fixed Dose Combination	**Yes**	**100**	**%**
Estimated HIV positive TB cases	**63.8**	**%**	Treatment in private sector Category 1: virtually all TB patients public sector Category 2: <15% in private sector Category 3: 15% or more in private sector	**Cat 1**		
			TB drugs available on the private market	**No**		

CHARACTERISTICS OF THE SURVEY/SURVEILLANCE PROGRAMME

Study Duration	**12 Months**
Target Area	**Gauteng Province**
Sampling Method	**Multistage stratified cluster sampling**
Culture Media	**Löwenstein-Jensen**
DST Method	**Indirect proportion**
Supranational Reference Laboratory	**Medical Research Council (MRC) National TB Research Programme, South Africa**

*Notations to accompany profile: Retreatment indicates sputum smear positive pulmonary cases only

*For survey settings where less than 100% of cases are sampled, combined estimates are based on the rates of new and previously treated cases obtained in the survey, but weighted by the absolute number of new and previously treated sputum positive TB cases, as published by the national authorities.

COUNTRY PROFILES

PREVALENCE OF DRUG RESISTANCE

Gauteng Province: 2001-2002

	New		Previous		Combined	
	N	%	N	%	N	%
Total number of strains tested	592	100.0	165	100.0		100.0
SUSCEPTIBLE TO ALL 4 DRUGS	**553**	**93.4**	**144**	**87.3**		**92.4**
ANY RESISTANCE	**39**	**6.6**	**21**	**12.7**		**7.6**
- Isoniazid (INH)	26	4.4	16	9.7		5.3
- Rifampicin (RMP)	10	1.7	10	6.1		2.4
- Ethambutol (EMB)	2	0.3	8	4.8		1.1
- Streptomycin (SM)	23	3.9	13	7.9		4.5
MONORESISTANCE	**24**	**4.1**	**5**	**3.1**		**3.9**
- Isoniazid (INH)	11	1.9	1	0.6		1.7
- Rifampicin (RMP)	2	0.3	0	0.0		0.3
- Ethambutol (EMB)	0	0.0	0	0.0		0.0
- Streptomycin (SM)	11	1.9	4	2.4		2.0
MULTIDRUG RESISTANCE	**8**	**1.4**	**9**	**5.5**		**2.0**
- INH + RMP	3	0.5	2	1.2		0.6
- INH + RMP + EMB	0	0.0	2	1.2		0.2
- INH + RMP + SM	4	0.7	2	1.2		0.8
- INH + RMP + EMB + SM	1	0.2	3	1.8		0.4
OTHER PATTERNS	**7**	**1.2**	**7**	**4.2**		**1.7**
- INH + EMB	0	0.0	2	1.2		0.2
- INH + SM	6	1.0	4	2.4		1.2
- INH + EMB + SM	1	0.2	0	0.0		0.1
- RMP + EMB	0	0.0	1	0.6		0.1
- RMP + SM	0	0.0	0	0.0		0.0
- RMP + EMB + SM	0	0.0	0	0.0		0.0
- EMB + SM	0	0.0	0	0.0		0.0
NUMBER OF DRUGS RESISTANT TO:						
susceptible to 4 drugs	553	93.4	144	87.3		92.4
resistant to 1 drug	24	4.1	5	3.1		3.9
resistant to 2 drugs	9	1.5	9	5.5		2.2
resistant to 3 drugs	5	0.8	4	2.5		1.1
resistant to 4 drugs	1	0.2	3	1.8		0.4

COUNTRY PROFILES

SOUTH AFRICA

Free State Province: 2001-2002

PROFILE OF THE COUNTRY AND ITS CONTROL PROGRAMME

Population in year of survey	**2,834,519**		Year N.T.P was established	**1996** **(revised programme)**		
Notification all cases (rate)	**423**	**/100,000**	Year of Rifampicin introduction	**1979**		
Estimated incidence (all cases)	**530**	**/100,000**	Year of Isoniazid introduction	**1968**		
Notification new sputum smear +	**6455**		Use of Standardized Regimens	**Yes**		
Notification new sputum smear + (rate)	**228**	**/100,000**	% Use of Short Course Chemotherapy	**Yes**	**100**	**%**
Treatment Success	**69.3**	**%**	Use of Directly Observed Therapy	**Yes**	**70**	**%**
Retreatment cases	**1891**		During continuation phase	**Variable**		
Retreatment as % of NTP	**16**	**%**	Use of Fixed Dose Combination	**Yes**	**100**	**%**
Estimated HIV positive TB cases	**71.9**	**%**	Treatment in private sector Category 1: virtually all TB patients public sector Category 2: <15% in private sector Category 3: 15% or more in private sector	**Cat 1**		
			TB drugs available on the private market	**No**		

CHARACTERISTICS OF THE SURVEY/SURVEILLANCE PROGRAMME

Study Duration	**12 Months**
Target Area	**Free State Province**
Sampling Method	**Multistage stratified cluster sampling**
Culture Media	**Löwenstein-Jensen**
DST Method	**Indirect proportion**
Supranational Reference Laboratory	**Medical Research Council (MRC) National TB Research Programme, South Africa**

*Notations to accompany profile: Retreatment indicates sputum smear positive pulmonary cases only

*For survey settings where less than 100% of cases are sampled, combined estimates are based on the rates of new and previously treated cases obtained in the survey, but weighted by the absolute number of new and previously treated sputum positive TB cases, as published by the national authorities.

COUNTRY PROFILES

PREVALENCE OF DRUG RESISTANCE

Free State Province: 2001-2002

	New		Previous		Combined	
	N	%	N	%	N	%
Total number of strains tested	454	100.0	174	100.0		100.0
SUSCEPTIBLE TO ALL 4 DRUGS	**415**	**91.4**	**158**	**90.8**		**91.3**
ANY RESISTANCE	**39**	**8.6**	**16**	**9.2**		**8.7**
- Isoniazid (INH)	29	6.4	12	6.9		6.5
- Rifampicin (RMP)	11	2.4	5	2.9		2.5
- Ethambutol (EMB)	3	0.7	1	0.6		0.6
- Streptomycin (SM)	18	4.0	5	2.9		3.7
MONORESISTANCE	**25**	**5.5**	**11**	**6.3**		**5.7**
- Isoniazid (INH)	15	3.3	7	4.0		3.5
- Rifampicin (RMP)	3	0.7	2	1.1		0.8
- Ethambutol (EMB)	0	0.0	0	0.0		0.0
- Streptomycin (SM)	7	1.5	2	1.1		1.5
MULTIDRUG RESISTANCE	**8**	**1.8**	**3**	**1.8**		**1.8**
- INH + RMP	1	0.2	2	1.1		0.4
- INH + RMP + EMB	2	0.4	0	0.0		0.3
- INH + RMP + SM	4	0.9	0	0.0		0.7
- INH + RMP + EMB + SM	1	0.2	1	0.6		0.3
OTHER PATTERNS	**6**	**1.3**	**2**	**1.1**		**1.3**
- INH + EMB	0	0.0	0	0.0		0.0
- INH + SM	6	1.3	2	1.1		1.3
- INH + EMB + SM	0	0.0	0	0.0		0.0
- RMP + EMB	0	0.0	0	0.0		0.0
- RMP + SM	0	0.0	0	0.0		0.0
- RMP + EMB + SM	0	0.0	0	0.0		0.0
- EMB + SM	0	0.0	0	0.0		0.0
NUMBER OF DRUGS RESISTANT TO:						
susceptible to 4 drugs	415	91.4	158	90.8		91.3
resistant to 1 drug	25	5.5	11	6.3		5.7
resistant to 2 drugs	7	1.5	4	2.3		1.7
resistant to 3 drugs	6	1.3	0	0.0		1.0
resistant to 4 drugs	1	2.2	1	0.5		0.3

COUNTRY PROFILES

SOUTH AFRICA

Western Cape Province: 2001-2002

PROFILE OF THE COUNTRY AND ITS CONTROL PROGRAMME

Population in year of survey	4,255,743		Year N.T.P was established	1996 (revised programme)		
Notification all cases (rate)	632	/100,000	Year of Rifampicin introduction	1979		
Estimated incidence (all cases)	932	/100,000	Year of Isoniazid introduction	1968		
Notification new sputum smear +	15264		Use of Standardized Regimens	Yes		
Notification new sputum smear + (rate)	359	/100,000	% Use of Short Course Chemotherapy	Yes	100	%
Treatment Success	70.9	%	Use of Directly Observed Therapy	Yes	80	%
Retreatment cases	7553		During continuation phase	Variable		
Retreatment as % of NTP	21	%	Use of Fixed Dose Combination	Yes	100	%
Estimated HIV positive TB cases	28.2	%	Treatment in private sector	Cat 1		

Category 1: virtually all TB patients public sector
Category 2: <15% in private sector
Category 3: 15% or more in private sector

TB drugs available on the private market — **No**

CHARACTERISTICS OF THE SURVEY/SURVEILLANCE PROGRAMME

Study Duration	**12 Months**
Target Area	**Western Cape Province**
Sampling Method	**Multistage stratified cluster sampling**
Culture Media	**Löwenstein-Jensen**
DST Method	**Indirect proportion**
Supranational Reference Laboratory	**Medical Research Council (MRC) National TB Research Programme, South Africa**

*Notations to accompany profile: Retreatment indicates sputum smear positive pulmonary cases only

*For survey settings where less than 100% of cases are sampled, combined estimates are based on the rates of new and previously treated cases obtained in the survey, but weighted by the absolute number of new and previously treated sputum positive TB cases, as published by the national authorities.

PREVALENCE OF DRUG RESISTANCE

Western Cape Province: 2001-2002

	New		Previous		Combined	
	N	%	N	%	N	%
Total number of strains tested	427	100.0	228	100.0		100.0
SUSCEPTIBLE TO ALL 4 DRUGS	**403**	**94.4**	**210**	**92.1**		**93.6**
ANY RESISTANCE	**24**	**5.6**	**18**	**7.9**		**6.4**
- Isoniazid (INH)	22	5.2	15	6.6		5.6
- Rifampicin (RMP)	4	0.9	9	3.9		1.9
- Ethambutol (EMB)	0	0.0	3	1.3		0.4
- Streptomycin (SM)	10	2.3	8	3.5		2.7
MONORESISTANCE	**13**	**3.0**	**8**	**3.5**		**3.2**
- Isoniazid (INH)	11	2.6	5	2.2		2.4
- Rifampicin (RMP)	0	0.0	0	0.0		0.0
- Ethambutol (EMB)	0	0.0	0	0.0		0.0
- Streptomycin (SM)	2	0.5	3	1.3		0.7
MULTIDRUG RESISTANCE	**4**	**0.9**	**9**	**3.9**		**1.9**
- INH + RMP	3	0.7	4	1.8		1.1
- INH + RMP + EMB	0	0.0	1	0.4		0.1
- INH + RMP + SM	1	0.2	2	0.9		0.4
- INH + RMP + EMB + SM	0	0.0	2	0.9		0.3
OTHER PATTERNS	**7**	**1.6**	**1**	**0.4**		**1.2**
- INH + EMB	0	0.0	0	0.0		0.0
- INH + SM	7	1.6	1	0.4		1.2
- INH + EMB + SM	0	0.0	0	0.0		0.0
- RMP + EMB	0	0.0	0	0.0		0.0
- RMP + SM	0	0.0	0	0.0		0.0
- RMP + EMB + SM	0	0.0	0	0.0		0.0
- EMB + SM	0	0.0	0	0.0		0.0
NUMBER OF DRUGS RESISTANT TO:						
susceptible to 4 drugs	403	94.4	210	92.1		93.6
resistant to 1 drug	13	3.0	8	3.5		3.2
resistant to 2 drugs	10	2.3	5	2.1		2.3
resistant to 3 drugs	1	0.2	3	1.3		0.6
resistant to 4 drugs	0	0.0	2	0.8		0.3

SOUTH AFRICA

Limpopo Province: 2001-2002

PROFILE OF THE COUNTRY AND ITS CONTROL PROGRAMME

Population in year of survey	**5,683,605**		Year N.T.P was established	**1996 (revised programme)**	
Notification all cases (rate)	**166**	**/100,000**	Year of Rifampicin introduction	**1979**	
Estimated incidence (all cases)	**443**	**/100,000**	Year of Isoniazid introduction	**1968**	
Notification new sputum smear +	**4717**		Use of Standardized Regimens	**Yes**	
Notification new sputum smear + (rate)	**83**	**/100,000**	% Use of Short Course Chemotherapy	**Yes**	**100 %**
Treatment Success	**59**	**%**	Use of Directly Observed Therapy	**Yes**	**60 %**
Retreatment cases	**1097**		During continuation phase	**Variable**	
Retreatment as % of NTP	**4**	**%**	Use of Fixed Dose Combination	**Yes**	**100 %**
Estimated HIV positive TB cases	**52.4**	**%**	Treatment in private sector	**Cat 1**	
			Category 1: virtually all TB patients public sector Category 2: <15% in private sector Category 3: 15% or more in private sector		
			TB drugs available on the private market	**No**	

CHARACTERISTICS OF THE SURVEY/SURVEILLANCE PROGRAMME

Study Duration	**12 Months**
Target Area	**Limpopo Province**
Sampling Method	**Multistage stratified cluster sampling**
Culture Media	**Löwenstein-Jensen**
DST Method	**Indirect proportion**
Supranational Reference Laboratory	**Medical Research Council (MRC) National TB Research Programme, South Africa**

*Notations to accompany profile: Retreatment indicates sputum smear positive pulmonary cases only

*For survey settings where less than 100% of cases are sampled, combined estimates are based on the rates of new and previously treated cases obtained in the survey, but weighted by the absolute number of new and previously treated sputum positive TB cases, as published by the national authorities.

PREVALENCE OF DRUG RESISTANCE

Limpopo Province: 2001-2002

	New		Previous		Combined	
	N	%	N	%	N	%
Total number of strains tested	451	100.0	88	100.0		100.0
SUSCEPTIBLE TO ALL 4 DRUGS	**419**	**92.9**	**73**	**83.0**		**91.0**
ANY RESISTANCE	**32**	**7.1**	**15**	**17.0**		**9.0**
- Isoniazid (INH)	25	5.6	11	12.5		6.9
- Rifampicin (RMP)	11	2.4	9	10.2		3.9
- Ethambutol (EMB)	10	2.2	2	2.3		2.2
- Streptomycin (SM)	18	4.0	3	3.4		3.9
MONORESISTANCE	**13**	**2.9**	**8**	**9.0**		**4.1**
- Isoniazid (INH)	6	1.3	4	4.5		1.9
- Rifampicin (RMP)	0	0.0	3	3.4		0.6
- Ethambutol (EMB)	0	0.0	0	0.0		0.0
- Streptomycin (SM)	7	1.6	1	1.1		1.5
MULTIDRUG RESISTANCE	**11**	**2.4**	**6**	**7.0**		**3.3**
- INH + RMP	3	0.7	3	3.4		1.2
- INH + RMP + EMB	1	0.2	2	2.3		0.6
- INH + RMP + SM	2	0.4	1	1.1		0.6
- INH + RMP + EMB + SM	5	1.1	0	0.0		0.9
OTHER PATTERNS	**8**	**1.8**	**1**	**1.1**		**1.7**
- INH + EMB	4	0.9	0	0.0		0.7
- INH + SM	4	0.9	1	1.1		0.9
- INH + EMB + SM	0	0.0	0	0.0		0.0
- RMP + EMB	0	0.0	0	0.0		0.0
- RMP + SM	0	0.0	0	0.0		0.0
- RMP + EMB + SM	0	0.0	0	0.0		0.0
- EMB + SM	0	0.0	0	0.0		0.0
NUMBER OF DRUGS RESISTANT TO:						
susceptible to 4 drugs	419	92.9	73	83.0		91.0
resistant to 1 drug	13	2.9	8	9.0		4.1
resistant to 2 drugs	11	2.4	4	4.5		2.8
resistant to 3 drugs	3	0.6	3	3.4		1.2
resistant to 4 drugs	5	1.1	0	0.0		0.9

COUNTRY PROFILES

SOUTH AFRICA

North West Province: 2001-2002

PROFILE OF THE COUNTRY AND ITS CONTROL PROGRAMME

Population in year of survey	3,625,924		Year N.T.P was established	1996 (revised programme)		
Notification all cases (rate)	337	/100,000	Year of Rifampicin introduction	1979		
Estimated incidence (all cases)	486	/100,000	Year of Isoniazid introduction	1968		
Notification new sputum smear +	8136		Use of Standardized Regimens	Yes		
Notification new sputum smear + (rate)	224	/100,000	% Use of Short Course Chemotherapy	Yes	100	%
Treatment Success	68	%	Use of Directly Observed Therapy	Yes	75	%
Retreatment cases	1639		During continuation phase	Variable		
Retreatment as % of NTP	9	%	Use of Fixed Dose Combination	Yes	100	%
Estimated HIV positive TB cases	66	%	Treatment in private sector	Cat 1		

Category 1: virtually all TB patients public sector
Category 2: <15% in private sector
Category 3: 15% or more in private sector

TB drugs available on the private market	No	

CHARACTERISTICS OF THE SURVEY/SURVEILLANCE PROGRAMME

Study Duration	**12 Months**
Target Area	**North West Province**
Sampling Method	**Multistage stratified cluster sampling**
Culture Media	**Löwenstein-Jensen**
DST Method	**Indirect proportion**
Supranational Reference Laboratory	**Medical Research Council (MRC) National TB Research Programme, South Africa**

*Notations to accompany profile: Retreatment indicates sputum smear positive pulmonary cases only

COUNTRY PROFILES

*For survey settings where less than 100% of cases are sampled, combined estimates are based on the rates of new and previously treated cases obtained in the survey, but weighted by the absolute number of new and previously treated sputum positive TB cases, as published by the national authorities.

PREVALENCE OF DRUG RESISTANCE

North West Province: 2001-2002

	New		Previous		Combined	
	N	%	N	%	N	%
Total number of strains tested	631	100.0	188	100.0		100.0
SUSCEPTIBLE TO ALL 4 DRUGS	**580**	**91.9**	**152**	**80.9**		**90.1**
ANY RESISTANCE	**51**	**8.1**	**36**	**19.1**		**9.9**
- Isoniazid (INH)	37	5.9	21	11.2		6.8
- Rifampicin (RMP)	17	2.7	18	9.6		3.8
- Ethambutol (EMB)	8	1.3	2	1.1		1.2
- Streptomycin (SM)	28	4.4	23	12.2		5.7
MONORESISTANCE	**28**	**4.4**	**16**	**8.5**		**5.1**
- Isoniazid (INH)	14	2.2	1	0.5		1.9
- Rifampicin (RMP)	3	0.5	5	2.7		0.8
- Ethambutol (EMB)	0	0.0	0	0.0		0.0
- Streptomycin (SM)	11	1.7	10	5.3		2.3
MULTIDRUG RESISTANCE	**14**	**2.2**	**13**	**6.9**		**3.0**
- INH + RMP	3	0.5	6	3.2		0.9
- INH + RMP + EMB	3	0.5	1	0.5		0.5
- INH + RMP + SM	3	0.5	5	2.7		0.8
- INH + RMP + EMB + SM	5	0.8	1	0.5		0.7
OTHER PATTERNS	**9**	**1.4**	**7**	**3.7**		**1.8**
- INH + EMB	0	0.0	0	0.0		0.0
- INH + SM	9	1.4	7	3.7		1.8
- INH + EMB + SM	0	0.0	0	0.0		0.0
- RMP + EMB	0	0.0	0	0.0		0.0
- RMP + SM	0	0.0	0	0.0		0.0
- RMP + EMB + SM	0	0.0	0	0.0		0.0
- EMB + SM	0	0.0	0	0.0		0.0
NUMBER OF DRUGS RESISTANT TO:						
susceptible to 4 drugs	580	91.9	152	80.9		90.1
resistant to 1 drug	28	4.4	16	8.5		5.1
resistant to 2 drugs	12	1.9	13	6.9		2.7
resistant to 3 drugs	6	0.9	6	3.2		1.3
resistant to 4 drugs	5	0.8	1	0.5		0.7

COUNTRY PROFILES

SPAIN

Galicia: 2001-2002

PROFILE OF THE COUNTRY AND ITS CONTROL PROGRAMME

Population in year of survey	**2,724,809**		Year N.T.P was established	**1995**		
Notification all cases (rate)	**50.72**	**/100,000**	Year of Rifampicin introduction	**1968**		
Estimated incidence (all cases)	**50.72**	**/100,000**	Year of Isoniazid introduction	**1952**		
Notification new sputum smear +	**446**		Use of Standardized Regimens	**Yes**		
Notification new sputum smear + (rate)	**16.36**	**/100,000**	% Use of Short Course Chemotherapy	**Yes**	**88.4**	**%**
Treatment Success	**89.2**	**%**	Use of Directly Observed Therapy	**Yes**	**13.07**	**%**
Retreatment cases	**47**		During continuation phase	**Yes**		
Retreatment as % of NTP	**8.8**	**%**	Use of Fixed Dose Combination	**Yes**	**79.5**	**%**
Estimated HIV positive TB cases	**6.17**	**%**	Treatment in private sector	**Cat 1**		

Category 1: virtually all TB patients public sector
Category 2: <15% in private sector
Category 3: 15% or more in private sector

TB drugs available on the private market	**No**

CHARACTERISTICS OF THE SURVEY/SURVEILLANCE PROGRAMME

Study Duration	**12 Months**
Target Area	**Statewide**
Sampling Method	**All cases**
Culture Media	**Middlebrook 7H12**
DST Method	**BACTEC 460**
Supranational Reference Laboratory	**Servicio de Microbiologia, Hospital Universitaris Vall d'Hebron, Barcelona, Spain**

*Notations to accompany profile: Retreatment indicates sputum smear positive pulmonary cases only

*For survey settings where less than 100% of cases are sampled, combined estimates are based on the rates of new and previously treated cases obtained in the survey, but weighted by the absolute number of new and previously treated sputum positive TB cases, as published by the national authorities.

COUNTRY PROFILES

PREVALENCE OF DRUG RESISTANCE

Galicia: 2001-2002

	New		Previous		Combined	
	N	%	N	%	N	%
Total number of strains tested	360	100.0	40	100.0	400	100.0
SUSCEPTIBLE TO ALL 4 DRUGS	**318**	**88.3**	**31**	**77.5**	**349**	**87.3**
ANY RESISTANCE	**42**	**11.7**	**9**	**22.5**	**51**	**12.7**
- Isoniazid (INH)	16	4.4	7	17.5	23	5.8
- Rifampicin (RMP)	5	1.4	3	7.5	8	2.0
- Ethambutol (EMB)	8	2.2	3	7.5	11	2.8
- Streptomycin (SM)	26	7.2	7	17.5	33	8.3
MONORESISTANCE	**35**	**9.7**	**4**	**10.**	**39**	**9.8**
- Isoniazid (INH)	9	2.5	2	5.0	11	2.8
- Rifampicin (RMP)	0	0.0	0	0.0	0	0.0
- Ethambutol (EMB)	2	0.6	0	0.0	2	0.5
- Streptomycin (SM)	24	6.7	2	5.0	26	6.5
MULTIDRUG RESISTANCE	**5**	**1.4**	**3**	**7.5**	**8**	**2.0**
- INH + RMP	0	0.0	0	0.0	0	0.0
- INH + RMP + EMB	4	1.1	0	0.0	4	1.0
- INH + RMP + SM	0	0.0	1	2.5	1	0.3
- INH + RMP + EMB + SM	1	0.3	2	5.0	3	0.8
OTHER PATTERNS	**2**	**0.6**	**2**	**5.0**	**4**	**1.0**
- INH + EMB	1	0.3	0	0.0	1	0.3
- INH + SM	1	0.3	1	2.5	2	0.5
- INH + EMB + SM	0	0.0	1	2.5	1	0.3
- RMP + EMB	0	0.0	0	0.0	0	0.0
- RMP + SM	0	0.0	0	0.0	0	0.0
- RMP + EMB + SM	0	0.0	0	0.0	0	0.0
- EMB + SM	0	0.0	0	0.0	0	0.0
NUMBER OF DRUGS RESISTANT TO:						
susceptible to 4 drugs	318	88.3	31	77.5	349	87.3
resistant to 1 drug	35	9.7	4	10.0	39	11.3
resistant to 2 drugs	2	0.6	1	2.5	3	0.8
resistant to 3 drugs	4	1.1	2	5.0	6	1.6
resistant to 4 drugs	1	0.3	2	5.0	3	0.8

COUNTRY PROFILES

COUNTRY PROFILES

SPAIN

Barcelona: 2001

PROFILE OF THE COUNTRY AND ITS CONTROL PROGRAMME

Population in year of survey	**1,508,952**		Year N.T.P was established	**1982**		
Notification all cases (rate)	**31.6**	**/100,000**	Year of Rifampicin introduction	**1968**		
Estimated incidence (all cases)	**34.9**	**/100,000**	Year of Isoniazid introduction	**1954**		
Notification new sputum smear +	**210**		Use of Standardized Regimens	**Yes**		
Notification new sputum smear + (rate)	**13.9**	**/100,000**	% Use of Short Course Chemotherapy	**Yes**	**>90**	**%**
Treatment Success	**74.0**	**%**	Use of Directly Observed Therapy	**Yes**	**21.3**	**%**
Retreatment cases	**30**		During continuation phase	**Yes**		
Retreatment as % of NTP		**%**	Use of Fixed Dose Combination	**Yes**	**>90**	**%**
Estimated HIV positive TB cases	**14.8**	**%**	Treatment in private sector	**Cat 1**		

Category 1: virtually all TB patients public sector
Category 2: <15% in private sector
Category 3: 15% or more in private sector

TB drugs available on the private market

CHARACTERISTICS OF THE SURVEY/SURVEILLANCE PROGRAMME

Study Duration	**12 Months**
Target Area	**Citywide**
Sampling Method	**Cluster**
Culture Media	**Löwenstein-Jensen & MB/BacT Alert 3D**
DST Method	**Proportion and BACTEC**
Supranational Reference Laboratory	**Servicio de Microbiología, Hospital Universitario Vall d'Hebron, Barcelona, Spain**

*Notations to accompany profile: Retreatment indicates sputum smear positive pulmonary cases only

*For survey settings where less than 100% of cases are sampled, combined estimates are based on the rates of new and previously treated cases obtained in the survey, but weighted by the absolute number of new and previously treated sputum positive TB cases, as published by the national authorities.

PREVALENCE OF DRUG RESISTANCE

Barcelona: 2001

	New		Previous		Combined	
	N	%	N	%	N	%
Total number of strains tested	133	100.0	32	100.0		100.0
SUSCEPTIBLE TO ALL 4 DRUGS	**119**	**89.5**	**22**	**68.8**		**87.1**
ANY RESISTANCE	**14**	**10.5**	**10**	**31.3**		**12.9**
- Isoniazid (INH)	8	6.0	9	28.1		8.5
- Rifampicin (RMP)	2	1.5	4	12.5		2.8
- Ethambutol (EMB)	0	0.0	3	9.4		1.1
- Streptomycin (SM)	9	6.8	6	18.8		8.1
MONORESISTANCE	**10**	**7.5**	**4**	**12.5**		**8.1**
- Isoniazid (INH)	5	3.8	3	9.4		4.4
- Rifampicin (RMP)	0	0.0	0	0.0		0.0
- Ethambutol (EMB)	0	0.0	0	0.0		0.0
- Streptomycin (SM)	5	3.8	1	3.1		3.7
MULTIDRUG RESISTANCE	**1**	**0.8**	**4**	**12.5**		**2.1**
- INH + RMP	0	0.0	1	3.1		1.1
- INH + RMP + EMB	0	0.0	0	0.0		0.0
- INH + RMP + SM	1	0.8	0	0.0		0.7
- INH + RMP + EMB + SM	0	0.0	3	9.4		1.1
OTHER PATTERNS	**3**	**2.3**	**2**	**6.3**		**2.7**
- INH + EMB	0	0.0	0	0.0		0.0
- INH + SM	2	1.5	2	6.3		2.0
- INH + EMB + SM	0	0.0	0	0.0		0.0
- RMP + EMB	0	0.0	0	0.0		0.0
- RMP + SM	1	0.8	0	0.0		0.7
- RMP + EMB + SM	0	0.0	0	0.0		0.0
- EMB + SM	0	0.0	0	0.0		0.0
NUMBER OF DRUGS RESISTANT TO:						
susceptible to 4 drugs	119	89.5	22	68.8		87.1
resistant to 1 drug	10	7.5	4	12.5		8.1
resistant to 2 drugs	3	2.3	3	9.4		3.1
resistant to 3 drugs	1	0.8	0	0.0		0.7
resistant to 4 drugs	0	0.0	3	9.4		1.1

COUNTRY PROFILES

SWEDEN

Countrywide: 2000

PROFILE OF THE COUNTRY AND ITS CONTROL PROGRAMME

Population in year of survey	**8,861,426**		Year N.T.P was established	**NA**		
Notification all cases (rate)	**5.2**	**/100,000**	Year of Rifampicin introduction	**1970**		
Estimated incidence (all cases)		**/100,000**	Year of Isoniazid introduction	**1950s**		
Notification new sputum smear +	**118**		Use of Standardized Regimens	**Yes**		
Notification new sputum smear + (rate)	**1.3**	**/100,000**	% Use of Short Course Chemotherapy	**Yes**	**54**	**%**
Treatment Success	**78**	**%**	Use of Directly Observed Therapy	**No**		**%**
Retreatment cases	**NA**		During continuation phase	**No**		
Retreatment as % of NTP		**%**	Use of Fixed Dose Combination	**No**		**%**
Estimated HIV positive TB cases	**2.53**	**%**	Treatment in private sector Category 1: virtually all TB patients public sector Category 2: <15% in private sector Category 3: 15% or more in private sector	**Cat 1**		
			TB drugs available on the private market	**Rx only**		

CHARACTERISTICS OF THE SURVEY/SURVEILLANCE PROGRAMME

Study Duration	**12 Months**
Target Area	**Countrywide**
Sampling Method	**All cases**
Culture Media	**Löwenstein-Jensen and BACTEC**
DST Method	**BACTEC**
Supranational Reference Laboratory	**Swedish Institute for Infectious Disease Control (SIIDC), Stockhom, Sweden**

*Notations to accompany profile: Estimated HIV positive TB cases is a WHO estimate
The combined column includes patients with unknown treatment history

*For survey settings where less than 100% of cases are sampled, combined estimates are based on the rates of new and previously treated cases obtained in the survey, but weighted by the absolute number of new and previously treated sputum positive TB cases, as published by the national authorities.

COUNTRY PROFILES

PREVALENCE OF DRUG RESISTANCE

Countrywide: 2000

	New		Previous		Combined	
	N	%	N	%	N	%
Total number of strains tested	344	100.0	22	100.0	366	100.0
SUSCEPTIBLE TO ALL 4 DRUGS	**308**	**89.5**	**19**	**86.4**	**327**	**89.3**
ANY RESISTANCE	**36**	**10.5**	**3**	**13.6**	**39**	**10.7**
- Isoniazid (INH)	35	10.2	2	9.1	37	10.1
- Rifampicin (RMP)	4	1.2	1	4.5	5	1.4
- Ethambutol (EMB)	2	0.6	0	0.0	2	0.6
- Streptomycin (SM)	8	0.3	1	4.5	9	2.5
MONORESISTANCE	**25**	**7.3**	**2**	**9.1**	**27**	**7.4**
- Isoniazid (INH)	24	7.0	1	4.5	25	6.8
- Rifampicin (RMP)	0	0.0	0	0.0	0	0.0
- Ethambutol (EMB)	0	0.0	0	0.0	0	0.0
- Streptomycin (SM)	1	0.3	1	4.5	2	0.6
MULTIDRUG RESISTANCE	**4**	**1.2**	**1**	**2.4**	**5**	**1.4**
- INH + RMP	2	0.6	1	2.4	3	0.8
- INH + RMP + EMB	2	0.6	0	0.0	2	0.6
- INH + RMP + SM	0	0.0	0	0.0	0	0.0
- INH + RMP + EMB + SM	0	0.0	0	0.0	0	0.0
OTHER PATTERNS	**7**	**2.0**	**0**	**0.0**	**7**	**1.9**
- INH + EMB	0	0.0	0	0.0	0	0.0
- INH + SM	7	2.0	0	0.0	7	1.9
- INH + EMB + SM	0	0.0	0	0.0	0	0.0
- RMP + EMB	0	0.0	0	0.0	0	0.0
- RMP + SM	0	0.0	0	0.0	0	0.0
- RMP + EMB + SM	0	0.0	0	0.0	0	0.0
- EMB + SM	0	0.0	0	0.0	0	0.0
NUMBER OF DRUGS RESISTANT TO:						
susceptible to 4 drugs	308	89.5	19	86.4	327	89.3
resistant to 1 drug	25	7.3	2	9.1	27	7.4
resistant to 2 drugs	9	2.6	1	4.5	10	2.7
resistant to 3 drugs	2	0.6	0	0.0	2	0.5
resistant to 4 drugs	0	0.0	0	0.0	0	0.0

SWITZERLAND

Countrywide: 2000

PROFILE OF THE COUNTRY AND ITS CONTROL PROGRAMME

Population in year of survey	7,173,000		Year N.T.P was established			
Notification all cases (rate)	8	/100,000	Year of Rifampicin introduction	1967		
Estimated incidence (all cases)		/100,000	Year of Isoniazid introduction	1952		
Notification new sputum smear +	118		Use of Standardized Regimens	Yes		
Notification new sputum smear + (rate)	1	/100,000	% Use of Short Course Chemotherapy	Yes	50	%
Treatment Success		%	Use of Directly Observed Therapy	Yes	3	%
Retreatment cases	NA		During continuation phase	Rarely		
Retreatment as % of NTP		%	Use of Fixed Dose Combination	Yes	85	%
Estimated HIV positive TB cases	12.53	%	Treatment in private sector	95		

Category 1: virtually all TB patients public sector
Category 2: <15% in private sector
Category 3: 15% or more in private sector

TB drugs available on the private market — **Yes**

CHARACTERISTICS OF THE SURVEY/SURVEILLANCE PROGRAMME

Study Duration	**12 Months**
Target Area	**Countrywide**
Sampling Method	**All cases**
Culture Media	**Various**
DST Method	**Various**
Supranational Reference Laboratory	**Health Protection Agency Mycobacterium Reference Unit (HPA MRU), London, United Kingdom**

*Notations to accompany profile: Estimated HIV positive TB cases is a WHO estimate
The combined column includes patients with unknown treatment history

*For survey settings where less than 100% of cases are sampled, combined estimates are based on the rates of new and previously treated cases obtained in the survey, but weighted by the absolute number of new and previously treated sputum positive TB cases, as published by the national authorities.

PREVALENCE OF DRUG RESISTANCE

Countrywide: 2000

	New		Previous		Combined	
	N	%	N	%	N	%
Total number of strains tested	330	100.0	57	100.0	492	100.0
SUSCEPTIBLE TO ALL 4 DRUGS	**312**	**94.5**	**54**	**94.7**	**467**	**94.9**
ANY RESISTANCE	**18**	**5.5**	**3**	**5.3**	**25**	**5.1**
- Isoniazid (INH)	18	5.5	2	3.5	24	4.9
- Rifampicin (RMP)	0	0.0	2	3.5	3	0.6
- Ethambutol (EMB)	0	0.0	0	0.0	0	0.0
- Streptomycin (SM)	-	-	-	-	-	-
MONORESISTANCE	**18**	**5.5**	**2**	**3.5**	**23**	**4.7**
- Isoniazid (INH)	18	5.5	1	1.8	22	4.5
- Rifampicin (RMP)	0	0.0	1	1.8	1	0.2
- Ethambutol (EMB)	0	0.0	0	0.0	0	0.0
- Streptomycin (SM)	-	-	-	-	-	-
MULTIDRUG RESISTANCE	**0**	**0.0**	**1**	**1.8**	**2**	**0.4**
- INH + RMP	0	0.0	1	1.8	2	0.4
- INH + RMP + EMB	0	0.0	0	0.0	0	0.0
- INH + RMP + SM	-	-	-	-	-	-
- INH + RMP + EMB + SM	-	-	-	-	-	-
OTHER PATTERNS	**0**	**0.0**	**0**	**0.0**	**0**	**0.0**
- INH + EMB	0	0.0	0	0.0	0	0.0
- INH + SM	-	-	-	-	-	-
- INH + EMB + SM	-	-	-	-	-	-
- RMP + EMB	0	0.0	0	0.0	0	0.0
- RMP + SM	-	-	-	-	-	-
- RMP + EMB + SM	-	-	-	-	-	-
- EMB + SM	-	-	-	-	-	-
NUMBER OF DRUGS RESISTANT TO:						
susceptible to 4 drugs	312	94.5	54	94.7	467	94.9
resistant to 1 drug	18	5.5	2	3.5	23	4.7
resistant to 2 drugs	0	0.0	1	1.8	2	0.4
resistant to 3 drugs	0	0.0	0	0.0	0	0.0
resistant to 4 drugs	-	-	-	-	-	-

THAILAND

Countrywide: 2001

PROFILE OF THE COUNTRY AND ITS CONTROL PROGRAMME

Population in year of survey	**63,584,000**		Year N.T.P was established	**1949**		
Notification all cases (rate)	**76**	**/100,000**	Year of Rifampicin introduction	**1985**		
Estimated incidence (all cases)	**110**	**/100,000**	Year of Isoniazid introduction	**1949**		
Notification new sputum smear +	**28363**		Use of Standardized Regimens	**Yes**		
Notification new sputum smear + (rate)	**45**	**/100,000**	% Use of Short Course Chemotherapy	**Yes**	**100**	**%**
Treatment Success	**77**	**%**	Use of Directly Observed Therapy	**Yes**	**76**	**%**
Retreatment cases	**1405**		During continuation phase	**Yes**		
Retreatment as % of NTP	**4.95**	**%**	Use of Fixed Dose Combination	**Yes**	**20**	**%**
Estimated HIV positive TB cases	**7.12**	**%**	Treatment in private sector	**Cat 1**		

Category 1: virtually all TB patients public sector
Category 2: <15% in private sector
Category 3: 15% or more in private sector

TB drugs available on the private market	**All 1st line**

CHARACTERISTICS OF THE SURVEY/SURVEILLANCE PROGRAMME

Study Duration	**24 Months**
Target Area	**Countrywide**
Sampling Method	**Proportional cluster**
Culture Media	**Ogawa and Löwenstein-Jensen**
DST Method	**Proportion**
Supranational Reference Laboratory	**Korean Institute of Tuberculosis (KIT), Seoul, Republic of Korea**

*Notations to accompany profile: Estimated HIV positive TB cases is a WHO estimate

COUNTRY PROFILES

*For survey settings where less than 100% of cases are sampled, combined estimates are based on the rates of new and previously treated cases obtained in the survey, but weighted by the absolute number of new and previously treated sputum positive TB cases, as published by the national authorities.

PREVALENCE OF DRUG RESISTANCE

Countrywide: 2001

	New		Previous		Combined	
	N	%	N	%	N	%
Total number of strains tested	1,505	100.0	172	100.0	1,677	100.0
SUSCEPTIBLE TO ALL 4 DRUGS	**1,282**	**85.2**	**105**	**61.0**	**1,387**	**82.7**
ANY RESISTANCE	**223**	**14.8**	**67**	**39.0**	**290**	**17.3**
- Isoniazid (INH)	143	9.5	53	30.8	196	11.7
- Rifampicin (RMP)	21	1.4	39	22.7	60	3.6
- Ethambutol (EMB)	17	1.1	26	15.1	43	2.6
- Streptomycin (SM)	124	8.2	42	24.4	166	9.9
MONORESISTANCE	**158**	**10.5**	**20**	**11.6**	**178**	**10.6**
- Isoniazid (INH)	80	5.3	7	4.1	87	5.2
- Rifampicin (RMP)	5	0.3	3	1.7	8	0.5
- Ethambutol (EMB)	1	0.1	1	0.6	2	0.1
- Streptomycin (SM)	72	4.8	9	5.2	81	4.8
MULTIDRUG RESISTANCE	**14**	**0.9**	**35**	**20.3**	**49**	**2.9**
- INH + RMP	5	0.3	7	4.1	12	0.7
- INH + RMP + EMB	1	0.1	4	2.3	5	0.3
- INH + RMP + SM	4	0.3	8	4.7	12	0.7
- INH + RMP + EMB + SM	4	0.3	16	9.3	20	1.2
OTHER PATTERNS	**51**	**3.4**	**12**	**7.0**	**63**	**3.8**
- INH + EMB	5	0.3	2	1.2	7	0.4
- INH + SM	40	2.7	7	4.1	47	2.8
- INH + EMB + SM	4	0.3	2	1.2	6	0.4
- RMP + EMB	2	0.1	1	0.6	3	0.2
- RMP + SM	0	0.0	0	0.0	0	0.0
- RMP + EMB + SM	0	0.0	0	0.0	0	0.0
- EMB + SM	0	0.0	0	0.0	0	0.0
NUMBER OF DRUGS RESISTANT TO:						
susceptible to 4 drugs	1,282	85.2	105	61.0	1,387	82.7
resistant to 1 drug	158	10.7	20	11.6	178	10.6
resistant to 2 drugs	52	3.4	17	9.9	69	4.1
resistant to 3 drugs	9	0.4	14	8.1	23	1.4
resistant to 4 drugs	4	0.3	16	9.3	20	1.2

COUNTRY PROFILES

TURKMENISTAN

Dashoguz Velayat (Aral Sea Region): 2001-2002

PROFILE OF THE COUNTRY AND ITS CONTROL PROGRAMME

Population in year of survey	**1,141,900**		Year N.T.P was established	**1999**		
Notification all cases (rate)	**166.5**	**/100,000**	Year of Rifampicin introduction	**NA**		
Estimated incidence (all cases)	**92.9**	**/100,000**	Year of Isoniazid introduction	**NA**		
Notification new sputum smear +	**366**		Use of Standardized Regimens	**Yes**		
Notification new sputum smear + (rate)	**32.3**	**/100,000**	% Use of Short Course Chemotherapy	**Yes**	**>80**	**%**
Treatment Success	**82**	**%**	Use of Directly Observed Therapy	**Yes**		**%**
Retreatment cases	**425**		During continuation phase	**Yes**		
Retreatment as % of NTP	**44**	**%**	Use of Fixed Dose Combination	**Yes**	**100**	**%**
Estimated HIV positive TB cases	**NA**	**%**	Treatment in private sector	**Cat 2**		

Category 1: virtually all TB patients public sector
Category 2: <15% in private sector
Category 3: 15% or more in private sector

TB drugs available on the private market — **All 1st line, some 2nd line**

CHARACTERISTICS OF THE SURVEY/SURVEILLANCE PROGRAMME

Study Duration	**9 Months**
Target Area	**4 districts**
Sampling Method	**All cases**
Culture Media	**Löwenstein-Jensen**
DST Method	**Absolute concentration**
Supranational Reference Laboratory	**National Reference Center for Mycobacteria, Borstel, Germany**

*Notations to accompany profile: Retreatment indicates sputum smear positive pulmonary cases only

*For survey settings where less than 100% of cases are sampled, combined estimates are based on the rates of new and previously treated cases obtained in the survey, but weighted by the absolute number of new and previously treated sputum positive TB cases, as published by the national authorities.

COUNTRY PROFILES

PREVALENCE OF DRUG RESISTANCE

Dashoguz Velayat (Aral Sea Region): 2001-2002

	New		Previous		Combined	
	N	%	N	%	N	%
Total number of strains tested	105	100.0	98	100.0		100.0
SUSCEPTIBLE TO ALL 4 DRUGS	**73**	**69.5**	**37**	**37.8**		**52.5**
ANY RESISTANCE	**32**	**30.5**	**61**	**62.2**		**47.5**
- Isoniazid (INH)	16	15.2	47	47.9		32.8
- Rifampicin (RMP)	4	3.8	19	19.4		12.2
- Ethambutol (EMB)	2	1.9	15	15.3		9.1
- Streptomycin (SM)	26	24.8	50	51.0		38.9
MONORESISTANCE	**22**	**20.9**	**23**	**23.5**		**22.3**
- Isoniazid (INH)	6	5.7	9	9.2		7.6
- Rifampicin (RMP)	0	0.0	1	1.0		0.5
- Ethambutol (EMB)	0	0.0	0	0.0		0.0
- Streptomycin (SM)	16	15.2	13	13.3		14.2
MULTIDRUG RESISTANCE	**4**	**3.8**	**18**	**18.4**		**11.6**
- INH + RMP	0	0.0	0	0.0		0.0
- INH + RMP + EMB	0	0.0	0	0.0		0.0
- INH + RMP + SM	3	2.9	10	10.2		6.8
- INH + RMP + EMB + SM	1	1.0	8	8.2		4.8
OTHER PATTERNS	**6**	**5.7**	**20**	**20.4**		**13.6**
- INH + EMB	0	0.0	1	1.0		0.5
- INH + SM	5	4.8	13	13.3		9.3
- INH + EMB + SM	1	0.9	6	6.1		3.7
- RMP + EMB	0	0.0	0	0.0		0.0
- RMP + SM	0	0.0	0	0.0		0.0
- RMP + EMB + SM	0	0.0	0	0.0		0.0
- EMB + SM	0	0.0	0	0.0		0.0
NUMBER OF DRUGS RESISTANT TO:						
susceptible to 4 drugs	73	69.5	37	37.8		52.5
resistant to 1 drug	22	20.9	23	23.5		22.3
resistant to 2 drugs	5	4.8	14	14.3		9.9
resistant to 3 drugs	4	3.8	16	16.3		10.5
resistant to 4 drugs	1	0.9	8	8.2		4.8

COUNTRY PROFILES

UNITED KINGDOM (WITHOUT SCOTLAND)

Countrywide: 2000

PROFILE OF THE COUNTRY AND ITS CONTROL PROGRAMME

Population in year of survey		Year N.T.P was established	**NA**	
Notification all cases (rate)	**/100,000**	Year of Rifampicin introduction	**1969**	
Estimated incidence (all cases)	**/100,000**	Year of Isoniazid introduction		
Notification new sputum smear +		Use of Standardized Regimens	**Yes**	
Notification new sputum smear + (rate)	**/100,000**	% Use of Short Course Chemotherapy	**Yes**	**100 %**
Treatment Success	**%**	Use of Directly Observed Therapy	**No**	**%**
Retreatment cases		During continuation phase	**No**	
Retreatment as % of NTP	**%**	Use of Fixed Dose Combination	**Yes**	**%**
Estimated HIV positive TB cases	**3.56 %**	Treatment in private sector	**Cat 1**	

Category 1: virtually all TB patients public sector
Category 2: <15% in private sector
Category 3: 15% or more in private sector

TB drugs available on the private market

CHARACTERISTICS OF THE SURVEY/SURVEILLANCE PROGRAMME

Study Duration	**12 Months**
Target Area	**Countrywide**
Sampling Method	**All cases**
Culture Media	**Löwenstein-Jensen and BACTEC**
DST Method	**Resistance Ratio**
Supranational Reference Laboratory	**Health Protection Agency Mycobacterium Reference Unit (HPA MRU), London, United Kingdom**

*Notations to accompany profile: Estimated HIV positive TB cases is a WHO estimate
The combined column includes patients with unknown treatment history, SM is not routinely tested for in the UK

*For survey settings where less than 100% of cases are sampled, combined estimates are based on the rates of new and previously treated cases obtained in the survey, but weighted by the absolute number of new and previously treated sputum positive TB cases, as published by the national authorities.

PREVALENCE OF DRUG RESISTANCE

Countrywide: 2000

	New		Previous		Combined	
	N	%	N	%	N	%
Total number of strains tested	2,312	100.0	237	100.0	3,004	100.0
SUSCEPTIBLE TO ALL 4 DRUGS	**2,117**	**91.6**	**201**	**84.8**	**2,735**	**91.0**
ANY RESISTANCE	**195**	**8.4**	**36**	**15.2**	**269**	**9.0**
- Isoniazid (INH)	139	6.0	25	10.5	192	6.4
- Rifampicin (RMP)	28	1.2	13	5.5	48	1.6
- Ethambutol (EMB)	11	0.5	5	2.1	19	0.6
- Streptomycin (SM)	84	3.6	19	8.0	120	4.0
MONORESISTANCE	**148**	**6.4**	**20**	**8.4**	**196**	**6.5**
- Isoniazid (INH)	92	4.0	9	3.8	119	4.0
- Rifampicin (RMP)	7	0.3	3	1.3	11	0.4
- Ethambutol (EMB)	0	0.0	0	0.0	0	0.0
- Streptomycin (SM)	49	2.1	8	3.4	66	2.2
MULTIDRUG RESISTANCE	**21**	**0.9**	**10**	**4.2**	**37**	**1.2**
- INH + RMP	5	0.2	2	0.8	8	0.3
- INH + RMP + EMB	6	0.3	2	0.8	9	0.3
- INH + RMP + SM	7	0.3	4	1.7	13	0.4
- INH + RMP + EMB + SM	3	0.1	2	0.8	7	0.2
OTHER PATTERNS	**26**	**1.1**	**6**	**2.5**	**36**	**1.2**
- INH + EMB	1	0.1	1	0.4	2	0.1
- INH + SM	24	1.0	5	2.1	33	1.1
- INH + EMB + SM	1	0.1	0	0.0	1	0.1
- RMP + EMB	0	0.0	0	0.0	0	0.0
- RMP + SM	0	0.0	0	0.0	0	0.0
- RMP + EMB + SM	0	0.0	0	0.0	0	0.0
- EMB + SM	0	0.0	0	0.0	0	0.0
NUMBER OF DRUGS RESISTANT TO:						
susceptible to 4 drugs	2,117	91.6	201	84.8	2,735	91.0
resistant to 1 drug	148	8.4	20	8.4	196	6.5
resistant to 2 drugs	30	1.3	8	3.4	43	1.4
resistant to 3 drugs	14	0.6	6	2.5	23	0.8
resistant to 4 drugs	3	0.1	2	0.8	7	0.2

COUNTRY PROFILES

UNITED KINGDOM

Scotland: 2000

PROFILE OF THE COUNTRY AND ITS CONTROL PROGRAMME

Population in year of survey	**5,064,200**		Year N.T.P was established	**NA**		
Notification all cases (rate)	**7.9**	**/100,000**	Year of Rifampicin introduction	**1969**		
Estimated incidence (all cases)	**7.9**	**/100,000**	Year of Isoniazid introduction	**NA**		
Notification new sputum smear +	**118**		Use of Standardized Regimens	**Yes**		
Notification new sputum smear + (rate)	**2.3**	**/100,000**	% Use of Short Course Chemotherapy	**Yes**	**100**	**%**
Treatment Success	**NA**	**%**	Use of Directly Observed Therapy	**No**		**%**
Retreatment cases	**18**		During continuation phase	**No**		
Retreatment as % of NTP	**NA**	**%**	Use of Fixed Dose Combination	**Yes**	**100**	**%**
Estimated HIV positive TB cases	**NA**	**%**	Treatment in private sector	**Cat 1**		

Category 1: virtually all TB patients public sector
Category 2: <15% in private sector
Category 3: 15% or more in private sector

TB drugs available on the private market — **Rx required**

CHARACTERISTICS OF THE SURVEY/SURVEILLANCE PROGRAMME

Study Duration	**12 Months**
Target Area	**Countrywide**
Sampling Method	**All cases**
Culture Media	**BACTEC**
DST Method	**BACTEC**
Supranational Reference Laboratory	**Health Protection Agency Mycobacterium Reference Unit (HPA MRU), London, UK**

*Notations to accompany profile:

*For survey settings where less than 100% of cases are sampled, combined estimates are based on the rates of new and previously treated cases obtained in the survey, but weighted by the absolute number of new and previously treated sputum positive TB cases, as published by the national authorities.

COUNTRY PROFILES

PREVALENCE OF DRUG RESISTANCE

Scotland: 2000

	New		Previous		Combined	
	N	%	N	%	N	%
Total number of strains tested					302	100.0
SUSCEPTIBLE TO ALL 4 DRUGS					290	96.0
ANY RESISTANCE					12	4.0
- Isoniazid (INH)					11	3.6
- Rifampicin (RMP)					0	0.0
- Ethambutol (EMB)					0	0.0
- Streptomycin (SM)					1	0.3
MONORESISTANCE					12	4.0
- Isoniazid (INH)					11	3.6
- Rifampicin (RMP)					0	0.0
- Ethambutol (EMB)					0	0.0
- Streptomycin (SM)					1	0.3
MULTIDRUG RESISTANCE					0	0.0
- INH + RMP					0	0.0
- INH + RMP + EMB					0	0.0
- INH + RMP + SM					0	0.0
- INH + RMP + EMB + SM					0	0.0
OTHER PATTERNS					0	0.0
- INH + EMB					0	0.0
- INH + SM					0	0.0
- INH + EMB + SM					0	0.0
- RMP + EMB					0	0.0
- RMP + SM					0	0.0
- RMP + EMB + SM					0	0.0
- EMB + SM					0	0.0
NUMBER OF DRUGS RESISTANT TO:						
susceptible to 4 drugs					290	96.0
resistant to 1 drug					12	4.0
resistant to 2 drugs					0	0.0
resistant to 3 drugs					0	0.0
resistant to 4 drugs					0	0.0

COUNTRY PROFILES

UNITED STATES

Countrywide: 2001

PROFILE OF THE COUNTRY AND ITS CONTROL PROGRAMME

Population in year of survey	**284,796,887**		Year N.T.P was established	**1953**		
Notification all cases (rate)	**6**	**/100,000**	Year of Rifampicin introduction	**1971**		
Estimated incidence (all cases)	**5.6**	**/100,000**	Year of Isoniazid introduction	**1952**		
Notification new sputum smear +	**5600**		Use of Standardized Regimens	**Yes**		
Notification new sputum smear + (rate)	**2.0**	**/100,000**	% Use of Short Course Chemotherapy	**Yes**	**90**	**%**
Treatment Success	**76**	**%**	Use of Directly Observed Therapy	**Yes**	**49**	**%**
Retreatment cases	**NA**		During continuation phase	**Yes**		
Retreatment as % of NTP		**%**	Use of Fixed Dose Combination	**Yes**		**%**
Estimated HIV positive TB cases	**9.0**	**%**	Treatment in private sector	**Cat 3**		

Category 1: virtually all TB patients public sector
Category 2: <15% in private sector
Category 3: 15% or more in private sector

TB drugs available on the private market	**Rx required**

CHARACTERISTICS OF THE SURVEY/SURVEILLANCE PROGRAMME

Study Duration	**12 Months**
Target Area	**Countrywide**
Sampling Method	**All cases**
Culture Media	**Various**
DST Method	**Various**
Supranational Reference Laboratory	**Centers for Disease Control and Prevention (CDC), Atlanta, United States of America**

*Notations to accompany profile: Estimated HIV positive TB cases is a WHO estimate

*For survey settings where less than 100% of cases are sampled, combined estimates are based on the rates of new and previously treated cases obtained in the survey, but weighted by the absolute number of new and previously treated sputum positive TB cases, as published by the national authorities.

COUNTRY PROFILES

PREVALENCE OF DRUG RESISTANCE

Countrywide: 2001

	New		Previous		Combined	
	N	%	N	%	N	%
Total number of strains tested	9,751	100.0	537	100.0	10,288	100.0
SUSCEPTIBLE TO ALL 4 DRUGS	**8,516**	**87.3**	**436**	**81.2**	**8,952**	**87.0**
ANY RESISTANCE	**1,235**	**12.7**	**101**	**18.8**	**1,336**	**13.0**
- Isoniazid (INH)	753	7.7	75	14.0	828	8.0
- Rifampicin (RMP)	142	1.5	35	6.5	177	1.7
- Ethambutol (EMB)	154	1.6	19	3.5	173	1.7
- Streptomycin (SM)	718	7.4	46	8.6	764	7.4
MONORESISTANCE	**859**	**8.8**	**59**	**11.0**	**918**	**8.9**
- Isoniazid (INH)	391	4.0	35	6.5	426	4.1
- Rifampicin (RMP)	23	0.2	6	1.1	29	0.3
- Ethambutol (EMB)	43	0.4	1	0.2	44	0.4
- Streptomycin (SM)	402	4.1	17	3.2	419	4.0
MULTIDRUG RESISTANCE	**112**	**1.1**	**28**	**5.2**	**140**	**1.4**
- INH + RMP	31	0.3	9	1.7	40	0.4
- INH + RMP + EMB	9	0.1	3	0.6	12	0.1
- INH + RMP + SM	20	0.2	5	0.9	25	0.2
- INH + RMP + EMB + SM	52	0.5	11	2.1	63	0.6
OTHER PATTERNS	**264**	**2.7**	**14**	**2.6**	**278**	**2.7**
- INH + EMB	16	0.2	1	0.2	17	0.2
- INH + SM	212	2.2	9	1.7	221	2.1
- INH + EMB + SM	22	0.2	2	0.4	24	0.2
- RMP + EMB	4	0.1	0	0.0	4	0.1
- RMP + SM	2	0.1	1	0.2	3	0.1
- RMP + EMB + SM	1	0.1	0	0.0	1	0.1
- EMB + SM	7	0.1	1	0.2	8	0.1
NUMBER OF DRUGS RESISTANT TO:						
susceptible to 4 drugs	8,516	87.3	436	81.2	8,952	87.0
resistant to 1 drug	859	8.8	59	11.0	918	8.9
resistant to 2 drugs	272	2.8	21	3.9	293	2.8
resistant to 3 drugs	52	0.5	10	1.9	62	0.6
resistant to 4 drugs	52	0.5	11	2.0	63	0.6

COUNTRY PROFILES

URUGUAY

Countrywide: 1999

PROFILE OF THE COUNTRY AND ITS CONTROL PROGRAMME

Population in year of survey	**3,313,000**		Year N.T.P was established	**1980**	
Notification all cases (rate)	**19**	**/100,000**	Year of Rifampicin introduction	**1970**	
Estimated incidence (all cases)		**/100,000**	Year of Isoniazid introduction		
Notification new sputum smear +	**392**		Use of Standardized Regimens	**Yes**	
Notification new sputum smear + (rate)	**12**	**/100,000**	% Use of Short Course Chemotherapy	**Yes**	**100** %
Treatment Success	**83**	**%**	Use of Directly Observed Therapy	**Yes**	**87** %
Retreatment cases	**40**		During continuation phase	**Yes**	
Retreatment as % of NTP		**%**	Use of Fixed Dose Combination	**No**	**%**
Estimated HIV positive TB cases	**1.11**	**%**	Treatment in private sector	**Cat 2**	

Category 1: virtually all TB patients public sector
Category 2: <15% in private sector
Category 3: 15% or more in private sector

TB drugs available on the private market

CHARACTERISTICS OF THE SURVEY/SURVEILLANCE PROGRAMME

Study Duration	**Months**
Target Area	**Countrywide**
Sampling Method	**All cases**
Culture Media	**Löwenstein-Jensen**
DST Method	**Proportion**
Supranational Reference Laboratory	**Instituto de Salud Pública de Chile, Santiago, Chile**

*Notations to accompany profile: Estimated HIV positive TB cases is a WHO estimate

*For survey settings where less than 100% of cases are sampled, combined estimates are based on the rates of new and previously treated cases obtained in the survey, but weighted by the absolute number of new and previously treated sputum positive TB cases, as published by the national authorities.

COUNTRY PROFILES

PREVALENCE OF DRUG RESISTANCE

Countrywide: 1999

	New		Previous		Combined	
	N	%	N	%	N	%
Total number of strains tested	315	100.0				
SUSCEPTIBLE TO ALL 4 DRUGS	**305**	**96.8**				
ANY RESISTANCE	**10**	**3.2**				
- Isoniazid (INH)	5	1.6				
- Rifampicin (RMP)	1	0.3				
- Ethambutol (EMB)	0	0.0				
- Streptomycin (SM)	5	1.6				
MONORESISTANCE	**9**	**2.8**				
- Isoniazid (INH)	4	1.3				
- Rifampicin (RMP)	0	0.0				
- Ethambutol (EMB)	0	0.0				
- Streptomycin (SM)	5	1.6				
MULTIDRUG RESISTANCE	**1**	**0.3**				
- INH + RMP	1	0.3				
- INH + RMP + EMB	0	0.0				
- INH + RMP + SM	0	0.0				
- INH + RMP + EMB + SM	0	0.0				
OTHER PATTERNS	**0**	**0.0**				
- INH + EMB	0	0.0				
- INH + SM	0	0.0				
- INH + EMB + SM	0	0.0				
- RMP + EMB	0	0.0				
- RMP + SM	0	0.0				
- RMP + EMB + SM	0	0.0				
- EMB + SM	0	0.0				
NUMBER OF DRUGS RESISTANT TO:						
susceptible to 4 drugs	305	96.8				
resistant to 1 drug	9	2.8				
resistant to 2 drugs	1	0.3				
resistant to 3 drugs	0	0.0				
resistant to 4 drugs	0	0.0				

COUNTRY PROFILES

UZBEKISTAN

Karakalpakstan (Aral Sea Region): 2001-2002

PROFILE OF THE COUNTRY AND ITS CONTROL PROGRAMME

Population in year of survey	**1,527,009**		Year N.T.P was established	**1998**		
Notification all cases (rate)	**477.8**	**/100,000**	Year of Rifampicin introduction	**NA**		
Estimated incidence (all cases)	**267.4**	**/100,000**	Year of Isoniazid introduction	**NA**		
Notification new sputum smear +	**643**		Use of Standardized Regimens	**Yes**		
Notification new sputum smear + (rate)	**94.4**	**/100,000**	% Use of Short Course Chemotherapy	**Yes**	**>90**	**%**
Treatment Success	**68**	**%**	Use of Directly Observed Therapy	**Yes**		**%**
Retreatment cases	**651**		During continuation phase	**Yes**		
Retreatment as % of NTP	**44**	**%**	Use of Fixed Dose Combination	**Yes**	**100**	**%**
Estimated HIV positive TB cases	**NA**	**%**	Treatment in private sector	**Cat 2**		
			Category 1: virtually all TB patients public sector Category 2: <15% in private sector Category 3: 15% or more in private sector			
			TB drugs available on the private market	**All 1st line, some 2nd line**		

CHARACTERISTICS OF THE SURVEY/SURVEILLANCE PROGRAMME

Study Duration	**7 Months**
Target Area	**4 districts**
Sampling Method	**All cases**
Culture Media	**Löwenstein-Jensen**
DST Method	**Absolute concentration**
Supranational Reference Laboratory	**National Reference Center for Mycobacteria, Borstel, Germany**

*Notations to accompany profile: Retreatment indicates sputum smear positive pulmonary cases only

*For survey settings where less than 100% of cases are sampled, combined estimates are based on the rates of new and previously treated cases obtained in the survey, but weighted by the absolute number of new and previously treated sputum positive TB cases, as published by the national authorities.

COUNTRY PROFILES

PREVALENCE OF DRUG RESISTANCE

Karakalpakstan (Aral Sea Region): 2001-2002

	New		Previous		Combined	
	N	%	N	%	N	%
Total number of strains tested	106	100.0	107	100.0		100.0
SUSCEPTIBLE TO ALL 4 DRUGS	**55**	**51.9**	**22**	**20.6**		**36.1**
ANY RESISTANCE	**51**	**48.1**	**85**	**79.4**		**63.9**
- Isoniazid (INH)	39	36.8	74	69.2		53.1
- Rifampicin (RMP)	14	13.2	43	40.2		26.8
- Ethambutol (EMB)	16	15.1	37	34.6		24.9
- Streptomycin (SM)	47	44.3	76	71.0		57.8
MONORESISTANCE	**16**	**15.1**	**19**	**17.8**		**16.4**
- Isoniazid (INH)	4	3.8	8	7.5		5.6
- Rifampicin (RMP)	0	0.0	0	0.0		0.0
- Ethambutol (EMB)	0	0.0	0	0.0		0.0
- Streptomycin (SM)	12	11.3	11	10.3		10.8
MULTIDRUG RESISTANCE	**14**	**13.2**	**43**	**40.2**		**26.8**
- INH + RMP	0	0.0	1	0.9		0.5
- INH + RMP + EMB	0	0.0	0	0.0		0.0
- INH + RMP + SM	5	4.7	10	9.3		7.0
- INH + RMP + EMB + SM	9	8.5	32	29.9		19.3
OTHER PATTERNS	**21**	**19.8**	**23**	**21.5**		**20.7**
- INH + EMB	0	0.0	0	0.0		0.0
- INH + SM	14	13.2	18	16.8		15.0
- INH + EMB + SM	7	6.6	5	4.7		5.6
- RMP + EMB	0	0.0	0	0.0		0.0
- RMP + SM	0	0.0	0	0.0		0.0
- RMP + EMB + SM	0	0.0	0	0.0		0.0
- EMB + SM	0	0.0	0	0.0		0.0
NUMBER OF DRUGS RESISTANT TO:						
susceptible to 4 drugs	55	51.9	22	20.6		36.1
resistant to 1 drug	16	15.1	19	17.8		16.4
resistant to 2 drugs	14	13.2	19	17.8		15.5
resistant to 3 drugs	12	11.3	15	14.0		12.7
resistant to 4 drugs	9	8.5	32	29.9		19.3

COUNTRY PROFILES

295

VENEZUELA

Countrywide: 1998-1999

PROFILE OF THE COUNTRY AND ITS CONTROL PROGRAMME

Population in year of survey	**23,242,435**		Year N.T.P was established	**1936**		
Notification all cases (rate)	**26.3**	**/100,000**	Year of Rifampicin introduction	**1982**		
Estimated incidence (all cases)	**42.0**	**/100,000**	Year of Isoniazid introduction	**1950**		
Notification new sputum smear +	**3450**		Use of Standardized Regimens	**Yes**		
Notification new sputum smear + (rate)	**14.8**	**/100,000**	% Use of Short Course Chemotherapy	**Yes**	**100**	**%**
Treatment Success	**80**	**%**	Use of Directly Observed Therapy	**Yes**	**80**	**%**
Retreatment cases	**336**		During continuation phase	**Yes**		
Retreatment as % of NTP	**5.2**	**%**	Use of Fixed Dose Combination	**Yes**	**100**	**%**
Estimated HIV positive TB cases	**1.64**	**%**	Treatment in private sector	**Cat 2**		
			Category 1: virtually all TB patients public sector Category 2: <15% in private sector Category 3: 15% or more in private sector			
			TB drugs available on the private market	**Rifampicin only**		

CHARACTERISTICS OF THE SURVEY/SURVEILLANCE PROGRAMME

Study Duration	**9 Months**
Target Area	**Countrywide**
Sampling Method	**Proportionate cluster**
Culture Media	**Löwenstein-Jensen**
DST Method	**Proportion**
Supranational Reference Laboratory	**Instituto de Salud Pública de Chile, Santiago, Chile**

*Notations to accompany profile: Estimated HIV positive TB cases is a WHO estimate
Retreatment indicates sputum smear positive pulmonary cases only

*For survey settings where less than 100% of cases are sampled, combined estimates are based on the rates of new and previously treated cases obtained in the survey, but weighted by the absolute number of new and previously treated sputum positive TB cases, as published by the national authorities.

COUNTRY PROFILES

PREVALENCE OF DRUG RESISTANCE

Countrywide: 1998-1999

	New		Previous		Combined	
	N	%	N	%	N	%
Total number of strains tested	769	100.0	104	100.0		100.0
SUSCEPTIBLE TO ALL 4 DRUGS	**711**	**92.5**	**72**	**69.2**		**90.4**
ANY RESISTANCE	**58**	**7.5**	**32**	**30.8**		**9.6**
- Isoniazid (INH)	30	3.9	24	23.1		5.6
- Rifampicin (RMP)	8	1.0	19	18.3		2.6
- Ethambutol (EMB)	8	0.9	8	7.7		1.6
- Streptomycin (SM)	36	0.7	16	15.4		5.6
MONORESISTANCE	**38**	**4.9**	**12**	**11.5**		**5.5**
- Isoniazid (INH)	13	1.7	6	5.8		2.1
- Rifampicin (RMP)	3	0.4	3	2.9		0.6
- Ethambutol (EMB)	1	0.1	0	0.0		0.1
- Streptomycin (SM)	21	2.7	3	2.9		2.7
MULTIDRUG RESISTANCE	**4**	**0.5**	**14**	**13.5**		**1.7**
- INH + RMP	2	0.3	4	3.8		4.3
- INH + RMP + EMB	0	0.0	2	1.9		0.2
- INH + RMP + SM	1	0.1	5	4.8		0.5
- INH + RMP + EMB + SM	1	0.1	3	2.9		0.4
OTHER PATTERNS	**16**	**2.1**	**6**	**5.8**		**2.4**
- INH + EMB	2	0.3	1	1.0		0.3
- INH + SM	10	1.3	3	2.9		1.4
- INH + EMB + SM	1	0.1	0	0.0		0.1
- RMP + EMB	1	0.1	0	0.0		0.1
- RMP + SM	0	0.0	0	0.0		0.0
- RMP + EMB + SM	0	0.0	2	1.9		0.2
- EMB + SM	2	0.3	0	0.0		0.2
NUMBER OF DRUGS RESISTANT TO:						
susceptible to 4 drugs	711	92.5	72	69.2		90.4
resistant to 1 drug	38	4.9	12	11.5		5.5
resistant to 2 drugs	17	2.2	8	7.7		2.7
resistant to 3 drugs	2	0.3	9	8.7		1.0
resistant to 4 drugs	1	0.1	3	2.9		0.4

COUNTRY PROFILES

ZAMBIA

Countrywide: 2000

PROFILE OF THE COUNTRY AND ITS CONTROL PROGRAMME

Population in year of survey	**1,421,000**		Year N.T.P was established	**1964**	
Notification all cases (rate)		**/100,000**	Year of Rifampicin introduction	**1989**	
Estimated incidence (all cases)	**475**	**/100,000**	Year of Isoniazid introduction	**1964**	
Notification new sputum smear +	**13024**		Use of Standardized Regimens	**Yes**	
Notification new sputum smear + (rate)	**125**	**/100,000**	% Use of Short Course Chemotherapy	**Yes**	**100** %
Treatment Success		**%**	Use of Directly Observed Therapy	**Yes**	**<10** %
Retreatment cases	**1522**		During continuation phase	**No**	
Retreatment as % of NTP		**%**	Use of Fixed Dose Combination	**Yes**	**100** %
Estimated HIV positive TB cases	**43.4**	**%**	Treatment in private sector	**Cat 1**	

Category 1: virtually all TB patients public sector
Category 2: <15% in private sector
Category 3: 15% or more in private sector

TB drugs available on the private market	**All 1st line**

CHARACTERISTICS OF THE SURVEY/SURVEILLANCE PROGRAMME

Study Duration	**14 Months**
Target Area	
Sampling Method	**Cluster**
Culture Media	**Löwenstein-Jensen**
DST Method	**Proportion**
Supranational Reference Laboratory	**Medical Research Council (MRC) National TB Research Programme, South Africa**

*Notations to accompany profile: Estimated HIV positive TB cases is a WHO estimate
Retreatment indicates sputum smear positive pulmonary cases only

*For survey settings where less than 100% of cases are sampled, combined estimates are based on the rates of new and previously treated cases obtained in the survey, but weighted by the absolute number of new and previously treated sputum positive TB cases, as published by the national authorities.

PREVALENCE OF DRUG RESISTANCE

Countrywide: 2000

	New		Previous		Combined	
	N	%	N	%	N	%
Total number of strains tested	445	100.0	44	100.0		100.0
SUSCEPTIBLE TO ALL 4 DRUGS	**394**	**88.5**	**37**	**84.0**		**88.1**
ANY RESISTANCE	**51**	**11.5**	**7**	**15.9**		**11.9**
- Isoniazid (INH)	28	6.3	3	6.8		6.3
- Rifampicin (RMP)	8	1.8	1	2.3		1.8
- Ethambutol (EMB)	9	2.0	1	2.3		2.0
- Streptomycin (SM)	24	5.4	2	4.5		5.3
MONORESISTANCE	**38**	**8.5**	**5**	**11.4**		**8.8**
- Isoniazid (INH)	15	3.4	2	4.5		3.5
- Rifampicin (RMP)	0	0.0	0	0.0		0.0
- Ethambutol (EMB)	3	0.7	1	2.3		0.8
- Streptomycin (SM)	20	4.5	2	4.5		4.5
MULTIDRUG RESISTANCE	**8**	**1.8**	**1**	**2.3**		**1.8**
- INH + RMP	4	0.9	1	2.3		8.5
- INH + RMP + EMB	3	0.7	0	0.0		0.6
- INH + RMP + SM	0	0.0	0	0.0		0.0
- INH + RMP + EMB + SM	1	0.2	0	0.0		0.2
OTHER PATTERNS	**5**	**1.1**	**0**	**0.0**		**1.0**
- INH + EMB	2	0.4	0	0.0		0.4
- INH + SM	3	0.7	0	0.0		0.6
- INH + EMB + SM	0	0.0	0	0.0		0.0
- RMP + EMB	0	0.0	0	0.0		0.0
- RMP + SM	0	0.0	0	0.0		0.0
- RMP + EMB + SM	0	0.0	0	0.0		0.0
- EMB + SM	0	0.0	0	0.0		0.0
NUMBER OF DRUGS RESISTANT TO:						
susceptible to 4 drugs	394	88.5	37	84.0		88.1
resistant to 1 drug	38	8.5	6	13.6		9.1
resistant to 2 drugs	9	2.0	1	2.3		2.0
resistant to 3 drugs	3	0.7	0	0.0		0.6
resistant to 4 drugs	1	0.2	0	0.0		0.2

COUNTRY PROFILES

Design and typesetting: JOTTO ASSOCIATI - Italy